2/98

Second Edition Revised & Updated

The SIDS Survival Guide

*Information and Comfort
for Grieving Family and Friends
and Professionals Who Seek To Help Them*

Joani Nelson Horchler
& Robin Rice Morris

Foreword by Actor Lloyd Bridges

Introduction by Thomas G. Keens, M.D.
SIDS Researcher, University of Southern California

SIDS Educational Services
Hyattsville, Maryland
1997

Library of Congress Cataloging-in-Publication Data

Horchler, Joani Nelson, 1956–
    The SIDS survival guide: information and comfort for grieving family and friends and professionals who seek to help them / Joani Nelson Horchler and Robin Rice Morris; foreword by Lloyd Bridges; introduction by Thomas G. Keens, M.D.—Rev. and updated 2nd ed.
        p.   cm.
    Includes bibliographical references (p.   ).
    ISBN 0-9641218-8-3
    1. Sudden infant death syndrome—Psychological aspects. 2. Bereavement—Psychological aspects. I. Morris, Robin Rice, 1962–   . II. Title.
    RJ320.S93H63   1997
    618.92—dc21   97-16269
                                                            CIP

© 1997 by SIDS Educational Services Inc., a nonprofit, charitable corporation

Published in 1997 by

    SIDS Educational Services Inc.
    P.O. Box 2426
    Hyattsville, MD 20784

Additional copies may be ordered through bookstores or by using the forms on the last pages of this book. If you need information, call 301-773-9671 or fax 301-322-2620.

Cover photo: Photri/G. Schoolfield
Cover and book design: Pam Page Cullen

"I cannot tell you how this book affected me.
But let me just say that the Kleenex® box is half full, where
it was once full. I don't mean to suggest that
The SIDS Survival Guide is overly sad, but it made me
think of many things and reinforced my belief (and trust)
in the wonder of life, and what we all value, and why
we are, indeed, such a remarkable species.
The SIDS Survival Guide is not just a 'SIDS' book.
It is one of the most life-affirming, informative, and moving books
that I have ever read. The writings of SIDS survivors
are nothing less than inspirational and the best
illustrations of how, even in the aftermath of tragedy,
our most precious emotions of joy and hope can be reclaimed.
I cannot think of a single group touched by SIDS,
or who worry about SIDS, or who need to be reminded of
the power of love, who will not derive comfort and insight
from this remarkable book. It is unprecedented
in the degree to which it successfully integrates and bridges
both human and scientific dimensions of SIDS."

— *James J. McKenna, Ph.D.,*
SIDS Researcher and Professor of Anthropology
Pomona College, Claremont, California

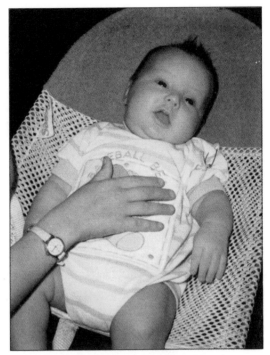

Christian Gabriel Horchler
3/8/91–5/9/91

Dedication

For Christian Gabriel Horchler and all babies who have died of SIDS. Their spirits will live on forever, in our hearts and in all that we achieve in their honor.

For Christian's baby sisters, Genevieve Désirée and Stephanie Laura, and all other so greatly desired "healing babies."

For Christian's big sisters, Ilona Dora, Gabrielle Christine, and Julianna Henriette.

For my hero and the father of all my children, Gabe.

And for all the other courageous SIDS survivors who give us comfort and reasons to hope and endure.

—Joani Nelson Horchler

For my favorite babysitter, Roxanne; my childhood friends, Nelle and JoAnne; my little brother, Ricky; my college buddy, Dick; and my father, David. Each one died far too young, thus becoming my silent mentors in grief.

—Robin Rice Morris

"We lost our first son, Mikey, on New Year's Eve, 1989. As SIDS survivors, this is the most comprehensive, cleansing, uplifting, soul-searching book we've ever read on SIDS. We'll share it with family and friends who have seen us go through this tragedy but can't begin to comprehend the power of the anger, guilt, and depression we must go through in order to assimilate the fact that our baby died into our life history."

—Kathy and Steve Whelan

"We lost our son, Chase, to SIDS in 1994. He was a normal, healthy, three-month-old. There were no warning signs. From the initial shock, to the unending questions, to dealing with the loss as an individual, a spouse, and a parent (our daughter was two at the time), this book has played an essential role in the healing we have begun to experience. We initially gave 15 copies to family members, friends, and our minister, and recently sponsored 16 more to be donated in Chase's memory to newly bereaved parents, hospitals, libraries, emergency responders, and others who need to know about SIDS.

—Doug and Elise Brammer

Table of Contents

Chapter 1
What Everyone Should Know about SIDS 1

Chapter 2
The Nightmare Begins 19

Chapter 6
Children Grieving Children 103

Chapter 7
Grandparents: A Grief Doubled 124

Chapter 8
When a Baby Dies at the Child-Care Provider's ..133

Chapter 9
How To Be a Friend to a SIDS Survivor 143

Chapter 10
Planning a Funeral and the Role of the Clergy......154

Chapter 11
Learning To Live Again..170

Chapter 12
Happy Birthday? Merry Christmas? 187

Missing Danny at the Beach   by Janice John Roper
Surviving Anniversaries and Holidays   by Shelley A. LeDroux
Portraits for Easter   by Cheryl Radich
Kathy's Day   by William C. Ermatinger
Marking the Milestones When You Have Lost Your Only Child
  by Michelle Morgan Spady
Portraits for Easter   by Cheryl Radich

Chapter 13
Peer Contact and Professional Help 196

A Peer Contact Answers the Question: "Are You Still Doing That?"
  by Debbie Gemmill
Untitled   by H. Thurman
A SIDS Parent Counseling SIDS Survivors   by Carla Hosford, LCSW-C
Finding Friends Among Other SIDS Families   by Nancy Maruyama, RN
Home Visits by Public Health Nurses
  by Linda Esposito, RN, MPH, CNS, CNA
Hitting It Off with a Counselor   An Interview with Mike Hitch
My Lifeline   An Interview with Gwen Robinson

Chapter 14
Emergency Medical Responders
and the Authorities 212

Dos and Don'ts for Emergency Responders   by Kerry Day
When Emergency Responders Lose Their Own Baby   by Michelle Grogan
SIDS and the Homicide Detective
  An Interview with J. Richard Salen and Steve Kerpelman
How NOT To Treat a SIDS Survivor   by Darlene Buth
The "Suspicious" Loss of Twins   by Joani Nelson Horchler
The Role of the Medical Examiner   by John E. Smialek, M.D.

Chapter 19

Foreword

We wanted four children, that is, if we were lucky enough to have them and the money to support them. After a few years of marriage we were blessed with our son, Beau.

Two years later, we decided it was time for child number two. But unluckily, my wife had developed an infertility problem and for five years went through every known test and procedure to correct it.

We'd just about considered adoption when the miracle happened and she again became pregnant. With a special joy and thankfulness, we prepared for this truly blessed event.

It seemed especially appropriate that another son, Garry, chose to arrive on June 14th because it was Flag Day, a celebration date on the calendar. He weighed in at 10 pounds and was instantly declared handsome because he sported two dimples in his cheeks. It's inadequate to say we were overjoyed. At his six-week checkup, the pediatrician joked, "What a guy! He looks like a fullback already!" We puffed up with pride.

The next morning, my wife nursed him and came downstairs for her breakfast. "What a good baby," she said. "He went right to sleep so Mommy could have her breakfast."

Then she went back upstairs, and I heard her screaming. I rushed there and saw why. Our baby was lying limply in her arms, lifeless.

We ran with him to the car, stopped at the first "Doctor" sign we saw, and burst into the doctor's examining room. While the doctor did what he could, the paramedics were called. All to no avail. Our baby, our beautiful boy, was declared dead.

We lived through the next days, the next weeks and months, with agonizing grief. Whatever philosophies we had in our brains, whatever religion in our hearts, were knocked for a loop. No person we talked to, no books we read, could do much to help.

But gradually, inexorably, the rays of reason and hope, and thankfulness for Beau, for all the good and wonderful things that were part of our life, began to sift through our gloom. And it is true that time heals.

Not that you ever forget. Not that sometimes you don't relive the terror of that awful event. If you are as fortunate as we were and are given two more children to love, you are so much more anxiety-ridden with them because you know that the brink of danger is ever present.

When people ask us how many children we have, we want to say "four" because Garry, our little lost one, is always part of our lives. But then they say, "But we know about Beau and Jeff and Cindy. Who else is there?" We're then required to state what we've never wanted to believe, that our son Garry died when he was a baby. But that's lying because he's always with us, even if beyond our horizon, and every June 14th—when the flags are flying—we know it's for Garry's birthday.

— Lloyd Bridges

Preface

*"Life is something that happens to you while you're making
other plans."*

—Margaret Millar

Until my midthirties, I felt I was writing the script of my life. It
wasn't that nothing bad had ever happened to me. Both my father
and my brother had died when I was very young. Still, I felt basically
in control of my life and was probably one to show some scorn for
people who felt fate or God were in charge.

So, on my 35th birthday, I sat back in my easy chair, opening gifts
and gazing at the husband I love, my three beautiful daughters, and
my strong and handsome six-week-old son. "Wow," I thought with
pride, "I must have done things right because here I am with my
perfect family and my perfect life." Still, I had a vague feeling of
uneasiness: Was our luck too good to last?

Two weeks later, our baby boy, Christian, was inexplicably dead
and my perfect world was shattered. I was no longer in control; no
longer writing the story of my life. I felt the best part of me--the
"career mom" with the breast-feeding baby—had been amputated.
I suddenly thought I must be the most horrible, incompetent person
alive because I couldn't keep my baby alive. Even though everyone
said I wasn't to blame for my son's death from SIDS, I couldn't shake
the feeling that I must have done something wrong. Babies can't die
from nothing, so I must be to blame, I constantly thought. What an
awful burden it was to take on all the responsibility for destroying
my entire family's happiness. As the guilt began to subside, I experienced whirlwinds of anger against fate and God and people who said
stupid things. I was even angry with my baby for leaving us. I was
often depressed.

I share this with you, newly bereaved families, because I know you
are feeling many of these same emotions. I also know that most of the

people surrounding you are well-intentioned but cannot even begin to imagine what you are going through (unless they have themselves lost a child). How can you explain to someone how terrified you are to try to imagine your life five to ten years down the road? You can't even envision getting through the minutes, hours, and days—let alone the weeks, months, and years—of your despair. You think your life will always be plagued by anger, guilt, and bitterness. You suffer deep, cutting pains in your heart and your gut that seem intolerable and everlasting. You don't need people who have never experienced the death of their own child telling you they understand. They don't and they can't. What you need are people who can tell you, "I survived my baby's death, and I have some practical suggestions that can help you cope, too." This is the reason this book was written—to try to give you comfort and hope through the stories and experiences of SIDS survivors.

What you may need most of all initially is validation of the reasons for your depths of despair. Our children are "something like our own humanness or our reasons for being on earth," says Ann Finkbeiner in *After the Death of a Child*, a book that is cited in this book's suggested reading list. "If children are part of parents, they are not arms or legs but bone and breath," Ms. Finkbeiner writes.

Moreover, when an infant dies in our society, "the family usually grieves with little recognition and support for its profound loss," state Joan Hagan and Penelope Gemma in *A Child Dies: A Portrait of Family Grief*, another book on our suggested reading list. Our infants, our greatest treasures, "are all too insignificant in society's eyes," say Hagan and Gemma. Because most people in our society will not give you the strong support you need, you must seek help elsewhere. Through *The SIDS Survival Guide*, you will gain information, comfort, and courage from the only people who truly understand what you are experiencing—others who have lost a baby to SIDS. We wish we could tell you that your pain will go away completely, but unfortunately we cannot tell that lie. Our collective experience is that the pain never goes away completely but that the raging fire of grief does soften and the pain becomes easier to live with. Moreover, many of the people in this book have grown from their tragedies; have come to a greater appreciation for all that they do have; and now give more to others because of what they have learned. Many find that they have a changed set of priorities because the death has put into perspective what is really important. Many find themselves more sensititve to others who are hurting.

Of course, we'd all much rather have our babies back than anything good that could come from losing them. But that choice is not given to us. The only real options are 1) to commit suicide (which we do not advise); 2) to feel angry, guilty, or bitter all our lives (an easy but very sad option); or 3) to forge ahead with our lives as best we can while honoring our babies' memories. The last choice is the one we believe that our babies would want us to make. It is also the only choice that makes the rest of our lives worth living.

I have to admit that even six years after Christian died, I'm still angry sometimes. The month that he would have started kindergarten was awful. It was tough when my husband saved a three-year-old boy from drowning the year Christian would have been three. I was happy for the parents, but envious of their luck. As much as I adored my mother, her death in 1994 (after a truck with inoperative brakes hit her car) was not nearly as difficult to accept as our son's. I dreaded her death, but expected to someday have to endure it. Who can fathom the death of a healthy infant? SIDS is horribly unfair. I feel cheated out of having a son, and I feel that having something so vital to my well-being—my parenthood of a healthy little boy—ripped out of me means that I can never be completely whole again.

Still, the open, bleeding wound in my heart is now healing, and I have begun to fill the empty space that remains with all the fabulous memories and love that I will always have for Christian. Whereas at first it was only painful to remember those perfect days with Christian, I can now usually feel joy when I think of them. Time really does help. When I am doing something fun with my other children, I can now actually feel some pleasure—not only pain—in thinking that Christian would have loved doing this with us. I don't believe one can ever "let go" of a child. I have never let go of Christian because I want to keep him a part of me forever; however, I do believe it is important to let go of as much of the pain associated with his death as possible. I feel that Christian is always with us spiritually, and I am not saying this from a religious standpoint. I work at preserving my spiritual relationship with Christian by making time to do my grief work; by listening to and talking with newly bereaved families; and by helping to keep this book in print.

When we wrote the first edition of this book in 1994, we were almost unable to publish it for lack of funding. Fortunately, the University of Maryland SIDS Institute (through its now retired director Dr. M. John O'Brien) came to the rescue with $4,000 from a Baltimore Harbor Cruises fund-raiser, and Healthdyne Technologies chipped in as the largest of the other group donors. Also important were small donations from many individuals.

Many small-press books like this one die because of high printing, marketing, and distribution costs and because of the large number of volunteer hours needed to keep the publisher-distributor, SIDS Educational Services (SIDS-ES), going. These are the reasons we set up a nonprofit, charitable organization, which achieved 501(c) (3) status in 1994. We needed to be able to accept tax-deductible donations to publish the book and keep it going. Unfortunately, the book cannot survive on sales revenues alone. Our goal is to get preferably free books into the hands of newly bereaved families immediately after a death. As Jennifer Banowsky, area coordinator of SIDS Support for San Antonio, says, "I first read the book two and a half years after my son Zachary's death, and it was still such a help to me. I only wish I could have read it sooner." Now, Jennifer says, "we are so pleased that we will be able to provide this book to all our newly bereaved parents." Her organization is one of many SIDS support groups around the country that use donations or grants to buy books at large discount from SIDS-ES to give to every newly bereaved family in their areas. (Groups and individuals that sponsor books in this way are mentioned in the acknowledgments.) This not only provides SIDS-ES with enough money to keep this important limited edition book in print, but ensures that families receive as soon as possible after the death the most comprehensive support book available on SIDS. Book donations to SIDS support groups, hospitals, doctors' offices, libraries, emergency responders, day-care facilities, and other organizations are tax-deductible. Sponsoring books is a wonderful way to honor your baby's memory (through personalized tributes on labels that SIDS-ES makes for you to place on the inside cover of each book) while educating the general public about SIDS and ensuring that newly bereaved families receive information and comfort immediately after the death of their babies.

Besides being grateful to book sponsors, I will forever be indebted to the contributors to this book. By baring their souls through often deeply personal testimonials, they exemplify bravery and generosity and give us valuable insights into how to deal with what is likely life's most searing loss—the death of one's own child. Much of what we learn from them can also be applied to other losses that we all constantly suffer throughout life, for no one is immune from loss. Although there is nothing worse than losing a child, everyone experiences grief, whether it be through death, separation, divorce, or deep disappointment.

As you, too, do your tough grief work, please write to me and let me know how you're progressing. I'd like to know what suggestions from this book helped you and what other survival strategies you've found. Send me your stories and poems. It is therapeutic for you to write them, and we will try to publish them in a future edition. While it is, unfortunately, impossible to publish all of the large number of submissions we receive, we will help you identify other publication vehicles, such as state SIDS newsletters and local and national newspapers and magazines. I can be reached through our small, nonprofit, charitable organization, SIDS-ES, at Post Office Box 2426, Hyattsville, MD 20784. (Please note that this is the new address as of 1997; our old post office closed.)

Please call me any time you need emotional support as it helps me honor my son's memory and makes me feel better to be able to provide peer counseling to you. A mission of our nonprofit is to provide free peer support to bereaved families from me and a group of volunteer parents throughout the country who are honored to listen to you and provide practical suggestions for coping with SIDS. We also provide referrals to your area SIDS support groups and free lists of resources. (Phone: 301-773-9671 or fax 301-322-2620.)

If you have suggestions for obtaining positive publicity about the whole issue of SIDS and about this book, please contact me. I have often been asked why we don't get this book better known by going on the talk show circuit. Here's why: I was invited, when the first edition was published in 1994, to discuss *The SIDS Survival Guide* on a nationwide talk show. As I started packing my bags for Los Angeles, an assistant producer called me back to 'uninvite' me. Her boss, she said, had decided 'to focus on more sensationalist topics.' It is infuriating that a huge and serious public health problem like SIDS must constantly take a backseat to monsters who drown their own babies and slimebags who have sex with their girlfriend's teenage daughter or whoever else happens to be handy. Even worse, when talk shows *have* addressed the issue of SIDS, they have often dredged up a few extremely rare cases to imply that SIDS cases are really murder cases. We did have a positive experience discussing SIDS on Broadcast House Live-WUSA, a Washington, DC talk show, but our overall experience has taught us to beware of press attention.

To conclude, I probably never would have garnered the enormous emotional energy it took to write and edit this book without the deep understanding and support that I received from other SIDS parents. They became my "survival guides," walking beside me on the dark path of grief and gently steadying me the many times that I stumbled. For example, Sandy Lamb, who lost her only son about a year before I did, guided me in my grief work by relating a dream she had about a year after Christian died. At that time, I had become stuck behind the roadblocks of guilt and anger. Sandy's baby, my baby, and two other infants who had died of SIDS were spirits who had grown older since their deaths. In Sandy's dream, these three- to five-year-olds were on a softball field. My son, Christian, the youngest, was dressed in a baseball suit and cap but was sitting out the game on a log. In her dream, Sandy asked Christian why he was not out on the field playing ball. He replied, "I can't go out and play until my mother does."

This book is my way of going out to play.

—Joani Nelson Horchler

Acknowledgments

The publication of the second edition of this book would not have been possible without contributions of $500 or more from the SIDS Network; the CJ Foundation for SIDS; Healthdyne Technologies (makers of the infant SmartMonitor™); the New England Hi-Tech Charity Foundation (in memory of Brianna Opal Lawrence); Dr. Stuart Tomares, president of ChildSecure Inc. (makers of the video "SIDS: Reducing the Risks"); Dr. M. John O'Brien; Kee Schuth Marshall and family (in memory of Margaret Hood Schuth); The Maryland SIDS Information and Counseling Program; Margaret Fischer (in memory of her husband Dr. John Fischer); Janice and Bruce Roper and employees of Greenhorne and O'Mara (in memory of Daniel C. Roper IV); Joani and Gabe Horchler and Kathy and Darrel Gustin and family (in memory of Christian Horchler and his grandmother Doris Guhin Nelson); and federal workers who contributed through the Nation's Capital Area Combined Federal Campaign.

The SIDS Network donation listed above resulted from a fundraising drive by Chuck and Deb Mihalko (parents of Margaret, who died of SIDS) of the SIDS Network, which raised $4,000 over the Internet in memory of the individual babies listed later in a Special Memory Section in these acknowledgment pages. We will be forever grateful to Chuck, Deb, and the SIDS Network for their continuing support.

Many thanks also for the continuing generous donation of accounting services to our nonprofit SIDS-ES by David Zack, independent CPA, and Michael Gellman, CPA at Rubino and McGeehin of Bethesda, Maryland, and to Jesse Torgerson and Laura Jean Torgerson for their help with data entry.

Janice John Roper, mother of Daniel C. Roper IV (9/9/95–12/4/95), deserves a big thank you for many hours of help in establishing the book sponsorship program that is helping to ensure the survival of this book. Without Janice's invaluable work in memory of her son, funds to print the second edition of this book would not have been available.

Many thanks also to Darlene and Jim Buth, who have volunteered many hours making beautiful, personalized color photo labels (for book sponsors to place on the inside cover of each book they donate in memory of their babies). Darlene and Jim volunteer in memory of their son, Peter James-Alan (7/23/95–10/3/95).

We are deeply grateful for the services of top-notch professional copy editor Paula Bérard and professional graphic designer Pam Page Cullen. (Paula says she had to read each writing twice, since the first time was blurred by her tears.) Other friends who helped a lot were Christine Fackler Salemi, Amadeo Szaszdi, Nikki Greco, Nancy and Ed Gant, Carla Hosford, Cathy Smith, Vicki Yokota, and Lee Hackel. (Lee is with the Georgia SIDS/Other Infant Death Information and Counseling Program.)

Thanks also to the current board of directors of SIDS-ES: Kee Schuth Marshall, vice-president of NationsBank; Patrick T. Hand, Esq., of the law firm of Crowley, Hoge, & Fein; Sandra Graben of the Alliance of Grandparents Against SIDS Tragedy; Dr. M. John O'Brien; Janice John Roper; Sheri Laigle; and Carla Hosford, LCSW.

I personally thank my brother, D. Bradley Nelson, for serving as an early writing mentor to me. (Brad, who in his mid-twenties penned a lovely book of poetry, was killed in an auto accident at age 28 when I was 15.) I also thank my mother, Doris Guhin Nelson, who was killed in 1994 when a truck without operating brakes hit her car. My mom was always there to support my dreams, and she is still with me in spirit. I can't imagine surviving without the support of my sister, Kathy Gustin, the only person outside our immediate family who never fails to remember Christian's anniversaries.

There is not room here to thank all of the SIDS parents who have helped me greatly in my grief work. However, I must mention the dozens of hours that Ruth Skopek, Sandy Lamb, Marie Pascale-Hill, and Joanne Hill spent on the phone with me in those early days.

Of course, my biggest thanks go to my husband, Gabe, and my oldest children, Ilona, Gabrielle, and Julianna, for helping with our two younger children so I could work on this book. Special thanks to Nancy Gant and Rachel Gabel, my best babysitters outside of my family.

Book Sponsors (Groups):

We would like to thank the following organizations for helping us pay the printing costs of this second edition by in one way or another supporting our book sponsorship program. Through this program, many of the mentioned groups buy books at discount to give to each newly bereaved family in their localities. Other mentioned groups buy multiple copies to donate to public libraries, police facilities, local health departments, or a variety of other organizations that need to know about SIDS. Some, like the national SIDS Alliance (Baltimore, Maryland) and the American SIDS Institute (Atlanta, Georgia), help publicize the sponsorship program and refer newly bereaved parents who ask about a book to SIDS-ES, the publisher of *The SIDS Survival Guide*. Special thanks to the CJ Foundation for SIDS (address and phone number in the appendix of this book) for providing grants to several of the following organizations so that they could afford to buy books at discount to give to newly bereaved families.

The state and local organizations that support the book sponsorship program are: Arizona SIDS Alliance; California SIDS Program; Guild for Infant Survival of Orange County, California; ParentsPlace; Colorado SIDS Program; Connecticut SIDS Center; State Health Office of Tallahassee, Florida; Georgia SIDS/Other Infant Death Information and Counseling Program; Hawaii SIDS Information and Counseling Program; SIDS Alliance of Illinois; Caring and Hope of Slidell, Illinois; Iowa SIDS Alliance; Bill McCawley Enterprises and Re/Max of Bowie, Maryland; Massachusetts SIDS Center; SIDS Resources Inc. of St. Louis; New Hampshire SIDS Alliance; SIDS Information and Counseling Program of New York City; SIDS Alliance of Western New York; Cabarrus County Health Department of Concord, North Carolina; North Carolina SIDS Alliance; SIDS Support Network of Greater Toledo, Ohio; Miami Valley SIDS Alliance of Dayton, Ohio; Northeastern Ohio SIDS Alliance; Wood County Women's Care of Bowling Green, Ohio; SIDS Resources of Oregon; SIDS Network—Pennsylvania Connection; Pennsylvania SIDS Alliance; Pediatric Care of York, Pennsylvaia; Pulmon Air Service/ SIDS Alliance of Chattanooga, Tennessee; Greater Houston Chapter of the SIDS Alliance; North Texas SIDS Alliance; Wichita Falls Branch of the North Texas SIDS Alliance; SIDS Support for San

Antonio; Vermont Department of Health; Northern Virginia SIDS Alliance; West Virginia Department of Health; Health Care Management Services Inc. of Fort Atkinson, Wisconsin.

The first and second editions of this book could not have been produced without the invaluable financial support and encouragement of Dr. M. John O'Brien and the University of Maryland Medical Center, Baltimore, Maryland.

Special Memories Section:

In memory of Cody Ledon Albritton (9/27/95–12/1/95): Gary Albritton.

In memory of Rachel Lorraine Andell (7/13/94–10/10/94): Karen and Jonathon Andell; Bette Jane Andell.

In memory of Maggie Clare Arcement (5/23/96–7/29/96): Leslie and Brian Arcement.

In memory of Austin Alan Archer (5/18/94–8/22/95): Allison and Dennis Archer.

In memory of Taylor Dorothy Atkinson (11/17/93–6/7/94): Beverly and Scott Atkinson.

In memory of Nicholas Atwood (8/7/92–2/2/93): Annie, George, and Caroline Atwood.

In memory of Tucker Brooks Baer (4/10/96–8/26/96): Debbie and Rich Baer.

In memory of Alexander Wayde Baldwin (who was lost to SIDS in August 1995): Dale and Sharon Baldwin.

In memory of William "Willie" David Stewart Balzer (11/10/92–3/10/93): Margie Stewart, Ned Balzer, and Benjamin Stewart Balzer.

In memory of Jake Arthur Bauroth: Craig and Janice Bauroth, Angela Bauroth, and the Moody family.

In memory of Ariel Miranda Bicklein (4/10/95–5/1/95): Deborah A. Bicklein.

In memory of Casey Boekenoogen (12/12/91–3/20/92): Kathy and Chuck Boekenoogen.

In memory of Katie Boggs (2/24/95–12/20/95): Brett and Marna Boggs; brother Vaughan; grandmother Ann Anderson; great-grandmother Mickey Nuttall.

In memory of Kaydee Sue Braaten (10/1/91–1/3/92): Becky Braaten; Tonia Bowden of The American SIDS Institute.

In memory of Chase Edward Brammer (5/27/94–9/2/94): Doug and Elise Brammer.

In memory of Emily Marie Brink (8/15/96–12/28/96): Todd and Chris Brink; Lee and Cathy Brink; Harlan and Lois Peterson.

In memory of Kali Alyssa Brown (4/12/96–4/12/96): Nancy A. Brown.

In memory of Peter James-Alan Buth (7/23/95–10/3/95): Darlene and James Buth.

In memory of Tanner James Carnell (3/15/96–9/5/96): Baba and Gido Carnell.

In memory of James Patrick Carney (6/27/89–7/23/89): Mary Ann and William Barta.

In memory of Joshua Abraham Chaidell: Sue Ellen Dodell and Joel Chaiken; Lynette Charboneau and Roger Morie.

In memory of Patrick Ryan Check (4/26/87–8/4/87): Alice Check.

In memory of Joshua Ralph Cipriano (4/15/96–6/12/96):Suzanne Cipriano.

In memory of Robyn Catherine Clendening (10/26/95–12/18/95): Denise Clendening.

In memory of Nicole Lynn Corson (1/14/92–4/15/92): Michelle Corson.

In memory of Harrison Dawes: Laura and Robert Dawes.

In memory of T. C. Dickey (8/31/94–12/9/94): Lori, Tom, and Trevor Dickey.

In memory of Catherine Christine Dietrich (9/20/94–2/20/96): Theresa Dietrich.

In memory of Kelly William Donnelly (7/14/61–9/9/61): Joan and William Donnelly.

In memory of Ryan Richard Downing-Todd (1/24/97–1/27/97): Sandie Todd and Michael Downing.

In memory of Avonlea Dutkiewicz (10/30/90–3/13/91): Aimee Dutkiewicz.

In memory of Cory Steven Eckert (2/22/85–5/24/85): Nancy Amodt Eckert.

In memory of Jacob Riley Elder (9/18/96–11/1/96): Matt and Becky Elder; Joe and Debbie Frankenfield (Jacob's day-care providers).

In memory of Devin Taylor Estes (7/3/95–9/11/95): Jan Estes.

In memory of Emily Francis Fallon: Nancy and Steve Fallon and the American SIDS Institute.

In memory of Madison Nicole Ferrell (7/9/95–10/24/95): Torie Ferrell.

In memory of Quentin Fischer (8/23/94–12/3/94): Eric Fischer.

In memory of Lane Jason Fontaine (10/11/96–1/3/97): Valerie Henry, Tonia Bowden of The American SIDS Institute.

In memory of Hannah Shae George (1/2/96–4/17/96): Alyssa George and family.

In memory of Daniel Gervais (8/6/91–4/29/93): Chris Gervais.

In memory of Scott Christopher Gomez, Jr. (9/10/95–11/13/95): Tina M. Ramirez and Scott C. Gomez.

In memory of Andrew Dalton Greco (10/17/95–1/2/96): Tracy and Victor Greco and Tony and Christopher.

In memory of Ellie Anna Elaine Gronseth (10/17/96–12/2/96) and her grandmother, Anna Elaine: Rhonda and Steve Gronseth.

In memory of Aaron Patrick Guttman (8/18/95–12/23/96): Dr. Michael D. and Dr. Mary Ann Guttman, and family.

In memory of Ashley Nicole Hallo (2/23/85–6/5/85): Christy Hallo.

In memory of Alexander P. Hance (9/3/93–12/11/93): Nevada L. Fuller; Bernice, James, and Jaime Hance.

In memory of Samantha Grace Harmon (2/22/96–2/22/96): Vicki Harmon.

In memory of Benjamin Dale Hayman (2/17/87–6/10/87) and his great-grandmother, Ann Birchenough: Jean Hulse-Hayman and Dale Hayman.

In memory of Jacquelyn M. Hoffman (6/11/96–10/4/96): Terrie and Duncan Hoffman.

In memory of Wesley Scott Holding, who was lost to SIDS in December 1996.

In memory of Tyler John Albert Hollinda (6/5/96–8/31/96): Heather and J. J. Hollinda.

In memory of Brennan Edward Hood (1/21/96–3/21/96): Laurie, Bill, Jordan, and Tanner Hood; Carol Hood.

In memory of Christian Gabriel Horchler (3/8/91–5/9/91) and his grandmother Doris Guhin Nelson: Joani and Gabe Horchler; Kathy and Darrel Gustin and family; Kenneth Edward Nelson; Garry and Vicky Nelson and Alyssa and Camilla; Amadeo Szaszdi; Lynette Charboneau and Roger Morie; Richard and Nancy Selle; Pam and Richard Bard of the Bard Family Foundation; Michelle Walz Stegeman; Jim and Henriette Leanos; office of Dr. A. J. Modlin.

In memory of Grady James Hughes (5/3/96–6/5/96): Chris Hanson-Hughes.

In memory of Kollin Michael Hughes (4/19/96–7/10/96): Tracy, Michael, and Jordyn Hughes.

In memory of Timothy David (T.J.) Hulme (1/17/89–7/31/89): Timothy and Catherine Hulme; David and Sandra Graben.

In memory of George Wayne Hunt (7/6/95–12/5/95): Sheryl and David Hunt.

In memory of Arianna Sherry Zola-Joe (10/20/95–2/20/96): Lorah L. Joe.

In memory of Tyler Robert Johnson (3/9/95–5/25/95): Tena and John and Ashley Johnson.

In memory of Jessica Miriam Kaplan (9/12/88–12/10/88): David Kaplan.

In memory of Peter Keeler: Dr. George Keeler, M.D., and Kay Keeler.

In memory of Katharine Rogers King (8/3/95–12/21/95): Joan and Carl King.

In memory of Kyle Austin Koen (9/19/94–12/14/94): Karl and Traci Koen; Floyd and Janette Koen.

In memory of Alex James Kratzer (12/13/95–8/16/96): Colleen and Kris Kratzer.

In memory of Alexis Lauren Landgraf (8/1/95–4/3/96): Richard and Kathy Floyd.

In memory of Brianna Opal Lawrence (11/14/95–2/13/96): Gina and Stephen Lawrence, D and D Querci; New England Hi-Tech Foundation.

In memory of Stephen T. Lawton (10/20/92–7/15/93): Susan and Steve Lawton.

In memory of Marisa Angel Ley (7/5/95–7/9/95): Cindy Ley.

In memory of Michael Jerome Lindow (2/24/95–6/13/95): Michelle Lindow.

In memory of Hunter Jay Logan (7/9/95–10/19/95): Mechelle M. Logan.

In memory of Brendan Nobuo Maruyama (6/1/85–10/18/85) and his grandmother Yvonne Kilcoyne: Nancy, Rod, Caitlin, and Jennifer Maruyama.

In memory of Jenny Pearl Matthews and William Ty Matthews (1/2/96–1/2/96): April Matthews.

In memory of Cameron McKinley (3/16/96–5/9/96): Robert and Amelia and Katie McKinley; the Beaton family; Mike and Mary Beth Wusk.

In memory of Shamus McLaughlin (8/6/89–1/2/90): Janet and Norman Gray, Marguerite C. Devine.

In memory of Neil Peter Miglin (5/3/91–10/6/91): Marie Miglin.

In memory of Margaret Joy Mihalko (9/15/89–10/23/89): Deb, Chuck, Jay, Jon, Timmy, and Dru Mihalko; Margaret Morris; Annabelle and Ron Dennis; Annie and Kedric Bartsch; Jacky and Don Cola; Nancy and Steve Brewer; Nancy and Greg Schneider.

In memory of Robert "Robby" Matthew Miller (10/17/94–3/20/95): Angie and Matt Miller.

In memory of Anna Mikala Mills (3/6/95–5/14/95): Mike, Donna, Joel, Andrew, and Benjamin Mills.

In memory of Jonathan Daniel Mitchell (6/24/95–6/24/95): Rebekah and Byron Mitchell.

In memory of Magdalena Lynn Moore (12/18/95–3/8/96): Nancy and John Moore; Hugh and Doris Weber.

In memory of Daniel Peter Munguia (7/11/95–9/26/96): Peter R. and Michelle Levario Munguia, Grandpa Edmund Ross Levario, and Peter Daniel Ross Munguia (due 2/25/97).

In memory of Jayce Nathaniel Muniz (7/18/96–11/7/96): Suzanne, Peter, and Brandon Muniz; Joyce Joblonski.

In memory of Jaden Ford Murray (10/12/96–10/20/96): Kim Murray.

In memory of Dennis Naranjo-Cardenas (1/5/97–3/1/97): Dennis, Cathy, and Michelle.

In memory of Tyler James Nelson (10/18/96–12/5/96): Jeannie and Donny Nelson.

In memory of Skyelar Jordan Neumann (3/10/92–6/5/92): Jennifer and Anthony Neumann.

In memory of Christopher Aaron Oda (1/26/96–4/25/96): Esther, Steven, and Matthew Oda; Jaikwan and Soonok Ahn; Elma and Sam Oda; Nancy, Joseph, and Jordan Ahn; Eunice and Tom Millar; Faith and Jim Holland; LeAnna and Gunther Martin; Jan and Richard Michalsen; Cindy and Gary Stephan.

In memory of Molly Katherine O'Neill (11/14/95–7/18/96): Kelly Priest and Tom O'Neil.

In memory of Rebecca Peckham (11/4/92–6/14/93): Susan and Amy Porter; Thomas and Alexander Peckham.

In memory of Lauren-Raye Pinkham (6/19/92–3/26/93): April Pinkham.

In memory of Amy Caroline Purcell (10/21/91–3/8/92): Kenneth and Nancy Purcell.

In memory of Nigel Christopher Radich (2/24/94–7/11/94): Cheryl and Jeff Radich; Henrietta and Richard Kistner.

In memory of Jeremy Paul Reiner (9/27/88–11/30/88): Carol J. Clark; Valley-Sierra Affiliate SIDS Alliance.

In memory of Joshua Christian Richmond (4/17/94–2/6/95): Emma and Chris Richmond.

In memory of Jacob Daniel Robinson (7/30/95–1/10/96): LaRue and Jerry Robinson.

In memory of Daniel C. Roper IV (9/9/95–12/4/95): Bruce and Janice Roper and the employees of the Rockville office of Greenhorne and O'Mara, Inc.

In memory of David Marc Zontar Rowe (4/30/89–5/20/91): Dana Siegel and Eric Rowe.

In memory of Ashley Lynne Rubira (5/6/96–7/12/96): Nancy Rubira.

In memory of Lucas Anthony Ruggiero (9/20/95–12/12/95): Debbie and Steve Ruggiero.

In memory of Jesse Andrew Merlin Russell (8/3/96–10/12/96): Joel and Jackie and Jordan Russell.

In memory of Andrew Patrick Sargent (6/30/95–11/27/95): Kerry and Peter Sargent.

In memory of Thomas Lee Schlomer (lost to SIDS 9/25/89): Donna and Dicki and Jennifer and Laura Ann Schlomer; Domenick and Jill Commisso; Duane and Dorothy Schlomer; Bob and Lisa Commisso; Danni Schlomer; Deena and Jose Garcia.

In memory of Franklin (Frank) Snow Schrimsher (11/9/95–3/13/96): Scott and Margaret Schrimsher.

In memory of Margaret Hood Schuth (10/18/91–1/14/92): Kee Schuth Marshall.

In memory of Susan Marie Sebok (10/16/95–1/1/96): Maureen and David Sebok. (Maureen and David are delighted to announce the birth of Matthew David 10 months after their loss of Susan Marie. They also have a 3-year-old son, John David.)

In memory of Andrew R. Selberg (6/13/89–10/15/89): Lynnae and Bill Selberg.

In memory of Kemper Logan Siadak (10/17/92–12/28/93): Aunt Muriel, Uncle Tony, and cousins Austin and Ian.

In memory of Angel Pauline Siembida (6/5/96–6/5/96): Nancy Siembida.

In memory of Edward David Siska (6/25/91–9/15/91): Ellen and David Siska.

In memory of Jacob Richard Sleater (4/3/95–5/29/95): Carroll and O. B. English; Else and Richard Sleater; Ray and Ellen Sleater.

In memory of Samantha Snell who died of SIDS on 9/4/96: Her family and friends.

In memory of Matthew Stred Sowers (12/29/94–4/10/95): Dawn and Bill Sowers; Wanda Rodriguez; Pixie, Dave, and Deanna Rodriguez; Lorelei White.

In memory of Teresa Dvorak Splaine (5/11/95–6/13/95): Carol and David Splaine.

In memory of Jasmine Ferne Stamps (10/29/90–3/22/91): Ron and Désirée Stamps.

In memory of Craig Willem Steadman (5/22/96–5/24/96): Patty, Lloyd, and Peter Steadman; Marion and John Murphy..

In memory of Wiley Evan Stewart (2/9/96–5/2/96): Shanan and Wesley Stewart.

In memory of Morgan Alicia Stottle (11/1/95–3/25/96): Patti and Kevin Stottle; Kathy and Frank Stottle; Eileen and Joe Greenleaf; Barbara and Ronald Kingsbury.

In memory of Homer Ragsdale Sturges (11/15/95–2/9/96): Mary A. Sturges.

In memory of Ethan Daniel Thibodeau (10/29/95–12/17/95): Clarissa Thibodeau.

In memory of Heidi Annette Valdario (12/28/90–2/1/91): John and Annette Valdario.

In memory of Matthew L. Valley (12/7/93–5/5/94): Tami Valley.

In memory of Ryan Vaudry (10/29/76–12/28/76): Jo-Ann Vaudry.

In memory of Jessica Kay Wall (3/18/95–10/3/95): Amy and Matt Wall; Dottie and Ed Jones.

In memory of Nathan Douglas Weber (7/13/95–11/26/95): Chris and Deb Weber.

In memory of Mikey Whelan (10/21/89–12/31/89): Kathy Whelan.

In memory of Jessica Lynn Marie Wilson (2/29/96–4/14/96): Anna, Pat, JP, and Mark Wilson.

In memory of Janey Lou Worley (10/7/94–4/30/95): Tina and Barry, big brother, Zachary, little brother, Baby Worley (due in early May '97); Mary Jane and Kenneth Morrell.

In memory of Rebecca Paige Young (4/24/96–8/20/96): Brian and Elizabeth Young and family and friends.

Other Sponsors: Dr. Joseph D. DeCristofaro, Infant Apnea Program, University Medical Center, Stony Brook, New York (in memory of all our families in Long Island who have suffered a SIDS loss); Georgia SIDS/OID Information and Counseling Program (in memory of the 1,600 Georgia babies who were lost to SIDS over the last decade.); Loren G. Land; Deborah A. Wyzatecki (in memory of all the angels who have passed through my hands and touched my heart).

Other donations: Mathew L. Baker, Damon J. Breckheimer, Cheryl Edwards, Pamela K. Esposito, Susan Gill, Mary Haddix, Bertrice C. Jones, Daniel M. Mahoney, James W. Redding, Nicole J. Rhodes, Joseph M. Rind, Michelle Sol, Sheri A. Steiner, Leslie Y. Thompson, Walter J. Vest, Linda Whitsett.

Along with Joani, Robin gives a hearty salute to everyone who has selflessly contributed to this project. Her most heartfelt thanks, of course, goes to her husband, John, son Richard, and daughter Taylor. "They sacrificed daily for almost a year, putting up with my divided passions, meagerly prepared meals, and constantly avoided laundry baskets. They have been a prod and a safety net, but most of all dear friends for allowing me this important self-expression," says Robin. Also deserving of her thanks, Robin says, is Elaine Butler, her part-time child-care provider. Knowing her children were safe and happy was a gift that enabled her to work in peace and good conscience. Finally, Robin thanks her dear friend, Edwina Peterson Cross, for donating her time and talents editing poetry for the book.

Introduction

"And this woman's son died in the night…"

—1 Kings 3.19 (950 B.C.)

"What happened?" My thoughts were racing as I ran down the halls of the hospital toward the emergency room. I had just arrived at work in the morning when I was beeped. When I answered the telephone, I was told that Michael, one of my patients, had arrested, and they were trying to resuscitate him. I ran faster.

"Dr. Keens, you're here to see the *baby*?" a nurse said to me, directing me toward a small room. It was crowded with people, three or four doctors and as many nurses. All were working feverishly on the small baby who lay motionless on the gurney. A respiratory therapist was ventilating Michael through a tube in his windpipe. A resident physician was performing CPR. Another resident and nurse were attempting to start IVs, one working on each foot. Nurses were drawing up medications. Another recorded everything that happened during the code. Michael had no heartbeat.

Children's Hospital Los Angeles is a teaching hospital. I was a faculty member there, and for several years, I had been involved in Sudden Infant Death Syndrome (SIDS) research and in providing medical care for infants at high risk for SIDS.

Michael, five months old, was one of my patients because he had had an apparently life-threatening event three months earlier. He had been found blue, limp, and not breathing by his mother. He required full CPR to resuscitate him, but he *was* revived. After a lengthy hospitalization, we were unable to find the cause of this episode, and so he was discharged on a home apnea–bradycardia monitor. This monitor sounds an alarm when the baby stops breathing, and the parents can then revive him, if necessary. We had treated a number of high-risk babies with these monitors.

The room was small and noisy. Michael was brightly lit by the harsh, high-intensity lights. The doctors and nurses worked with intensity, calling out the baby's status and asking for medications and supplies.

"Still no heartbeat," said the doctor in charge of the resuscitation. "Give me another dose of epinephrine down the breathing tube." Drawers on the red metal crash cart were slammed open and closed. Nurses shuffled medications about looking for the right ones. "Give me another angiocath," said the doctor trying to start an IV. There wasn't much for me to do. Helplessly, I watched the skilled resuscitation team perform its work. There was a steady din of voices.

"Heart rate is 30. Give me a dose of atropine, bicarb, and calcium." We still didn't have an IV line. Another resident placed an intraosseous line in Michael's left leg. We started running fluids and medications into Michael, but his heart rate did not improve.

"Does anyone know what happened?" I asked.

"I don't know, but the mother is right there," said a resident.

I knew Michael's mother well, but I hadn't noticed her in the room. She was sitting on a low stool in a corner, motionless and silent. No one was speaking to her. Her face had a blank, distant look. She was in shock and disbelief. She was still bundled in her coat, and she sat there almost as motionless as her son. It was unusual for a parent to be allowed to stay in the room while her child was being resuscitated. I wondered what was going through her mind. What was she thinking?

"Stop CPR." Everyone looked at the cardiac monitor. "Still no heartbeat. Start CPR again. Give me another round of epi, bicarb, and calcium."

I knelt down to speak to Michael's mother. "What happened?" I asked.

Tearfully, she explained to me that he had had some apnea alarms on his monitor the night before, indicating that he had had episodes when he stopped breathing. This morning, he had had another series of alarms, and she had brought Michael to the hospital.

He had a final episode just outside the emergency room. He was dark blue, limp, and lifeless. He was immediately taken into this room, and resuscitation was started.

"Still no heartbeat. He hasn't responded," said the doctor running the code. "How long has it been?"

"Thirty-five minutes," said the nurse. It hadn't seemed that long. It seemed as if only five minutes had passed. However, we all knew that further resuscitation attempts would be futile. "Let's call it. Time of death, 8:45."

The respiratory therapist stopped bagging. The doctor stopped CPR. There was no heartbeat on the monitor. Michael was dead.

The doctors left the room. Nurses began cleaning up the syringes, half-empty medication bottles, and needles. A nurse took the breathing tube out of Michael's throat and began to clean him off.

What was the impact of this moment for Michael's mother? Did she realize what lay ahead for her and her family as they would try to put their lives back together? How could she have any idea how bad things would get? How would they survive Michael's death? The nurse asked Michael's mother if she would like to hold her baby. As she sat alone, holding her lifeless infant in her arms, the reality of Michael's death set in. She cried inconsolably. Her pain was intense and raw, and it encompassed everyone in the room.

Michael had died suddenly and unexpectedly. Even though he was "at high risk for SIDS," his death was still unexpected and could not be predicted. He died from Sudden Infant Death Syndrome. But this diagnosis does not explain anything. SIDS is not new. It has been with us for thousands of years.

SIDS is defined as the sudden, unexpected death of an apparently healthy infant under one year of age, usually occurring during sleep, which remains unexplained after a thorough postmortem evaluation, including an autopsy, investigation of the death scene, and review of the medical history.

SIDS is the most common cause of death in infants between the ages of 1 month and 1 year, yet its cause remains unknown. It is a mysterious killer. The typical story is that the parents place their baby down to sleep, either overnight or for a daytime nap. Generally, the baby was healthy. Some time later, a parent comes back to find that the baby has died. In some cases, death has occurred with the parent in the next room, yet there was no sign of a struggle. Sometimes, parents have come back to check on their babies within 20 or 30 minutes of last seeing them alive, to find that they have died swiftly and quietly in that short period of time. SIDS cannot be predicted. SIDS cannot be prevented.

Michael's mother did everything right in raising Michael. She was a model mother. Michael slept on his back. He was breast-fed, he was never dressed too warmly, and he had not even had a cold in his short life. There were no cigarette smokers in Michael's family. Michael had been a healthy baby, except for the two spells he had, one of which took his life. Yet, he still died. His death could not be prevented by good parenting or medical technology. There is nothing SIDS parents did to cause the deaths of their babies. There is nothing we know that they could have done to prevent the deaths of their babies.

The cause of SIDS is unknown. Because a SIDS death cannot be explained, many SIDS parents relive the pregnancy and short life of the baby who died, looking for something they did that caused their precious baby to die.

As medical science has advanced, some of the greatest difficulties for parents who have already had a baby die from SIDS arise from SIDS research. Over the past several years, scientists have shown that the number of babies dying from SIDS has been reduced when babies sleep on their backs instead of their stomachs, when parents do not smoke cigarettes, when babies are not exposed to cigarette smoke, when babies are not overdressed and allowed to get too hot, when babies sleep on hard, firm mattresses, and (perhaps) if they are breast-fed. However, the implication of publicity around such "Back to Sleep" campaigns is that SIDS is preventable and that the only reason babies now die from SIDS is because the parents did something wrong; it was their fault.

It is important to emphasize that SIDS has not been eliminated or prevented completely, even when all of the "Back to Sleep" or "Reduce the Risk" strategies have been followed. SIDS remains with us. Even though we do not know the cause of SIDS, if these risk-reduction strategies can prevent even a few babies from dying of SIDS, we would all endorse them. And they should be endorsed as attempts to reduce the risk of babies dying from SIDS, even if they do not completely prevent SIDS. On the other hand, these recommendations are of little comfort to families who have had a baby die from

SIDS, whether or not they were followed. A challenge of our era is to use this information in a positive way, but not to batter SIDS families by using it as ammunition to suggest that their babies died because they did something wrong.

Unfortunately, Michael was not the first of my patients to die. And yet his death, and each death, forces me to face SIDS in a way that I have never desired. As a SIDS researcher, I work in the laboratory and hope for the day when we can put an end to SIDS. However, babies continue to die, and much remains to be done for those surviving family members, who are no less the victims of SIDS. Many SIDS parents knew little about SIDS before their babies died. Some SIDS parents were unaware of SIDS before their babies died. Where do they turn for help? Where can they find information about SIDS? Where can they find support from someone who really understands what they are going through? Where can they find the hope that the initial raw pain and devastation will evolve and lessen so that they can rebuild their lives?

There are no better teachers about SIDS than these parents. SIDS parents are the best teachers, listeners, and healers for each other. This book is written by surviving family members for surviving family members and for those who wish to be supportive friends of these survivors. It is written by those who have found ways to survive the devastating impact of SIDS. This book cannot tell each person how to survive his or her own baby's SIDS death. However, it is a place to start, for each SIDS survivor must find his or her own way. Each reader can benefit from guideposts along the way. This book lovingly and powerfully provides such guideposts for those who must make this journey. The inspiring stories of these courageous survivors bring the SIDS experience alive and make it real. Pragmatic information is intertwined with personal stories in a unique and powerful approach to guiding SIDS survivors.

What remains to be done for SIDS families? Research is ongoing to try to put an end to SIDS, but this may not happen in the near future. People need to be educated about SIDS. If parents who are freshly thrust into the agony of SIDS already have some knowledge of SIDS, it may reduce some of their guilt and anguish. Health professionals, clergy, first responders, and loving friends and relatives need to be educated about the impact of SIDS on the lives of surviving family members. To have a real understanding about what SIDS is and how it affects those family members and loving friends who are left behind, one must know how it changes the parents of these babies. One must learn that these babies are never forgotten and that these deaths change these parents forever. It is this need to which this book so powerfully responds.

I am not a SIDS parent, and I cannot truly put myself in their place. However, I have learned the most about SIDS by talking with SIDS parents and listening to the stories of their babies and their lives after SIDS. These SIDS parents are able to emerge courageously and rebuild their lives. Their stories help those who are touched by SIDS and inspire those of us who have not had our own babies die.

The human spirit has an incredible capacity to survive tragedy. Those SIDS parents and friends who unselfishly share their stories in *The SIDS Survival Guide* provide us with the surest proof that this is possible.

Thomas G. Keens, M.D.
Professor of Pediatrics
University of Southern California School of Medicine

Chapter 1

What Everyone Should Know about SIDS

Sudden Infant Death Syndrome is the most common cause of death for babies between the ages of one month and one year. Although figures differ, at least 4,000 babies in the United States die from SIDS each year. Yet according to Richard Salen, a police detective who has handled many SIDS deaths, more than three-fourths of the parents he encounters do not learn what SIDS is until after their baby has died.

When Joani Horchler found her son, Christian, dead in his crib, she was only vaguely aware of SIDS. She assumed Christian must have spit up in his sleep and somehow choked. How else could an apparently healthy and content baby have died so suddenly? The first time Joani saw printed literature about SIDS she was at a funeral home after viewing Christian in his coffin. She felt a mixture of regret and rage. "I couldn't understand why I'd never seen pamphlets like that before. I'd given birth four times, and not once did I read anything—not in the OB's office, not in pediatric offices, not in the hospital. No one said anything about potential breathing problems or sleeping positions."

It was 1991 when Christian died. Joani was told by her doctors that they routinely didn't mention SIDS to parents because they didn't want to scare them, especially because they did not feel SIDS could be predicted or prevented. But many SIDS survivors, including Joani, disagree with that rationale and believe that the lack of information creates an even deeper emotional pit out of which survivors must dig themselves. Today, in light of the American Academy of Pediatrics' 1992 recommendation that healthy infants be placed on their sides or backs for sleep, the controversy has sided with routinely talking about SIDS with all new parents. (In 1996 the AAP revised its recommendation, stating that the *back* position is the best position.) With sleeping position as an introduction to the subject of SIDS, health-care providers can go on to explain what SIDS is and what it is not.

Regardless of what they knew about SIDS before losing a baby, all survivors want to know as much as possible after a loss. There is much information (more than 3,000 documents in the National SIDS Resource Center), but there is little to answer the most pressing question: "Why?" Even so, this chapter is dedicated to providing the highlights of what is known about SIDS, including its history, causes, prevention, and who is at risk. Also within this chapter, and throughout the book, are the poems, essays, and stories of those who have lived through a SIDS loss. Through their eyes, we learn what is most important to know after a SIDS loss: how to travel the long road of grief to a place of rest and hope.

In Memory of Samuel Yves Lyman Laigle

by Sheri Laigle

> *there is no*
> *greater expression of love*
> *beauty innocence*
> *than the one   on a baby's face*
> *your face last night*
> *as I held you*

> *soft white skin*
> *mountains of cheeks and forehead*
> *pinky nose   leftover wrinkle*

> *eyelids paper-thin*
> *hide those searing blue eyes*
> *they make your face come alive with color*
> *earth nature*
> *your whole being reaching out*
> *seizing me*
> *still part of me*

> *tiny mouth open in awe and wonder*
> *mystery dreams*
> *lullaby*
> *zigzag tongue so pink and wet*

I would have thought you asleep my son
　　if not for the dark bruise
　　　　on your nose
　　tubes from your mouth and nostrils

　　　　white sheet

Defining SIDS

What Is SIDS?

SIDS is the sudden death of an infant under one year of age that
remains unexplained after a thorough case investigation, including a
complete autopsy, examination of the death scene, and review of the
clinical history.

Who Is at Risk?

Unfortunately, any baby can die of SIDS. It happens throughout the
world and does not pass over any social, economic, ethnic, or racial
group. However, age is a factor. About 70% of SIDS victims die before
four months of age. Another 20% die before six months of age. Race
has also been shown through studies to be a factor. For example, in the
United States, the overall SIDS rate for black infants is about two times
that of white infants. Gender also matters: Males are 50% more likely to
die of SIDS than females.

How Does SIDS Happen?

Most SIDS victims appear perfectly healthy before being put down for
a nap or the night. At most, there might be signs of a slight cold. Some
time later, be it 15 minutes or what appears to be a long night's sleep,
the baby is found dead. There typically is no telltale sound or indication
of a struggle. Babies have been known to die in a parent's arms while
being rocked, even when that parent is a physician.

　　SIDS can strike with a fury that baffles even medical experts.
In many cases, babies seem almost determined to die and cannot be
revived, even when someone immediately and correctly administers
CPR. An article in Chapter 16, "Against All Odds," tells the story of a
baby who suddenly arched back in her father's arm and started turning

gray. Her father immediately started CPR and paramedics arrived within minutes, yet she could not be revived.

How Many Babies Die of SIDS Each Year?

The good news is that the rate of SIDS decreased 30% between 1993 and 1995. This dramatic drop is thought to have resulted mainly from the decrease in the prevalence of prone sleeping from 70% in 1992 to 24% in 1996. The bad news is that SIDS still claims the lives of about 4,000 infants (or about 1 of every 1,000 babies) each year in the United States alone. Moreover, the drop in the SIDS rate for black infants has lagged behind that of whites; it dropped 10.4% for blacks and 16.7% for whites between 1993 and 1995.

SIDS rates are reliable only for about two dozen industrialized countries, says the National Center for Health Statistics, but in most of these countries the rates are not radically different from those in the United States, ranging from a low of 1 in 1,000 to a high of 2.5 in 1,000. Although the SIDS rate in Japan has always been reported to be very low, Dr. Thomas Keens quotes a leading Japanese researcher as stating that SIDS rates are comparable to North America in areas of Japan where SIDS is being actively sought as a cause of death and autopsies are being performed. (Autopsies are performed on only one-third of potential SIDS victims in Japan.)

SIDS is still the leading killer of all infants between one week and one year of age. More American children die of SIDS each year than all those who die of cancer, leukemia, heart disease, cystic fibrosis, and child abuse combined.

What Causes SIDS?

There are more than 400 theories about what causes SIDS. One of the two major schools of thought is that infants are vulnerable at certain phases of development. In *The Discovery of Sudden Infant Death Syndrome*[1], Dr. Abraham B. Bergman theorizes that SIDS is a developmental phenomenon stemming from a failure in the normal maturation of nervous system control centers. Dr. Bergman does not believe that any particular baby has a fixed abnormality that destines it for SIDS. Rather, he likens SIDS to a "nuclear explosion where a 'critical mass' must be attained for the event to occur."

Dr. J. Bruce Beckwith, who currently directs the division of pediatric pathology at Loma Linda University in California, shares the belief that babies are normal, not abnormal, when they die. For more than 20 years, Dr. Beckwith has researched SIDS. In a pamphlet written for the Colorado SIDS Program Inc.[2], Dr. Beckwith describes SIDS in part as an abnormal event that happens to a normal baby. "Virtually all of brain growth occurs in the first two years of life, and the growth rate in the first six months is the most rapid of any time in life," he writes. "During the time when these important control centers are in a period of transition, abnormal messages might come down to the organs of respiration, one of which is to 'close off' rather than to 'open up.' Normally, at the end of a breath, the throat collapses or closes, then opens up prior to a new breath being taken. But if the wrong message comes down from the brain, the throat may stay closed instead of opening. That wrong message isn't necessarily a result of this baby being abnormal, but occurs in a normal baby whose brain is growing at a tremendously rapid rate."

The other major (and growing) school of thought is that SIDS babies are not healthy before birth and are predisposed to SIDS because of some subtle problems beginning in the fetal period.

Studies led by Dr. Hannah C. Kinney of Children's Hospital in Boston have confirmed that many SIDS victims have abnormalities in their brain stems that help to explain apnea-related and sleep arousal deficiences. Specifically, Dr. Kinney has observed decreased development of a small area in the brain stem that is thought to be very important for arousal responsiveness from sleep. In another subset of SIDS victims, she observed diminished maturation of individual nervous tissue.

"Dr. Kinney's studies lend further support to the existence of multiple causes of sudden and unexpected death in infancy," states Dr. Carl E. Hunt, Chairman of Pediatrics at Medical College of Ohio, in a column for the Greater Toledo SIDS Support Network's newsletter. "In addition to her findings in subsets of SIDS victims, in other infants the brain appears entirely normal despite the use of state-of-the-art methods of analysis," Dr. Hunt notes.

Is SIDS Preventable or Avoidable?

SIDS is considered unpredictable and unpreventable because there are no sure ways to avoid it. In most cases in which babies die of SIDS, the mothers and babies have few or no apparent risk factors. Because SIDS happens to mostly low-risk people, there are few things that parents can do to protect their babies from SIDS. Breast-fed babies are, according to some studies, less likely to die of SIDS, although many breast-fed babies do die. Pregnant mothers should avoid cigarette smoking, alcohol and drug abuse, poor or belated prenatal care, low weight gain, anemia, sexually transmitted diseases, and urinary tract infections. However, because risk factors are not, in and of themselves, causes of SIDS, avoiding these risks will by no means guarantee avoiding SIDS.

Until the past few years, it was widely believed that virtually nothing could be done to lessen the risk of a baby dying of SIDS. However, that assumption has been challenged over the past decade by dozens of studies in more than 20 countries demonstrating that fewer babies die of SIDS while sleeping on their backs or sides. Despite the overwhelming evidence by the mid to late 1980s from Dr. Susan Beal of Australia and many others that prone sleeping was a major risk factor for SIDS, the American Academy of Pediatrics recommendation to place otherwise healthy babies to sleep on their backs was not published until 1992. The National Institutes of Health began its "Back to Sleep" campaign in 1994. Studies in other countries had indicated that SIDS rates declined approximately 50% concurrent with decreases in the prevalence of prone sleeping. In the United States, from 1992 to 1995, the SIDS rate declined 30% concurrent with a decrease in the prevalence of prone sleeping from 70% in 1992 to 24% in 1996. Although the prevalence of breast-feeding did not change substantially during the study period, birth certificate data indicate that from 1989 to 1994, the prevalence of cigarette smoking during pregnancy declined by approximately 25% (from 20% to 15%).

One important piece of advice to heed is to put a baby to sleep on her back rather than on the baby's side. "The available data lead to the clear conclusion that supine (back) should be the only recommended sleep position for infants," says Dr. Hunt. "Side sleeping is safer than prone sleeping, but the lowest risk is associated with supine sleeping."

It is not known why sleep position may be important, but one study suggested that sleeping face down leads to an accumulation of toxic bacteria in babies' airways. Among other theories are these:

■ Babies sleeping on their tummies become more easily overheated, which may inhibit their respiration.

■ Babies may rebreathe the oxygen-depleted air they've already exhaled.

■ Sleeping more deeply on one's stomach may make it more difficult to awaken if physiological mistakes occur.

■ The jaw may be pushed slightly backward when sleeping prone, leading to airway obstruction.

Will avoiding infant immunizations help avoid SIDS? No, according to Dr. Hunt. "Recent studies have shown conclusively that DPT immunization in early infancy does not increase the risk of SIDS," he says, adding, "Indeed, the SIDS rate is actually higher in infant groups that are not immunized compared to infant groups appropriately immunized."

The issue of the extent to which SIDS is avoidable is further discussed in Chapter 16.

What SIDS Is and What SIDS Is Not
by the National SIDS Resource Center

SIDS Is

■ The major cause of death in infants from one month to one year of age, with most deaths occurring between two and four months

■ Sudden and silent—Infants are seemingly healthy

■ Currently, unpredictable and unpreventable

■ A death that occurs quickly, often associated with sleep and with no signs of suffering

■ Determined only after an autopsy, an examination of the death scene, and a review of the clinical history

■ Designated as a diagnosis of exclusion

■ A recognized medical disorder listed in the International Classification of Diseases, 9th Revision (ICD-9)

■ An infant death that leaves unanswered questions, causing intense grief for parents and families

SIDS Is Not

■ Caused by vomiting and choking, or by minor illnesses such as colds or infections

■ Caused by the diphtheria, pertussis, tetanus (DPT) vaccines or other immunizations

■ Contagious

■ Child abuse

■ The cause of every unexpected infant death

A SIDS Expert's Perspective
by John G. Brooks, M.D.

SIDS is the leading cause of infant death between the end of the first month and the end of the first year of life, claiming approximately 4,000 lives each year in the United States. The good news is that the rate of SIDS is clearly dropping in this country and in many other areas of the world. Until about 1990, the SIDS rate was about 1.5–2.0 of every 1,000 babies, but in 1995, the rate fell below 1.0 of every 1,000 babies.

Most of the clearly established information about SIDS comes from the study of epidemiology, that is, the study of diseases in populations to describe the circumstances under which the problem occurs. As a result of multiple studies of this type, where carefully collected information about a group of SIDS infants is compared to similar information from a group of infants who did not die of SIDS and, in some investigations, by just studying SIDS infants, it has been established that SIDS occurs more frequently in the winter than in the summer and that the greatest risk of SIDS is between two and four months of age.

In other studies where comparison infants were also studied, certain characteristics of the mother, the infant, and the infant's environment have been found more frequently among the SIDS infants than among the surviving or control infants. These maternal risk factors include maternal smoking during or after the pregnancy (or both), young maternal age (teenage years), poverty, and maternal drug abuse. Each of these factors increases the risk of SIDS at least two- to threefold in comparison to infants born of mothers without these characteristics.

Infant factors associated with SIDS include being male, prematurity, low birth weight, and prone or side sleeping. The only consistently confirmed environmental risk factor is winter or the cold months of the year. Some factors such as soft bedding and an infant sharing a bed with an adult may increase the risk of SIDS, but this link is not clear at this time. Overheating an infant increases the risk of SIDS if the baby is sleeping on the stomach, but not in other sleeping positions. Babies with their heads covered by bedding or other material may be at increased risk of SIDS, although this fact is not yet firmly established.

In the past, it has been felt by many that breast-feeding would reduce the risk of SIDS, but newer information indicates that this effect was due to factors other than breast-feeding. So, although breast-feeding has many proven advantages, lowering the incidence of SIDS is not one of them.

Also not firmly established is the possibility that babies using pacifiers may be at slightly lower risk of SIDS. Because there is only limited information available about the relationship between SIDS and pacifier use, and because there are other important considerations with regard to the appropriateness of pacifier use, this finding regarding SIDS should not be interpreted as an indication that pacifier use should be encouraged to reduce the risk of SIDS.

Current SIDS Research

In many countries over the past five to eight years, public education campaigns directed at changing health behaviors to reduce the number of SIDS deaths have been implemented and have contributed to substantial decreases in SIDS rates. Most of these campaigns have focused on some combination of the hazards of maternal smoking, soft bedding, overheating infants, and the probable or possible benefits derived from supine sleeping position for infants and breast-feeding.

The only one of these health behaviors that has changed dramatically in response to the campaign is sleeping position practices. In most countries, the percentage of infants sleeping prone (on their stomachs) was 50–70% or higher before the campaigns and has dropped to less than 10% prone following the campaigns, except in the United States, where in 1996, 24% of infants are still sleeping prone.

There are many theories about why infants sleeping on their stomachs are at higher risk of SIDS, and much current research effort is being devoted to clarifying this issue. Most of the theories relate to the concept that babies on their stomachs, particularly on soft bedding, may get inadequate fresh air if their faces are straight into the mattress or if the weight of their heads produces a significant pocket in the bedding or mattress to limit their access to fresh air. Most babies will awaken and move their heads if they are in a situation with inadequate fresh air, but SIDS babies may, at least temporarily, lack some protective reflex that would trigger this arousal. The search for such an abnormality, particularly in the part of the brain responsible for maintaining normal breathing, heart rate, and arousal responses has been and continues to be the focus of significant research. Investigators from Dartmouth and Harvard recently reported that certain receptors that may be important in normal control of breathing and sensing an elevation in carbon dioxide are deficient in SIDS victims compared to infants dying suddenly of other causes.

Coping After the Death

The focus of this book is on helping SIDS families deal with their devastating losses. To conclude, I would like to include a few points that I think are especially important in this difficult process.

- After losing a baby to SIDS, almost every parent goes over and over the circumstances of the death and is likely to feel strong emotions of guilt, anger, or blame. Part of this is the "what if?" thinking that most people experience: "What if I had checked on him earlier?" "What if I had stayed home from work that day?" My response is that no one can be with his or her baby all the time. Even if you or someone else had been with the baby at the critical moment, it is quite likely that the baby would have died anyway, as it is clear that some infants die of SIDS in hospitals despite all appropriate efforts at resuscitation.

- Many newspaper writers and editors like to publish reports about SIDS, particularly breakthroughs in our understanding of SIDS based on new research. It is likely that friends and relatives will send SIDS families news clippings about such articles. We must be skeptical about "breakthroughs" that are reported first in the lay press. Some of them are true breakthroughs, but others are not, and may even be misleading. The best advice is to consult a SIDS expert, who can understand the scientific side of the research, for an opinion about the validity of this "breakthrough."

■ Another caution about interpretation of SIDS research results involves "SIDS risk factors" that are identified through epidemiological research. Such studies identify characteristics that are more common in SIDS babies than in babies who do not die of SIDS, but many babies who die of SIDS do not have any of the risk factors, and many babies with the risk factors do not die of SIDS. For this reason, risk factors are not useful in identifying who will die of SIDS. Some of them are useful, however, in identifying some environments or health behaviors that if avoided may lower any baby's risk of SIDS.

The good news is that the rate of SIDS is falling; the bad news is that many babies are still dying of this devastating problem. Good research has led to this reduction in SIDS rate; more good research is the key to further reduction in the rate and ultimately approaching our goal of eliminating SIDS.

Consider the Numbers

by Robin Rice Morris

Fearfully, and with an awful respect, I consider the numbers.
Four-thousand, at least, each year, in my country alone.
That means someone's baby died of SIDS today.
Probably more than a dozen.

How many people, then—be they mothers, fathers, sisters, brothers, grandparents, godparents, babysitters—how many were struck by death's powerful blow, dealt as if from a professional heavyweight boxer who allows his novice contender no handicap?

And how many funerals, full of well-intentioned people who grasped at meanings which were not there—are still not there—smacked of the unfairness of it all? After all, isn't death supposed to come to six-foot-tall old men a full lifetime before it claims twenty-six-inch-long baby boys?

Or what about the infant car seats that sat hauntingly empty? How many of them remained strapped in until, somehow, someone was able to summon the Herculean strength it required to move it to the basement, or closet, or someone else's car where someone else's baby will likely have the audacity to live long enough to outgrow it?

How many parents' arms felt heavy and yet hollow, useless save to run grief-thickened blood through, keeping life going whether they really wanted it to or not?

How many lockets of hair served as the only hard and fast proof that there really was a baby here, once, who smiled and cried and whose life made that house a home and those people a family?

How many pacifiers (or booties or rattles) were unexpectedly found behind a couch or under a chair, causing an unsuspecting father to buckle at the knees, and just when life's journey was haltingly yet courageously being undertaken again?

And who knows the number of imaginary cries and automatic wake-up calls for midnight feedings there were that drew a mother nearly to the nursery door before she remembered, and sunk to the floor in utter anguish?

How many future Little League players will never be suited up? And how many of tomorrow's dance recitals will be one angelic ballerina short, without anyone even knowing it?

And perhaps worst of all to consider: next year's batch. Next year's 4,000 or so who are in the womb as we speak, luring innocent parents-to-be into dreaming dreams and making plans clear through the college years—joyous dreams and important plans that will never be. Next year's 4,000, who will each be the world's most beautiful baby, and the world's most tragic death.

So, yes, as my own precious children quiet into lovely sleep, spared one more day from this and all the other possible deaths out there that could break me in a moment, I do consider the numbers. I consider the numbers, and I pray.

SIDS Then and Now: A Personal and Political History
by Carrie Griffin Sheehan

A simple child
That lightly draws its breath
And feels his life in every limb
What should it know of death?
— William Wordsworth

These words, written around the turn of the 18th century, no doubt reflected the high incidence of infant death at that time. Because so many forms of neonatal deaths and child disease have now been eradicated by medical discoveries, we in the United States, mid-century until now, do not expect infants to die. And yet infant mortality in our country remains high, with Sudden Infant Death Syndrome responsible for more deaths than any other cause in those one week to one year of age.

Perhaps one of the earliest available records of SIDS was in a diary dated February 13, 1686. It noted, "No symptom of overlaying," a reference to the biblical story of Solomon and the common belief that mothers smothered their infants by accident.

In spite of convent school education, I had no knowledge of what overlaying was. However, for the past 13 years, I have served as a regional director for the SIDS Foundation and, after its merger, with the SIDS Alliance. In a way, the position chose me. It was one of happenstance.

In the summer of 1954, I was 26 years old, married, and had three children. With my husband, a teacher and small-town winning basketball coach, we had just moved back to our native city, Seattle. We had nowhere to go but forward. So with our friends and neighbors we did our part to fill the rooms of the big old Capitol Hill homes with our "boomers."

Mary Caroline (Molly) came into the world on a glorious July 26 evening in 1955. It was a special birth because we used the methods of natural childbirth, with Tom (who was named the "tall mother") present for the birth. Seattle had one hospital that was beginning to experiment with natural childbirth, a process that was so unusual the hospital and its methods had been featured in Life *magazine. Having had the experience of birthing three infants in a drugged stupor, I decided to try this method that had the establishment embroiled in controversy.*

Our fourth child, a little strawberry blonde with a crooked smile, won everyone's heart. Summer days in the neighborhood rolled one into the other, with out-of-town guests, Seattle's Seafair, and the hydroplane races drawing the summer to a close. Not quite willing to give up the vacation feeling, we planned a "last of the season" holiday at our summer cabin on Whidbey Island. It was Columbus Day week-end, and everyone would be ready to roll Friday mid-afternoon. It was October 6, and Molly's godmother came by with her one-month-old, Judith. For the infants' afternoon naps, Judith was put in the down-stairs bassinet and Molly in the crib upstairs. Over coffee, Betti and I marveled at the world of the '50s, post World War II, college behind us, days filled with children's activities, caring and loving husbands, and volunteer white-glove-lady activities to challenge our creative and intellectual energies.

When the school children and Tom came home and Betti had left, it was time to get ready for the island. Our five-year-old went to check on Molly and came downstairs saying that Molly looked funny. Sensing her tension, I went upstairs, and as long as I live I will never forget the moment. Then and now it is as if in slow motion: I am turning her over, my eyes bringing to consciousness tiny legs that look like white and blue marble cherub limbs heavy as any statue. Nothing prepared me for the shock of her lifeless, blackened face. It was at that moment that I lost all innocence. Death came as evil to suffuse all that was beautiful. I called for Tom and phoned the fire department, while he attempted CPR. The children were taken away by kind friends and neighbors, and the siren sound echoing far off and moving closer confirmed what part of me wanted to deny. Tom left in the police car that transported Molly to the county hospital's emergency room. It was not until many years later that I found out about his own ordeal: He was locked in a room like a criminal until his background was checked.

Tom returned home to a house full of family and friends, and I remember a vague space and time when no one would tell me that our two-month-and-ten-day-old Molly had been declared dead on arrival.

I never saw Molly again. The autopsy report would read "acute virus pneumonia," and the next day there was a short news article in the paper. There were no hysterics. Numbness, rather than grief was expressed. The next day, choosing the casket (I had never seen such a small one) was followed by the burial with just Tom, myself, and the parish priest. Tom went back to teaching the next day, and the next week I moderated a benefit fashion show, which ironically benefited our Children's Hospital.

Do not misunderstand. Family and friends were kind and loving. The fact that the chief of staff at Children's Hospital, a lifelong friend of the family, called to extend sympathy lent an authoritative sense of support. There was a whole small town's outpouring of love for their former coach and his wife. It took a good part of my day just to tend the plants and flowers so thoughtfully sent. The cards and letters for the most part never mentioned death (Did no one else experience an infant death?), and for the most part spoke of God and what a blessing we had. Displays of sorrow were not common, and I remember someone telling me that "thoroughbreds cry in their hearts." Before long, as the shock wore off, I realized that I was not a horse. A stiff upper lip only served well for a short time. Denial, I found out, is only postponement, and my acute depression and suicidal feelings were resolved primarily through the compassion and wisdom of a dear priest who was also a psychologist and a friend. However, until other losses in my life several decades later, Molly's death was not fully dealt with.

It is difficult to believe, but in 1955 no one dealt directly with children's grief. Hindsight can bring wisdom. But along with it comes its twin, regret. With the exception of a friend who was kind enough to bring a cake to celebrate our four-year-old son's birthday, no one spoke openly or shared feelings with five-year-old Christie, four-year-old Tommy, or eighteen-month-old Patrick. Nor, for that matter, was Tom—"the tall mother"—the focus of concern. We hadn't known anyone who had the same experience as we did, so there really was no way to measure what was "normal." Interestingly, I had a friend whose daughter had been murdered. Both of us recall now the emotional games we played about who was suffering the most. I believe this came from the religious notion that suffering is good for you, which had been planted firmly in both of us from an early age. Though tinged with ego and black humor, it served as a kind of survival tactic.

In 1957, Timothy Daniel joined the Sheehan clan. Nursing students now ask me about my anxiety level at that time. My reply is that it was much more an age of faith than science. (Remember, SIDS still had not been designated as a medical entity.) Not to mention the irony of a subsequent child being born on April Fool's Day, which serves to increase one's faith in Providence. Tim's arrival did give strong emphasis to the meaning of a "wanted child." Then followed Mary, Michael, and Caroline, healthy, beautiful babies who helped bring our very grand total to eight.

What was happening on the national health scene about these mysterious deaths, sometimes called "the disease of theories"? Twentieth-century research in America was probably initiated with the documented studies of pathologist Jacob Werner and Irene Garrow, a husband-and-wife team in the medical examiner's office of Queens, New York. In the '40s, their studies ruled out suffocation as a cause of "crib deaths" and showed that natural inflammatory processes were involved in most deaths. In 1958, a Connecticut couple suffered the death of their son, Mark, and refused to accept the autopsy report of "acute bronchial pneumonia" as cause of death. In 1962, because they questioned the cause of their son's death and were committed to Mark's memory and a desire to prevent other such deaths, they developed and funded the Mark Addison Roe Foundation, which would later become the National SIDS Foundation. It would involve medical personnel, researchers, and those families affected by a "crib death."

Meanwhile, on the West Coast in Seattle, Fred and Mary Dore in 1961 became the victims of the sudden death of their infant daughter, Christine. At the time, Fred was a Washington state legislator. In 1963, as Chairman of the Appropriations Committee, he introduced a bill to require that all sudden deaths of children under three years of age be autopsied and studied at the University of Washington. In the fall of 1963, the university was contracted to conduct the First International Conference on the Causes of Sudden Death in Infancy. A first-time display regarding SIDS at the American Academy of Pediatrics was as recent as 1964. The following year marked a three-year epidemiology study of SIDS in Kings County, Washington, and in 1969, the Second

International Conference defined SIDS and described its pathology. It was not until April 22, 1974, that the National SIDS Act was signed. Research grants and federal contracts followed as the states implemented counseling projects. SIDS was finally coded in the International Classification of the Causes of Death and published by the World Health Organization.

Our baby boomers took over. The progression of grade school and high school filled calendar pages and, with seven teenagers in the '60s and '70s, there were times I questioned whether the Almighty had taken the wrong child. I went back to college when my older children did. I was a member of the Washington state chapter of the National Sudden Infant Death Syndrome Foundation (NSIDSF), which had been established in the '60s, and served on the board during the chapter reorganization in the late '70s. In an era when every board and commission needed a "token woman," I often was one. I served as the first woman on the Seattle Planning Commission and, after chairing it, decided to run for public office. I lost, but without too much disappointment, and, in retrospect, with joy, for that year (1980) was when I was elected to the national board of the SIDS Foundation and subsequently was asked to serve as a staff person in the position of regional director.

And so serve I did, for 13 years. Chapters were organized, and the program of support for the victims of SIDS became more comprehensive. In the '80s, SIDS moved into the mainstream, with audiences on Oprah Winfrey, LA Law, and an off-Broadway play. The 25-year anniversary of the SIDS Foundation also brought increased media attention. With the recognition of child abuse, SIDS became more prominent but also more confusing to officials and painful to families. Communities received training for the emergency responders, police, and fire departments. Fund-raising events brought attention to local chapters. Congressional hearings began to bring about an increase of research funding, from a half million dollars in 1985 to $15 million for 1994. A merger of many of the SIDS groups was formalized in 1991, resulting in the SIDS Alliance. Their Family Services Advisory Committee continues. Its goals are autopsies of all infants who die suddenly and unexpectedly, prompt notification of the results of the autopsy, the use of the term SIDS, and follow-up counseling and information for those affected by the deaths.

Fund-raising and advocacy efforts ensure the continuation of research. Concern about SIDS was for so long almost exclusively on the backs of the parents. Now there is an increase in enlightened community support, with the perception that one death touches 100 lives. Families have the resources of SIDS medical professionals, groups such as the SIDS Alliance, the Southwest SIDS Research Institute in Texas, Compassionate Friends, Association of SIDS Program Professionals, and SHARE, to mention a few who support with hope and healing.

Now, more than 40 years since our Molly's death, I can say I have resolved it. The loss of days and hours with her has been transcended not without bittersweet feelings, but with the knowledge that her coming and going have greatly enriched my life. I have had a supportive family, intimate friendships, and great depths of support given and taken. In 1987, with others of the world SIDS community, we formed SIDS Family International (now SIDS International). Meeting at Lake Como, Italy—on the shores that I learned about in my ancient history book, among centuries-old statuary and colonnades—I was struck with the knowledge that in my lifetime I had witnessed the beginning of hope. Perhaps the ancient pain of "overlaying" might be solved and, at least on this earth, no one ever need again suffer the isolation and guilt that comes when something so irrational as SIDS extinguishes the beauty and innocence of an "infant newly formed."

With the years have come grandchildren, among them another Molly. This pre-three-year-old's "wuv you" thrills like a burst of fireworks. But it also represents to me the truth of the words of Camus, the French philosopher, who wrote to his friend at the death of his son, "But what does it truly matter what we lack when what we have is not used up. So many things are susceptible of being loved, that surely no discouragement can be final."

Chapter 2

The Nightmare Begins

Probably the most stressful and anxiety-provoking act in human existence is the separation of a woman from her newborn infant. The response to this, which humans share with most of the animal kingdom, is an overwhelming combination of panic, rage, and distress.

— Dr. A.P. Ruskin

SIDS is a sudden, forced separation that will last forever. In the beginning, survivors are so shocked that their bodies and minds cannot even begin to comprehend all that has been lost. Their investment in such a tiny life is immense and deep-rooted, from the planning (that for many began in early childhood), to the lovemaking, to the first blessed cry. After birth, there is the excitement of seeing who the baby looks like; catching his first smile; taking her to Mom's or Dad's office to show off; monumental first trips to parks and grocery stores, or over the river and through the woods to Grandmother's house. There is the pride of having a growing, healthy baby and being a "good mom" or a "good dad."

And then, suddenly, nothing. Babies who ought to have woken up hungry and alert do not wake up at all. Shock and disbelief overtakes most survivors so that they can only vaguely feel their own empty arms and the rage that will eventually come full force.

In the dark nights after Christian died, Joani sometimes held her then two-year-old daughter's life-size doll. "It was the same size Christian had been, and I just needed to fill my aching arms. They were so empty, so void of anything. My nursing baby, who depended completely on me, had been like an appendage of me, and when he died it was like part of my own body was ripped off. When I could actually sleep, I'd wake up wishing I could die. The first thing I thought of every morning was, 'I can't believe it really happened.'"

What shook Joani most during those early days was the strong sense she had that the nightmare was only just beginning. She already felt like she wanted to die, and yet she sensed that somehow her feelings would plummet to yet lower and lower depths. "I was very afraid that I might take my own life," Joani says, "or just conveniently die in a car crash. It helped when my sister-in-law told me how devastating it had been when her own mother committed suicide. I realized that I was still Gabe's wife and my three daughters' mother. I had other people in my life who really needed me."

Other than stating that it is perfectly normal to feel depressed and even suicidal after a SIDS death, there is little anyone can say to ease the continuous, crashing waterfall of pain. Even so, Abraham Lincoln, who lost three sons, is quoted in this chapter as saying, "You are sure to be happy again." Of course, to get to the point Lincoln talks about involves a trek through grief—a strange and hostile territory that no one would ever pass through if given the choice.

Below are some common and normal experiences in the first few weeks and months of that journey:

A sensation of numbness. This is shock, and often it is what gets people through the first weeks. It is the way your mind and body protect you from the full force of the blow. Many people find it hard to do ordinary things like cooking a meal or getting organized for an outing. "I felt lost in a fog," recalls Martina Murphy, a mother of five who lost her first son to SIDS. "I went to a food store a few days after Jimmy died, and then I wouldn't go back because I remembered it as being totally disorganized. It wasn't until seven years later that I realized that it hadn't been the store that was a mess—It was me!"

A continuous inner dialogue of "if onlys". This is your mind's way of trying to make the tragedy "unhappen." As irrational as that is, it's a very normal thing to do. "If only" is really a way of trying to go back in time, to change things so that your baby does not die, but instead wakes up—just as you expected, just as he should have.

Flashbacks. These are strong mental images of poignant times with your baby, especially the moment of finding—or finding out—your baby has died. These may often cause tension, anxiety, nervousness, guilt, bad dreams, and the feeling that you're losing your mind. They are also normal, and should eventually soften in impact and dwindle in frequency to only rare occasions.

Hearing your baby cry. This can happen when you actually hear another's baby cry, or when there is not a baby for miles. When Terre Dohrman was on a business trip a few months after her son Zachary died, she kept "hearing" a baby crying in the bushes outside her motel room. She looked and looked for the baby and, at last, with utter anguish, she accepted the fact that there was no baby.

People commenting that you appear to be "handling it well." In the beginning stages of grief, it is just as normal to withdraw from others as it is to reach out for comfort. Many people, like Joani, hardly cry during the first few weeks. Yet this is no indication of how much they loved their baby or are devastated by their loss. Friends and relatives often mistake this stalwart behavior for tremendous emotional strength. Unfortunately, this assumption creates yet another burden, because you begin to wonder if you loved your baby enough (after all, if you really loved your baby, how could you be strong after her death?) or whether you are grieving "right." The truth is that you loved your baby deeply. You are in shock, and it will be a long time before you'll feel anything like "strong."

Extreme irritability, especially with the little things others consider important. After a SIDS loss, there is new meaning to the phrase "life-and-death matter." To you, nothing is important but the vitally important. So, intermingled with the great sadness of your loss, there is a low boiling rage, ready to explode at the slightest infraction of your idea of what should be. How dare that strange woman argue with a sales clerk over a price! Doesn't she know your world has stopped, your baby is dead? No, in fact, she does not know. Nor do most of the world's population. As unfair as it is, the world is going on without you both. And other people will continue to cry over stupid, little, unimportant things as you cry over a life—a whole life! What you are offended by is the unfairness of it all, and that, too, is perfectly normal.

But strangers are not the only ones who will displease you. Far worse are the family and friends who should know better. In utter frustration, you may become tempted to tell everyone to get lost and leave you alone forever. Instead, so as not to burn bridges you may one day need to cross, you might tell nonessential family and friends to make a note on their calendar to call you in a week or a month. And, if you can, remember the words "I'm sorry." Most people are quick to forgive the grieving, and an occasional "I'm sorry" can significantly lower the temperature of *their* boiling pot.

Indecision on the more practical baby matters. Many people feel somewhat frozen in time after their baby dies. What should I do with his clothes? Her room? The bottles? The car seat? The baby shampoo? Often, it's easier not to think about it for a while. Things are left just as they were the day their baby died. A door is closed, and kept closed, for a few months or even a few years. As long as it doesn't last a lifetime, thus impeding the grieving process, it's perfectly fine.

Snap decisions about the more practical baby matters. Not everyone feels frozen after a baby dies. In fact, they may feel just the opposite: as if they are overwound and can't stop doing things. These people want to clean out the room immediately and throw every reminder into a big box. That's okay, too, so long as the box goes into storage, and not out the door. It's best not to throw or give belongings away immediately because you may change your mind about how they affect you. Many SIDS parents keep a little bag of cherished clothes, pacifiers, or toys— often unwashed—to remind them in quiet times of the baby. Which items will be most cherished will be easier to discern after time, so that choosing a bag of keepsakes is best after some time has passed.

Dumb friends. By dumb we mean either stupid or silent, or both. There may be those, both in your neighborhood and at work, who are too overwhelmed or too uncomfortable to visit, call, or send a note at the time of your tragedy. Later, they may feel compelled to avoid crossing paths for fear of embarrassment. SIDS parent Jennifer Wilkinson found that "many people were awkward in the face of our pain and looked to us for help and guidance in social situations."

The truth is, most people in our society have not been taught about death, and they need guidance. You—the new "expert"—may have to take the initiative in talking about your child so others will know that it is appropriate. One SIDS parent was extremely upset when her co-workers ignored a picture of her baby that she displayed prominently on her desk. She thought they would take the hint that the picture meant she wanted them to ask about her baby. When they didn't, she became angry and resentful at their "insensitivity." After several weeks she acted upon a suggestion from a parent support group meeting that she bring up the subject. As a result, she found several of her co-workers very willing to talk.

Questions about your next baby. There is no good way to ask a SIDS parent if he or she is planning to have another child. Not only is it too personal, it always sounds like a replacement issue, as if your lost child was nothing more than a pair of shoes and you think you'll just head on out to the mall this afternoon for another. Yet many people ask anyway, so it is a good idea to have thought out your answer—or non-answer—in advance. Because almost any positive or negative answer will trigger an opinion, you might wish to simply say: "My husband and I are discussing that privately for the time being."

Tears, frequent and flowing. Some SIDS survivors wonder if they will ever stop crying, at least in the grocery store. You will, but not for a long time. One mother said she cried every day for 10 months before she had a day without tears. However long it takes, each survivor must be allowed as much time as they need. As uncomfortable as they feel, tears are healthy—and not only for those close to the baby. Many SIDS parents say they welcome the opportunity to cry with others who simply care about them and their hurt. It helps them express their grief and release built-up tensions. If you tell people that it's okay that you're crying or that you actually want to cry, you will be helping them to help you.

Other babies. No one spots a baby carriage like a pregnant woman. And no one notices each and every baby in sight like the recent SIDS survivor. Babies may draw you or send you running. Either reaction is considered normal. If you can express your feelings and reactions, they will usually be understood.

Poor job performance. SIDS parents who return to work shortly after the death often describe themselves as confused and disoriented on the job. It is also common to feel that your work has no value any more, that it doesn't contribute to society, that everything pales in importance when compared to the life and death of your child. If you feel this way, it might be helpful to have some frank discussions with your boss and co-workers. Let them know that you're having a rough time just now but that you're doing the best you can to work things out.

Or you may want to ask for a leave of absence to do your grief work, if that is possible.

Superior job performance. Many people use work as a distraction from their grief. This can be good. But if taken to an extreme, so that the grief process is avoided, it can be a trap that lasts a lifetime. In addition, it often cuts out not only grief work, but the growth of any or all close relationships. It is easy to become impatient with the long and often drawn-out process of grieving, but it's necessary to give oneself permission, time, and space to move through difficult emotions to a new and better place.

Greeting people who don't know. Condolences are tough to take, but belated congratulations are especially tormenting. Yet it is likely that not everyone will hear of your baby's death. These acquaintances and co-workers will often become very flustered and embarrassed when their "Congratulations" is met with the dark news. There is little you can do in awkward situations like these except to tell them about the death and let them know it's okay to talk with you about it (if that's how you feel). Be assured that in most cases, they feel almost as badly as you do about the encounter.

A disconnectedness with the world. After a SIDS loss, many parents really can't identify with the rest of the world for quite some time. Feelings of isolation and loneliness are common. This is the time to become involved with a parent-support group. Even if you can't solve your problems of inattentiveness, impatience, and forgetfulness, you are likely to feel better just knowing that others also feel or have felt the same way. Call the national SIDS Alliance for a referral to a SIDS support group in your area. (See the appendix of this book for the phone number.) If there is not a SIDS support group in your area, contact your local hospital to see if there is a Compassionate Friends group (for parents of any-aged children who have died) or a Miscarriage, Infant Death, and Stillbirth (MIS) group.

The opportunity to medicate feelings. Some doctors automatically prescribe medication to the bereaved. Some survivors reach for their own self-medications, such as excessive drink, food, work, gambling, exercise, or illegal drugs. Unless closely supervised, any of these "medications" can become addictions, and grief work is tough enough without addiction recovery work added to it. As painful as it is, work through your grief one day at a time and in time, it will ease.

Relationship difficulties. Everyone grieves differently, even couples who have known each other for years. The strain of two grieving partners is immense, and many people decide to enter counseling just to keep their marriage alive. (See "Hitting It Off with a Counselor" in Chapter 13.) Joani was helped greatly by the increased intimacy she shared with her husband Gabe as they clung to each other for survival. However, like virtually all couples, they found they grieved differently and had to learn to respect each other's different ways and timetables of grieving. Allowing a partner to grieve in the way that he or she needs is perhaps the most important key to making it through the first tragedy without a second.

A Mental Replay of Thursday, March 21, 1991
by Michelle Morgan Spady

When I think back on that awful Thursday, March 21, of '91, I wish I could just press...

ERASE (As you would on a VCR)

Memories of that whole day are so vivid in my mind. It started out so beautiful and normal. Armani had slept with us the night before, just as he had done all his life. We all awoke and played together as usual. I fed him and put him in a carrier on my back (something that usually made him smile). But he cried a little, so somebody please press...

PAUSE

He wouldn't eat much that morning, so I prepared extra food to be taken to the babysitter's house. I got him dressed. I couldn't really decide what to put on him that day, and I changed outfits maybe three times. I let him play with his father as I got dressed to take him to the babysitter. They played hide-n-go-seek. Armani crawled behind the sofa! Somebody please press...

PAUSE

When it was Dad's turn to get dressed, Armani and I stood in the doorway of the bathroom so that he could watch his Dad shave. I said "See, Armani, you're gonna shave too, one day when you are grown up." Armani stared at his father for the longest time. Somebody please press...

STOP (I want to save this moment.)

Once we got to the sitter's he was a little fretful, so I stayed with him for about 20 minutes. The sitter insisted that I leave, but I stayed, held him and tried to feed him. He wasn't hungry. I encouraged him to get down on the floor and play with the other baby named Allison. He crawled away from me three times but each time came back to hold onto my knee. Somebody please press...

STOP

The sitter said, "He's okay now. Why don't you go?" I turned and looked at him and said, "Bye, Armani." He didn't cry today for some reason. Somebody please press...

PAUSE

When I got home the question was asked, "What took you so long today?" I replied, "Armani didn't want me to leave so I stayed with him a while." I started my errands and was totally disoriented all day. I couldn't seem to make decisions and couldn't find my way home. I picked up several toys to buy for Armani and put them back, rationalizing, "He's got plenty of time to buy one of these." In the end I bought one anyway! Around 3:00 I thought I should call home. I got no answer. I decided to stop at the store on the way home to buy Armani some food and diapers, as I often do.

After going through the check-out I rushed over to the pay phone to call the sitter to tell her I was on my way to pick up Armani. This was always my favorite time of day. I always hated to leave him anytime, anywhere. The sitter always liked me to call before I picked Armani up, so that she could have him ready. Somebody please press...

ERASE

A male voice answered the phone. It was her husband, which was unusual for 5 pm.

Me: Hi. May I speak to Sophia?

Husband: Sophia can't come to the phone right now. Who is this?

Me: This is Michelle, Armani's mom. Just tell Sophia I'm around the corner at the store and I'm on my way to pick up Armani.

Husband: Michelle, what's the matter with you? You can't pick up Armani!

Me: Why?

Husband: Haven't you heard what happened today?

Me: No! What happened today? (Immediately I thought he had gotten sick.)

Husband: Armani is dead! He is dead! He died today! Everybody's been looking for you! (In an instant I tuned in to the sounds in the background and heard a woman crying.)

Me: What? Let me speak to your wife!

Husband: No!

Sophia: Let me please speak to Michelle! Michelle, Michelle!

Me: Sophia, where is my baby! Where is Armani? What happened to him?

Sophia: I don't know. He died today. I put him down for his nap around 1:30. He didn't eat much lunch and Allison wanted to play with him. She kept shaking his crib and I called out to him, "Armani, Armani, get up honey, Allison wants to play with you," and he didn't move. When I went over to pick him up, he was limp....Michelle, I'm so sorry. Your husband is waiting for you at the Arlington Hospital.

Me: Hang up! (Looking for another quarter to call home, I was nervous, shaking, and crying. I dialed the number, and my brother answered.) Steve, let me speak to Arnett!

Arnett: (sounding very solemn) Where are you? We'll come and get you!

Me: No! What happened to Armani? What are they talking about? Where is my baby?

Arnett: Where are you? We'll come and get you.

Me: NO! I'm at the store and I'm on my way home! Somebody please press. . .

ERASE (Take this dreadful day out my life!)

I run to the car…put the groceries into the car…I've gotta get to Armani…I get home, then go to the hospital:…The doctor says, "Ms. Morgan, calm down. There is no way we can let you into the emergency room to see Armani if you don't calm down. There are very sick people in the emergency room!"

Please let me see my baby…What happened to him?…He's lying on the gurney in a clean diaper…He doesn't look like anything's wrong with him!…I have to touch him!…This can't be so… Armani, please tell mommy what happened today…Someone says that Armani cannot tell me what happened, but they think it's something called SIDS. We won't know for sure until an autopsy is performed, but from all apparent indications, it looks like SIDS. Ms. Morgan, SIDS is…Would you like to hold Armani? Yes! Please, I say…Ms. Morgan, we highly suggest that you seek the support of the local SIDS group at your convenience… Please, just leave me alone with my baby…

So cold, so still, so peaceful…This morning so warm, bubbly, and full of life. SIDS? What is SIDS? Not my baby, he's eight-and-a-half months old. He's due for his nine-month check-up next week. We have an appointment. He's healthy. He's happy. He has two teeth. He's just starting to walk. He's had all his shots. No cold. No fever. No sign… What is this thing called SIDS? I had all the genetic testing done, amniocentesis, sonograms, blood tests…What went wrong? When did it go wrong? Nobody mentioned watch out for SIDS. He's going to be christened on his first birthday…This can't be real. It's an awful nightmare. Please wake me up!

Remembering Armani today on the one-year anniversary of his death and wishing, like a videotape recorder I could just press REWIND, ERASE, PLAY, and finally, FAST FORWARD on with our lives. I hoped that I could finally put the events of that awful day on paper and thus close the chapter. Now that I've done it, I doubt that I will ever be able to erase the vivid details from my mind.

The Day Begins
For Daniel C. Roper, IV: 9/9/95–12/4/95
by Janice John Roper

The day begins with a fiery circle,
painful to look at, creeping over the homes.
Laser feelers pierce the blinds,
slice my face. Another day
without Danny. Turn over
and pull the covers up.

The covers are warm and soft, and the place
where Danny used to cuddle is dark,
the place begins at my heart and ends with his
tiny feet touching my thigh. My arms encircle him.
His head rests in my hand.
He faces me. We are dreaming
of all the adventures yet to come.

Facing the inside of my eyelids, the kiss
of an angel is a puff of cloud, an invisible breeze.
It splits in two with a hug,
drifts away in the haze of denial,
before reality pierces through
like a laser. The laser is a sword I use
to cut the world in half, looking for
my Danny
to be warm and whole again, to wake up
pink and breathing, to have his
little feet on my thigh.

The laser is a sword fate uses
to cut me in half,
watching to see what I will do.

Half of me gets up and goes to work.
The other half cuddles
Danny.

My New Life

by Gina Sabella Lawrence

Four months ago, we buried my beautiful little girl, Brianna Opal.

Eight years after the birth of my son, my husband and I had decided to add to our family. Born November 14, 1995, Brianna was a healthy, nine-pound baby. I had invited my entire family to share in the delivery and, of course, wanting the perfect family, I wanted a girl. My dream came true!

When she was one day shy of three months old, my dream became a nightmare. I received a call at work from my day-care provider, Paula, that Brianna had stopped breathing during her nap and was being rushed by ambulance to the hospital. I truly thought she would be okay. Why wouldn't she be? Paula had administered CPR, and now Brianna was in professional medical hands. Surely I would have felt something in my body if she were not okay. I was wrong. On February 13, I lost my princess to SIDS. My life as I knew it died that day with her. The events of that day and those that followed are what I consider "My New Life." During those days we crawled through the grief. I share with you my experience not only to help me but to let you know that you are not alone.

My day started out like any other day, rushing as usual, packing my son up for school, dressing and trying to feed Brianna. She wasn't hungry that morning, and she turned her head when I tried to feed her. I wasn't worried. I knew that my day-care provider would feed her after her morning nap if she was hungry. Dropping off Brianna, I gave her my kisses and good-byes. Once at work I got into my daily routine and then went off to lunch as usual. I was at the grocery store picking up some things, when out of nowhere my brother walked up to me and led me outside with a cellular phone in his hand.

Something had happened to Brianna. She had stopped breathing and was on the way to the hospital. My husband was already there when I arrived, as was Paula, our day-care provider. I knew it wasn't good. Paula tried to explain what had happened. I assured her that I did not put blame on anyone but needed to see my daughter. I begged them to let me see her. When they finally let me into her room, the nurse prepared us for how she would look. She was white. The doctors were still trying to revive her, and I begged them not to stop. I leaned over my baby and spoke encouragement into her ear. She was cold. My baby was gone. I asked them to stop. We got a chance to hold her one last time. Her beautiful blue eyes were open. I always loved her eyes. I only saw her beauty at that moment. We held her for a long time, crying, my husband and I. Before long my sisters and brother joined us. We all cried for our loss.

The Wake

We had first decided on a closed casket. My husband, my son, and I went to the funeral home early so that we could say good-bye in private. She looked beautiful in her pantsuit that she had worn that Christmas. We placed her pacifier and some pictures of us in her casket. At the last moment, we decided to leave the casket open. I think a part of us could not bear to say good-bye yet. For more than an hour, a line of friends and family came through the door to offer their sympathy. Sometimes I found myself holding on to someone, crying with the little strength I had left. Then I would stop. I was on a roller coaster of emotions. How could my tears come so freely one moment and then dry up so quickly the next?

The Funeral

The funeral was held the next morning. I could not look at any of the many people who came. It had hit me even harder that morning. I was surprised at how little the casket looked. My first thoughts were to pick up the little white box and hold it. I knelt down to touch it. When I went to speak, my emotions came to a head. I walked away in a blur.

For days the sun rose and set. I couldn't believe the world was going on without us. The old saying was true: Time waits for no one.

Sympathy cards filled our mailbox day after day. We still felt alone. All I could think of was that I lost MY baby. I, I, I, me, me, me. I thought that no one could possibly know how I felt. I wanted to scream at everyone. My story is different, I thought. No one could love their baby as much as I loved mine.

People tried to comfort us with their well-meaning words. "You can have another baby," people would say. I thought, "Another baby? Are you crazy? No one could ever replace Brianna." Then they'd say, "God only gives us what we can handle." BULL. Or they would say, "When you go to heaven Brianna will be there waiting." For a quick moment I pondered that thought. I wanted Brianna in my arms again, but I knew that was not the answer.

Shock

What is shock? I thought this word meant that I would be in a trance, unable to move or speak. Instead, I saw myself from outside my body moving, speaking, brainlessly. I came in and out of shock those first few weeks. It really felt like my body was giving me reality in pieces. I remember one day feeling okay. I actually laughed with people that day and then felt guilty that I was enjoying myself. The next day you could have scraped me off the floor. I was told by a nurse that this is the way our bodies protect us because our bodies cannot handle so much sadness day after day.

For a few weeks my husband and I stayed out of work. We would leave the house just to try to cheer ourselves up, but we always found ourselves returning a short time later. Our home became our comfort zone. We were not ready to function. Weeks went by, and I found myself feeling worse. I didn't care about anyone or anything. The bills were going unpaid. My husband and I drifted farther apart, and for a short time I thought I didn't even care about my son. I was sad all the time and had no desire to take care of myself or anyone else. People laughing made me angry. And both my husband and I had a sudden urge to run away from it all. Where would we go?

For days I would play the "what if" game. What if I didn't work? What if she had been on her back and not her stomach? Did her cold play a part in her death? Why did I take her out? Why didn't I breast-feed? At least then her immune system would have been stronger. I have since read in *The SIDS Survival Guide* that you play the "what if" game to put blame on something specific. This way in your mind you can return to the moment and reverse the end result of death.

I wanted her back so bad it hurt. I started to feel that I had endured as much pain as anyone could stand. If this was God's test for me, I felt I had passed and I wanted Brianna returned. I could not accept her death. I started waiting for signs from her. I thought her spirit would come to me and let me know she was all right. The only sign I was willing to accept as a true sign was for Brianna to come to me face to face. This was my way of trying to keep her alive. Needless to say, that sign never came. I have accepted a few little signs since in its place. I knew it was time to start reaching out for help. I spoke with many people about Brianna. They would give me their advice or theory on why they think this happened. I learned to take what I wanted to believe and forget the rest. I also found a SIDS support group and a few new friends along the way.

Most helpfully, the Massachusetts SIDS Center had sent me a complimentary copy of *The SIDS Survival Guide*, and this more than anything else aided me in realizing that I was not alone.

First Times

The first time I went into a store, which was a few days after Brianna's death, I found myself drawn to the little girls' section. I couldn't help myself, although I knew I was only torturing myself. Sure enough, it broke my heart that I couldn't buy Brianna something. Then I became angry that I no longer had that choice.

Everything I did became a first, and each new "first" brought new pain. The first trip to the grocery store I cried, remembering the last time I was there. I wanted to scream to the teller that I had heard the devastating news of my daughter's death right here in this very store. My son's hockey practices that Brianna and I always watched together I now faced alone. The first time driving in the car I couldn't help feeling the empty backseat. It seemed to scream at me that there was someone missing. Without my baby each day became a challenge.

The days started to become warmer. Spring was coming, whether I wanted it to or not. I didn't want everything green and bright. The snowy, rainy days fit my mood better. Each flower that broke through the earth made me realize Brianna wasn't here to share in its beauty. Why did you leave me, Brianna? I was such a good mother. I loved you so much. Please come back to me. Please, Brianna.

Hope

It has been four months since Brianna's death. My husband and I have painfully survived the births of two nieces and a nephew, holidays, and monthly anniversaries of Brianna's passing. One of the hardest days was the day Brianna was gone longer than she was alive. I constantly wonder what she would be doing at this stage. Would she be crawling? We have left her room for now. I don't know when I will be ready to pack things away. It hurts too much to think about. I still go to Brianna's grave every day, and I still cry every day, but I can feel myself healing. We have talked about having another baby. I feel guilty at those thoughts at times, and at other times I am excited about a new birth. It's strange how time heals. I know I have a long way to go before I become adjusted to my new life, but already I feel I have come far.

From my journal five months after Brianna's death: *"I did it, Brianna. I put your special clothes away. I woke up this morning knowing it was time. I woke up in a happy mood this morning. I feel so happy to be happy. My last "down" was scary, and I didn't think I would pull myself through it. Now I know that when a "down" comes, an "up" will follow. Today I feel special for having had you, even for such a short time. You will continue to grow in my thoughts. I will see you in other little girls. Watch over us, Brianna."*

I can't have Brianna back. I can only accept her death, learn from it, and go on. For everyone reading this, I am sorry that a similar tragedy has probably happened to you. It stinks. Have faith, though. Believe in your family and friends, and use their strength to help get you through. Express every thought you have, whether in a journal or to a friend. I have learned that my husband grieves differently than I do. Talk to your husband and listen to how he feels. Most importantly, talk about your feelings. Your friends and family will help you through this.

Baby Ben

by Lynne S. H. Javier (condensed by Jean K. Hulse-Hayman)

It was Tuesday, June 9, 1987, at about 4 pm. I held my playful two-and-a-half-year-old, Melissa, in my arms as I answered the phone. The words spoken by the trembling voice on the other end chilled me to the bone.

"Oh, Lynne," said my youngest sister, Jean, sounding nearly out of control. "I'm at the hospital. Something's wrong with Benjamin. He stopped breathing at the babysitter's.... I can't reach Dale...and I can't reach Mom and Dad..." Her words were engulfed by tears.

"Oh…my…God…. It'll be okay, Jean." My mind raced as I struggled to maintain control. "Look," I said, "I'll be right there…don't worry…everything will be okay…I love you."

Baby Ben in the hospital? How could this be? Ben was a healthy, robust baby. I had just seen him 10 days before. He was such a mellow three-month-old—so alert and yet so calm and happy around people. He was blonde and blue-eyed, like my sister, Jean. Their first child, Ben, was the loving creation of a strong, six-year marriage.

I remember Benjamin Dale Hayman bursting into the world on the night of February 17 following an emergency Cesarean section. He emerged strong, sturdy, and thriving. And I remembered driving this same road to the same hospital the day after his birth. It was such a joyous occasion. My eyes filled with tears.

When I reached the hospital, I raced into the nearest door and looked for someone to tell me where Ben was. And then I saw Ben's father, Dale, who had just arrived and was also trying to find Jean and Ben. I will never forget the childlike look on his face. His eyes were full of fear and confusion as he grabbed my arm.

"Lynne, what the f... is going on?

"Oh, Dale…" I choked my words. "He stopped breathing at the babysitter's, and…"

I stopped. We both spotted Jean.

"Dale…" Jean said, and dissolved into tears as she held on to him. I stood back feeling awkward, not knowing what to do. A friend from Jean's school came up and hugged me.

Dale asked, "What in the world happened?"

"They called me at school. After lunch Patricia rocked him to sleep." She dabbed a tear. "Then she put him down to bed. About 2 pm Ben woke up, but he did not want a bottle. Patricia said he still seemed sleepy, so she put him back down. She checked on him about 15 minutes later…(more dabbing)… and he had stopped breathing…and his heart had stopped…she started CPR. Oh, Dale, I don't even know CPR!" She took a deep breath and tried to continue. "They got his heart started again. They won't let me see him…he's in there…" Jean pointed to a room at the end of the hall.

The hospital chaplain came over to us and said, "They're getting ready to take him down to Georgetown University Hospital. They have an excellent Pediatric Intensive Care Unit…"

"When can we see him?" interrupted Jean.

"As soon as they have him ready on the stretcher. The helicopter should be here any minute. His heart is beating now on its own," she answered. "I'll let you know."

Soon the chaplain waved to us. They were bringing Ben out. Jean and Dale ran to him. They kissed his forehead and whispered to him.

About 6:30 Tuesday night we pulled into the parking lot at Georgetown University Hospital. The man at the gate said a few words to Jean and then waved her over to the special parking area near the emergency room entrance. A nurse escorted us to a special family waiting room in the PICU.

Jean begged for information about how Ben was doing. The nurse said that the situation was very grave. We waited for a report from the doctors. The wait seemed unending as Ben lay behind a closed door. All we saw was an endless stream of people going in and out of the room. We paced around the halls. Some of Jean and Dale's closest friends followed us to Georgetown, and they walked with us and tried to say encouraging things. A woman I did not know was among the group. She stood off to the side and cried constantly. I later learned that her name was Patricia, and that it was at her home and under her care that Ben had stopped breathing. I told her that we all knew she had done everything that she could.

When the head doctor of the PICU finally came to the waiting room, her words were not reassuring. Ben was still far from stabilized. The next 12 hours would be crucial. If he could make it through the night that would be a good sign, but the medical team was not sure that he could. She told us the door to his room would now be open, and we could go in as often as we wanted.

We were all very anxious to see Ben and to be with him. As we hurried toward the open door, I glanced at my sister and her husband. Until this afternoon they had been a happy-go-lucky new family. Jean and Dale loved Baby Ben as much as they loved each other.

I tried to prepare myself for what I might see. I wanted to be strong for Jean and Dale. I took a deep breath as I slipped into the room behind them and found that I was not prepared at all. Ben lay uncovered on an adult-size bed. It made him look tiny and unprotected. He had tubes running everywhere: an IV, a catheter, monitors for his heart, a tube in his mouth, even clips to measure oxygen levels on his tiny blue fingers. His color, in other areas, looked good. But then I looked at his face, and it broke my heart. That sweet face! To keep the tube down his throat, they had taped it on his cheeks with adhesive tape. Oh, Lord, and his eyes! They had taped them closed so that his eyes would not dry out. I could hardly bear it!

The doctors told us we could touch Ben, and do anything that we felt would be comforting to him. Jean touched his hand and kissed him immediately, and tried to whisper reassuring words to him. We talked with the nurses and doctors who came in and out of the room. They were very open with us. They answered our questions as clearly as they could. They could not, however, answer our biggest question: Why? Why had this happened? He had just been to the doctor a week ago to treat a cold—nothing unusual. He was well earlier today. Why did a perfectly healthy baby stop breathing?

As the night wore on we tried to continue being optimistic. But I was starting to have my first real doubts about Ben's ability to survive. Each time they took that awful tape off of his eyelids and shone a light directly into his eyes, I'd hold my breath. Did I see something? Was there the tiniest movement? No, there was nothing. The doctor had told us that after such a trauma to the body, sometimes the eyes do not react for the first 12 hours. By 7 am, we were into the sixteenth hour and there was still no reaction.

At 11 am Wednesday, the doctor came to speak with us. "I want to give you the most recent status of Ben," she began. "His vital signs are not improving." She could see the pain in our hearts, and she tried to explain gently. "They must breathe on their own, they must have a heartbeat of their own, they must have a choking reflex, and they must have brain activity. Ben has only one of these responses—a heartbeat. To me, as a doctor, I feel there is no brain wave activity going on." She stopped and looked around at us. I could tell she felt our anguish. Then she added, "I want electronic tests done to show me truly if there is brain activity or not."

It was about this time that she first mentioned the word SIDS. I'd heard the term, but it never had much meaning to me. Now it meant much more than I was ready to comprehend.

My sister Jean asked, "I don't understand this. I thought he was caught in time. Why isn't he getting better?" It was a question we all had on our minds.

The doctor said slowly, "Yes, Ben was caught in time…He should have revived. Babies with SIDS don't revive."

There, she said it. Ben would not revive. All these tests were not for diagnosis—they were only to prove that he was dead. There was nothing we could do but wait. Oh, God…

By 4 pm Wednesday the electroencephalogram was completed. "The EEG showed basically a flat line," the doctor said, "meaning no brain activity. But there seemed to be random waves on occasion—like a spasm. I had expected a totally flat chart, but as it is not, I think you and I would feel better if we go to the blood profusion test."

She paused. "As a doctor I think Ben is clinically dead, but as a mother I would not accept that. So, I would suggest that we do another test again in 12 hours. Then, if the results are good, we'll do a CAT scan. I just don't think we should do a CAT scan until the end, as I think that the stress of moving him may induce heart failure. My feeling is that we have already lost him. I think his brain activity has really ceased. Would you like to hold him?" she asked suddenly. Jean and Dale almost jumped out of their chairs. Of course they wanted to hold him!

At 9:08 pm on Wednesday night Baby Ben's heart gave out. Jean and Dale stood by his bed as he died. The healthy, laughing little boy they had hugged and kissed only 30 hours before had ceased to exist. The families left Jean and Dale alone with Ben. Jean later told me that during their time alone with him they cut a lock of his hair. It was the only way they were able to leave him…by taking part of Ben with them.

The memorial service was held at a tiny, old Methodist church near Jean and Dale's house. In the vestibule were several pictures of Benjamin. Jean and Dale had picked out their favorites, and a friend who worked in graphic arts had had them enlarged. Few people went to their seats dry-eyed. We, the family, were at the church early to meet people and to cry with most of them.

The minister read the last entry from a journal that Jean kept for Ben, "Everything seemed fine on Tuesday, June 9, 1987, when I dropped you off, except for a little cold. When I called at 12:30 pm, you'd just gone down for a nap. At 3:10 pm, I got a call at school to come to the hospital. You had stopped breathing. Oh, Benjamin, I can't believe you are gone. How can I learn to live with empty arms? I loved you so. You died last night at 9:10 pm, Wednesday, June 10, 1987. I'm not sure that you ever really recovered from not breathing, so I don't think you felt any pain. Oh, baby, you are going to be sorely missed. I just want to pick you up and hug you. We would have had such a lovely summer, a lovely life together. Your Dad and I will need a long time to adjust. Nothing seems worthwhile anymore. All the projects—who cares? I have to live with empty arms."

The minister offered a prayer. Then Jean and Dale arose and slowly walked forward and out the back door of the church. The final gathering for Benjamin Dale Hayman was over. But Jean would continue to write for and about Ben in her journal...

August 10, 1987: I miss you, miss you, miss you. You were so happy, such a smiler, so loving. It's all so final. I can't get over how final it is. It doesn't matter if I cry forever, or laugh and skip. If I go on with my life or mourn it away, nothing can change the fact that you are gone. I won't see you grow up, I won't get to know you. I'll never hug you again. It happened so fast.

The last morning you were here I took you in to see your Daddy. He was still in bed. I said to him, "This is the most wonderful baby in the whole world!" I wish that you'd had your chance at life, Ben. We wanted to share it with you. I hope you are at peace. We miss you.

September 23, 1987: I have returned to my teaching job. It's very nice to be back, really. I do love my work. The staff is wonderful. They must have passed the word because no one asked me how I was doing (a question I dreaded). They all said, "Glad to see you back." They're a special bunch of people.

Everything reminds me of you—a spot on a person's couch where you laid, places in our house where you were, phrases in articles—everything!

I went to the NSIDSF (National Sudden Infant Death Syndrome Foundation) 25th anniversary meeting in Bethesda. It lasted three days. There were many others there who had lost babies. The speakers were great...

I'm feeling pretty good these days. I miss you like crazy, but I'm able to go on. I think of myself as fragile or wounded. Gosh, I'd love to be able to hug you again. I miss you, Ben.

December 1987: We missed you at Christmas. We kept ourselves very busy. It helped some. We had our first party since you died, a Christmas party. During the party, I noticed the dim glow of the Winnie-the-Pooh nightlight coming from your room. "That's funny," I thought as I went into your room. I found my friend, Bonnie. Bonnie had put her daughter, Rachel, who is 3 months old, in your crib.

"Oh...Hi, Jean...I hope this is okay..."

Hiding my surprise, I responded, "No, it's fine. It's there; we might as well make use of it." I walked out of the nursery thinking, "Gee, I haven't even washed the sheets since you slept there." It hurt and helped to see Rachel in your crib. I realized that my friend was gently nudging me on. Perhaps it was time to wash those sheets.

January 1988: A friend at work told me I was looking good. He said he could see a real change in me since September. Dale and I talk about you every day. Sometimes we cry, sometimes we just feel sad. As time goes on, I know we will smile when we remember. We planted an oak tree in the yard for you. We placed your pacifier in the roots. If you were only able to/meant to/whatever...be on this earth 15 weeks, then I am glad that I knew you for that time. You were such a precious, wonderful little guy. I miss you, Ben.

February 17, 1988: Today is your birthday, Ben. Your Dad and I hugged a lot this morning. I am going to send money to the SIDS Foundation and the church. I am going to tie a ribbon on your oak tree. We call it the "Ben Oak". We have received many "Thinking of You" cards today. A friend brought us flowers, and family and friends have made donations to SIDS organizations in your honor. It's wonderful to know that there are so many people supporting us and thinking about us. I wonder what you'd be doing now and how you'd look. What good times we would have had. I miss you, Ben! Happy first birthday!

Empty Arms
(in memory of my son, Zachary Adam)
by Stacy Parks

There is an emptiness within me
And an emptiness within my arms.

I close my eyes and reach out
and pull back in.
I can feel those quiet times again
When I held you so close and caressed
your tiny face.

I smell the air around me and you're there.
The baby powder, your blanket, your brush, you're
everywhere, but in my arms.

Untitled
by Abraham Lincoln, who lost three sons

In this sad world of ours, sorrow comes to all…
It comes with bittersweet agony…
Perfect relief is not possible, except with time…
You cannot now realize that you will ever feel better…
And yet this is a mistake.
You are sure to be happy again.
To know this, which is certainly true,
Will make you some less miserable now.
I have experienced enough to know what I say.

The Sitting Time

by Joe Digman

Don't listen to the foolish unbelievers
who say forget.
Take up your armful of roses and
remember them,
the flower and the fragrance.

When you go home to do your sitting
in the corner by the clock
and sip your rosethorn tea
It will warm your face and fingers
and burn the bottom of your belly.

But as his gone-ness piles in white,
crystal drifts,
It will be the blossom of his moment
the warmth on your belly,
the tiny fingers unfolding,
the new face you've always known,
That has changed you.

Take his moment, and hold it
As every mother does.
He will always be your son
And when the sitting is done you'll find
bitter grief could never poison
the sweetness of his time.

Chapter 3

"Coulda, Woulda, Shoulda": Dealing with Guilt and Anger

People are often surprised by how powerful [the feelings of grief] are. "It just pours out," a bereaved father said. "It's like a dam that breaks. It keeps coming and coming and you wonder, is this ever going to end?" Despite what people think, those feelings may not completely disappear. But that torrential flood of grief eventually forms a river, and the river imperceptibly becomes a stream, and although that stream narrows, it could meander through your life forever.

— Candy Lightner and Nancy Hathaway
Giving Sorrow Words [1]

Anger and guilt are the passionate emotions of a SIDS grief. They are often unexpected and often dismissed by others; yet they can be almost overwhelming to a survivor. Both have positive aspects. Anger can serve as an emotionally healthy outburst of frustration and rebellion at injustice. Guilt can guide us to do right. But both also have their negative aspects. As Frederick Buechner says in the book *Wishful Thinking: A Theological ABC* [2], "[Wallowing in anger is] a feast fit for a king. The chief drawback is that what you are wolfing down is yourself." Similarly, sometimes guilt goes beyond guidance, gnaws away at the survivor's conscience, and eats away at the spirit.

Sometimes a survivor must dig deep within to discover all the roots of their anger and guilt. Perhaps the adjustment to parenthood was tough, and a survivor found themselves occasionally angry at their baby. Perhaps, like Joani, the lifelong dream of a son (or daughter) must be set aside. Perhaps the grocery clerk was too slow the day of your baby's death, causing you to arrive home five minutes too late to try to save your child. Perhaps your spouse was not the kind of father or mother you thought he or she should be. These are powerful sources of guilt and anger, and discovering and attending to them are what the grief process is all about.

In the early months of Joani's grief, she wrote a very short and angry letter to her lost baby Christian that was published in a SIDS newsletter. She wrote about how she sometimes wished his life had never been so that she and her family would not have had to suffer so much. She questioned whether two months of perfect joy with him were worth so many, many days and nights of tears. The article seemed to scream at Christian for dying. It reeked of devastation, despair, frustration, and resentment.

A few of the newsletter readers voiced their outrage to Joani. "How could you even think those things? How could you be angry at your baby for dying? It wasn't his fault!" But another SIDS parent who lost her baby 15 years ago—and whose family had blamed her for her baby's death—could relate. "I was so relieved when I saw your letter," she told Joani. "I thought I was the only one in the world who had such rotten thoughts, and I thought I was the only one who was angry at my baby."

After three years, Joani is not angry and is mostly grateful for the two precious months she had with Christian. But even now she is not sorry she wrote the nasty note in those earlier days. "Anger is a necessary part of the grief process," she says. "Moreover, it's okay to be angry at your baby for dying. If he's listening, he'll understand. He knows how much you hurt, and he knows that being angry at him for a while is part of your necessary grief work."

Many people try to repress their anger at the baby. "It's irrational!" they say. Of course it's irrational…so is much that survivors feel in the early stages of grief. Even so, to get through the grief process you have to accept even the irrational and crazy feelings and work through them.

It's also acceptable to be angry at God. He's big enough to take it. You may feel a little scared; afraid of the proverbial lightning bolt that could strike you dead, too. Joani went to pastoral counselor Joanne Hill to help her handle her feelings about this. Joanne stressed that it's okay—maybe even healthy—to be angry at God. If you consider Him your father, think of yourself telling your father, "I hate you!" And know that He knows you don't mean it. And even if you do, you are in luck, because most people who believe in God also believe that He is in the business of forgiving.

Guilt is often considered to be anger turned inward. Essentially, we are angry at ourselves because we didn't or couldn't control what we wanted to control. We want to feel that we can manage and direct the important things in our lives. When our baby dies, we lose all sense of control and realize that we are completely vulnerable. Through blaming ourselves we try to regain a sense of control. We would even rather shoulder the blame, as terribly burdensome as it is, than accept the simple fact that many things are out of our command.

To purge ourselves of guilt, we must first understand why we feel guilty. William Ermatinger, who facilitates a SIDS support group in Maryland, has a good explanation: "We feel that if we could just find that *one* thing we did wrong, then we could magically go back and change things and have our baby back." This is irrational, of course, but as we have said before, much of the grief process is not rational. Nonetheless, it is real, important, and normal, and it needs attention.

Attending SIDS support groups can be especially effective in easing the pain of guilt. Surrounded by their peers, survivors find that just about everyone feels guilty about something. They often realize that they are much harder on themselves than they would ever be on anyone else. Survivors must find a way to make peace with themselves, even if there was some actual error or oversight. After all, the last thing we ever intended to do was to harm our babies. A SIDS support group can help with this.

It also may help to write a letter to your baby listing and explaining everything you did, think you did, or just might have done to cause or contribute to your baby's death. Then, sit back and read the letter as if it were from someone else, asking yourself these questions: Would I blame the person for the alleged atrocities mentioned in the letter? Is the writer an evil person who has no regard for the baby's welfare? Are these really such horrible crimes? Is the intensity of the guilt at all justified by the actions? Or was this person just an ordinary human being trying to do the best she could at the time?

Grief's Healing Rage

by Nancy Purcell

My youngest daughter, Amy Caroline, died on March 8, 1992, of SIDS. She was four and a half months old. The year after her death was one of conflict, turmoil, depression, questioning, and then, finally, acceptance and understanding. What haunted me most was the question, "Why?"— Why me and why our daughter? Why my children's sister? Why! I was angry and disgusted with those who could so easily dismiss our tragedy by saying that it was God's will or that it was meant to be. How could that be so? Amy's birth was a most wonderful and happy day for my husband and me. In fact, it caused us to decide that Amy would not be our last child. We had stars in our eyes and three beautiful children.

Michael and Jennifer, Amy's brother and sister, loved and accepted Amy immediately. To celebrate her birth, Michael and I had made butter cookies in the shapes of tiny hands and feet for him to share with his class at school, and we had started a book of his own about his new baby sister. Jennifer was home with Amy and me every morning. She helped me bathe Amy and imitated Mommy when she played with her dolls. Jenny even named all of her baby dolls "Amy." Amy was an adored little sister. She lent a perfect balance to our cozy family.

Amy was. Amy was meant to be. I cannot accept her death as God's will or what was destined to be. It could not be God's will to steal away someone so precious to us, someone so innocent. Yet, death came like a thief in the night—quickly, quietly, she was no more. Call it a ghastly mistake, a cruel joke, a foul deed, life at its worst, or unfair—but do not say that it was meant to be. To say that is to grasp at straws, to try desperately to defend an imperfect world and to reassure that there is order and reason even in the midst of tragedy. It is a simple explanation for something that is not simple at all.

The pain of grief is so complex that there is no simple answer. There is no magic formula to resolve it and make it go away. Grief permeates every crevice of life. C. S. Lewis opens his book, *A Grief Observed*[3], with this description of grief:

No one ever told me that grief felt so much like fear. I am not afraid, but the sensation is like being afraid. The same fluttering in the stomach, the same restlessness, the yawning. I keep on swallowing. At other times it feels like being mildly drunk, or confused. There is a sort of invisible blanket between the world and me... And no one ever told me about the laziness of grief. Except at my job— where the machine seems to run on as usual—I loathe the slightest effort. Not only writing but even reading a letter is too much.

I, too, felt grief's invisible blanket between me and the world. It was both a welcomed protection and a suffocating cover. It protected me by letting me feel my pain in solitude and by not letting in too much of the world. Perhaps I wanted to fool myself into thinking that the rest of the world couldn't go on without Amy either. For a while this illusion was helpful, yet **the world does go on**. And, at times, I felt that I wanted to go on, too. But grief's blanket was over me and I could not get out from under it.

The blanket was suffocating because it kept me from being the person I wanted to be. I wanted to have enough energy to enjoy life again, to enjoy the children I still have, to be a good wife, to take care of my home, and to make new friends. But all of these things had to wait. I could only take care of myself. In this way, the pain of losing Amy had brought living down to its most basic level. Some days just doing the grocery shopping was a challenge. The same could be said for many other responsibilities that I had always performed without much thought, including driving the children to school, preparing dinner, and keeping house. Now there was little of me to spare, which made my jobs as a wife and mother all the more difficult. They are the two jobs that I want and love the most, yet it was a daily struggle to fulfill them.

While grieving, we are incorporating the unthinkable change and loss that we have suffered into our lives. We are becoming new people—people familiar with the pain of loss. The body is listless, and tasks that were once done effortlessly are suddenly too tiresome. The mind is stuck, and thoughts spin like a broken record, returning to that same scene, the same face over and over. The soul is confused and emotions run rampant. At one moment they are high, at another they are low.

Grief allows us to reorganize our bodies, minds, and souls so that we can experience that new birth of self. It is a tedious reorganization—one that brings to the surface very painful feelings and emotions. For me, the strongest of these feelings was anger.

I remember one day about six months after Amy's death a friend asked me if I felt that I was getting over my loss. At this point, I felt that the pain was just beginning. I was angry and impatient with the seemingly endless grief process, and I told her so. "What are you angry at?" she asked, perplexed. "I am angry at life. I am angry that I no longer have Amy. That's what I'm angry at," I replied. She was as surprised as I was to learn that I had so much to be angry about.

Anger is a major contender for our feelings while in grief. It comes out in many ways, including yelling, impatience, snapping, crying, exhaustion, and confusion. It can even lead to more destructive behaviors, such as alcohol and drug abuse or reckless spending. Usually playing the role of the peacemaker, I have never been comfortable with anger. So when my grief yielded to the anger building up inside of me, I was startled and horrified. I became impatient with everything and found it especially difficult to care for my children, who were two and four years old. The whining, potty training, bedtime routines—all things I could easily handle before—became a sometimes unbearable strain. I yelled and screamed. I snapped and roared. I cried.

With grief taking up so much of me, there was little left for me to give the two children I still had and adored. I became spent, worn out, and weary of the battle. My patience was always too thin. As a result, I was not only missing the rest of Amy's life, but also part of Michael's and Jennifer's lives. While this certainly gave me yet another reason to be angry, it also gave me the best reason to learn to deal with this anger constructively.

Venting anger, and not avoiding it, is key to dealing with it well. There are many ways to let anger loose without taking it out on yourself or others. First, **engage in strenuous physical activity**. An aggressive workout is great for letting go of tension and anger. Take an aerobics class, jog, hit a bucket of balls at a driving range, or punch a punching bag or pillow. Do some heavy cleaning around the house.

Next, **take time to relax**. Physical activity is definitely beneficial, but sometimes I had no energy to get started. That's when I would need to rejuvenate quietly. Read a book. Take a long hot bath. Hire a babysitter and get out alone.

Finally, **be patient**. Grieving is hard work, and it always seems to take too long. I was impatient with myself and the whole grieving process. I needed constant reminders to let grief take its course in me. Although Amy was gone in the wink of an eye, I had carried her for nine months and had taken care of her for another four and a half. There was no reason to expect this to be a quick recovery. Give yourself time to heal, and be as gentle on yourself as you can be.

In between the moments of rage, there was silence and exhaustion. C. S. Lewis wrote: "On the rebound one passes into tears and pathos. Maudlin tears. I almost prefer the moments of agony." Lewis is speaking of the erratic pattern of grief. It often felt like for every two steps I went forward, I was sent back five. It is easy to become impatient with this process, but each passage has its purpose. In the moments of calm I learned to appreciate the anger and to see how it was helping me to move beyond my grief. I could accept anger's purpose and its validity. I was no longer afraid of being angry. I no longer felt that I had to hold it in. The death of my youngest child was definitely something to be angry about. For this reason, I can agree with Lewis and say that I, too, almost prefer the moments of agony. They are moments of progress. It was the venting of my anger and rage that allowed me to get out from under the blanket of grief. Now I am able to breathe again, live again, enjoy life again.

To the Man Upstairs

by Joani Nelson Horchler (in the early stages of her grief)

Dear God,

On March 8 of last year, You gave us the most wonderful gift in the world—a beautiful, healthy, almost-nine-pound baby boy, Christian. His three big sisters, his proud and loving daddy (Gabe), and I—his doting mother—would have thrown a big birthday bash for him and his baby friends, with bright balloons and little-boy toys. Now March 8 every year will be empty of celebration—a heartbreaking reminder of what could have been, what should have been. Now three-year-old sister Julianna says, "Big people don't die. Only babies die." And, she mourns, "I wish Christian could come back." Seven-year-old Gabrielle asks why God kidnapped our baby. And nine-year-old Ilona writes in her diary to Christian: "I'll always remember you and I'll always love you."

God, I have no answers and a lot of questions for You. Why did You allow Christian to die? Our only little boy, our most precious possession, snatched away by a seemingly unjust, uncaring God. God, why couldn't You have taken our money, our worldly possessions? Why didn't You take my life? You might as well have because our greatest joy in life is gone. Why did You have to take back Your one gift that meant the most? How could You take a little brother from the arms of loving big sisters who were never jealous of him and wanted him more than any toy, any pleasure? How could You inflict such pain on little children? Some say my baby is better off with You, but how could he be in more loving arms, on more loving breasts, than mine?

Christian smiled at us; he was content with us; he loved to nurse and he loved to watch his sisters take their baths and play. We would have done anything for him.

I'm angry at You, God, because You're supposed to be all-loving and all-powerful. If You are, why don't You use Your power to help those of us who try to help You on earth? Why are You rotten to Your friends at the same time Your churches tell us to be good to our neighbors? Why don't You punish those who do wrong and reward those who believe in You and try to live in goodness? Why do murderers and rapists go free while those who love You suffer? Perhaps, God, You took away our baby to test us, to make us better people. Well, I think all of us who have lost babies to SIDS would rather be our old rotten selves and have our babies back. And, besides, most of us weren't axe murderers to begin with. We're decent people who would have raised our babies to believe in You, to worship You.

If, as some believe, SIDS is an accident of nature that You can't control, then why do we bother praying to You to keep us safe? Other SIDS parents, who are better Christians and better human beings than I, tell me that praying isn't like going to a candy store and getting everything you want. They say I must seek nothing more than Your comfort in prayer. I'm sorry, God, but I just can't help wanting the candy store. I want my baby back, and NOW! And, I'm sorry, but I can't help hating

You sometimes for not looking out for my baby when I thought he was safe in his crib. I counted on You to protect my baby, and You let me down at the one moment I needed You most.

Oh God, Your followers say You'll give grace to those who merit it least. I am the least deserving of Your love and favor because I've thrown dishes at You, I've screamed at You, and now I'm coming out in public ranting and raving at you and asking You nasty questions. Maybe that's why I had the miscarriage after losing Christian. Maybe You were punishing me for not accepting my sorrowful fate with enough grace. But, God, how much do I have to accept? I feel I've already been pushed to the limit. Are You going to refuse to give us another little boy as another test or as a punishment for not being good enough? (Then, God, tell me why You give little boys to drug addicts, to child abusers?)

Grace: the freely given, unmerited favor and love of God... That's what I need; that's what I'm desperately trying to work toward. I say I hate You, God, but I really think I love You. I just don't understand how You operate. I don't deserve Your grace, God. I'm wretched— I'm groveling in the dirt, crying for my husband's and my flesh and blood that was torn from our breasts. Oh God, how can I ever accept my son's death? How can I get through his birthday every year, think-ing of how he would have grown taller than his father?

Please, God, on Christian's birthday in heaven, hold him in Your arms. Tell him his mom isn't really as bad as she sounds in this letter. Tell him she just can't help hurting all over and that she's too narrow-minded, too insignificantly human, to understand the big picture. And, God, I know that I'm unworthy to receive You, but I need You to com-fort me and lead me through this darkest time of my life so that some-day I can be with You and my beautiful little boy again. (And, while you're at it, God, couldn't You answer a few of my questions?)

How Can Therapy Help with Guilt?

by Patricia W. Dietz, LCSW

Discussions in therapy are free-flowing, uncensored, and not governed by the rules of ordinary social communication. Thus, deeply painful, frightening, and shameful perceptions can be aired, shared, reflected upon, and often perceived from a new vantage point. For example, many parents feel devastating guilt about their baby's death. Guilt is a complicated emotion that derives in large part from how we have learned—directly and subliminally—to manage responsibility. Guilt can often represent a conflict between what we chose to do and what, with hindsight, we feel we ought to have done. Addressing guilt in therapy helps us to take responsibility for our choices: If, in our best judgment, we went to work or didn't check the baby before going to bed, then we must recognize that we indeed, and irrevocably, chose to do those things. At the same time, it is important to recognize the enormous improbability that any of the parents' actions contributed to or caused the baby's death from SIDS. But parents can be overwhelmed by feelings of their own lack of power to protect their child from death. Owning the reality that human beings are not omnipotent, and indeed are vulnerable to tragedies from unknown sources, is part of the process of facing the feelings and fears that the guilt is concealing. Guilt is really a partner of the need to control: We feel we could have prevented an outcome by acting differently, but in fact we usually need to acknowledge our powerlessness.

In some situations, there may have been ambivalence about the pregnancy or the birth. Being unmarried or experiencing problems in marriage, having an unplanned pregnancy, considering abortion, feeling too old or too young to bear or raise a child, obtaining insufficient prenatal care, or maintaining unhealthy habits—all these can lead to less than joyful feelings at the baby's birth, and tremendous, even secretive, guilt when the baby dies. Recognizing the reality of the connection—or lack thereof—between the feelings we had, the actions we took, and the baby's death from SIDS can help in addressing the guilt that stems from ambivalent feelings.

People who generalize their feelings of guilt and regret into ongoing life can become overprotective of their other children and fearful about life's risks in general. Gradually, it is important to explore and get support for taking ordinary risks so that we do not become the prisoners of our guilt. Guilt is ultimately relieved when we can recognize that we cannot control everything in life and prevent every disaster to those we love, but that at the same time it is our human—and moral—duty to carry out our responsibilities with attention, information, and judgment.

The Women in My Family
by Margaret Polizos

the women
  in
my family

  have
dealt
  with death

they have
  pinched
his
scabby scalp
  and
sent him
packing

they have shaken
  his shoulders
  and rattled
  his
  ears

  the women
  in my
family know
  how to deal
  with old
  slobbering
  slithering
coming tail between
  the legs
death

they have circled
  their skirts
  and pulled in
  thick like
  wagons

But this death
  was bold
like the wind
  knocking down
  the door
  standing tall
  fighting 'em all
  bold
  death

now
  he has won
  chipped paint
  from their
  smiles
  forever
  turned babies blue
  and made
  these
  women
  old

when they
  were
  not
  lookin'

Grasping at Straws To Blame Ourselves

by Joani Nelson Horchler

From the moment I picked up my baby's dead body, I "knew" I had done something wrong. He must have choked on my breast milk after I put him down; I must not have burped him enough. I killed my own son, I thought frantically, wanting to kill myself, too.

My thoughts were not at all uncommon. One SIDS parent, upon finding her dead baby, screamed, "I suffocated him!" Later, her then four-year-old daughter repeated, "Mommy said she suffocated the baby." By that time, Mom had found out what SIDS was and that he had not suffocated, but the reverberations from her initial scream were still resounding. Jennifer Wilkinson—not understanding that a baby could die for no known reason—also thought at first that she had suffocated her baby.

Guilty thoughts are expressed through "If only…" and "What if…?" If only I had checked him more. If only I hadn't let him sleep so long. If only I hadn't gone to work that day. If only I hadn't taken medicine when I was pregnant. What if I laid her on her back? What if I had known CPR? What if he hadn't gotten a cold?

"Unspecific guilty feelings are almost always reported by or found in SIDS mothers," writes Luisella Zerbi Schwartz in a paper called "The Origin of Maternal Feelings of Guilt in SIDS."[4] This is true even in mothers for whom the sequence of events was such as to completely rule out any, even minor, responsibility for the infant's death," Ms. Schwartz adds. Guilty feelings are normal in every man and woman, she says, so the SIDS event "brings to the surface something that is already there."

In her book, *The Bereaved Parent*,[5] Harriet Sarnoff Schiff talks about several cases of SIDS parents who were convinced that they had killed their babies but actually had not. One deeply anguished mother told everyone that she had smothered her child despite a coroner's report to the contrary.

Why do we feel guilty? Guilt arises from our often desperate need to explain to ourselves and others why a dreadful event occurred. We need to explain things that happen to us so we can make sense of the present and attain guidance for dealing with the future. Psychologists say that an unexpected, unexplained death normally causes more feelings of shock, confusion, anger, and guilt than a death that is anticipated and understood. That is ironic because a SIDS verdict should relieve our consciences since doctors are telling us, in effect, that the death was unpredictable and unpreventable. How can you combat a disease whose first warning sign is death? "SIDS is not subject to interruption; it is not reversible despite timely and appropriate intervention," says Milda Dargis Ranney in *SIDS: Who Can Help and How.*[6]

Yet because ways of explaining SIDS deaths are not available, we delve into our past behavior for clues and often distort reality. SIDS deaths leave more room in our imaginations to invent reasons to blame ourselves.

The fact that SIDS almost always occurs at home or in the community seems to lend impetus to guilt feelings. Our home is our castle! We are supposed to defend it unfailingly. When we perceive that we have failed to protect our homes and our babies, we feel guilty.

Neighbors may add to our bewilderment and self-condemnation. One elderly neighbor said to me a few days after Christian died that "SIDS is when babies suffocate in their bedclothes." Fortunately, most other people in the community did not think that and did not condemn us, but even one such statement can cause a SIDS parent to feel confused, embarrassed, and guilty.

Guilt also rears its ugly head when a person's self-esteem is at a low point. SIDS tends to happen at a time when we mothers are very vulnerable: We are often still recovering from a pregnancy; often overweight; often exhausted from nightly feedings; and sometimes we've complained about all these inconveniences. Then, when the baby dies, we think, "God must have struck me down for not being grateful enough."

Many of us who had a third or fourth child die think, "If only I hadn't been so laid back, so relaxed, with this baby. If only I'd been more vigilant I might have checked on him in time."

In fact, one of the most common "what ifs" is "What if I had checked on her more often?" Well, say you *had* checked your baby every 10 minutes around the clock, which is practically impossible to do. Even if you had, you might not have caught her in time to try to resuscitate her. A baby's brain can live for only about four to five minutes without oxygen. Even if you had begun resuscitation attempts before those four minutes were up, there is no guarantee that you would have been able to save your baby. There have been documented cases of babies dying of SIDS even when resuscitation efforts were begun almost immediately after a baby's breathing or heart stopped. (This is discussed further in Chapter 15.)

Yet as parents, we believe it is our responsibility above all to ensure our baby's survival. I felt guilty not only that I had "let" my baby die, but also that I had "let" a branch break off our family tree. Not only Christian, but all his prospective descendants had died, and I felt a responsibility to carry on the family heritage.

Our self-esteem can also suffer when we compare ourselves to other young mothers at church or the park or the pool who have not lost babies: "She has four healthy kids. She must be doing everything right, and I must have done something wrong."

I felt guilty for assuming that my baby was healthy. I thought that even though he looked healthy, I should have sensed that something was wrong with him. I think I would have felt less guilty if I had known what SIDS was so I would not have immediately assumed he choked to death. In all the education I'd had, I had never heard that babies could die of "nothing"!

As time goes on, other guilt feelings tug at your gut. You feel afraid and guilty that you can't remember exactly how your baby looked, how he felt, the funny things he did.

If the United States "Back to Sleep" campaign—launched in June 1994 to change the sleep position of babies—results in lives saved, those of us who put our babies to sleep on their bellies are likely to feel distress. "If only" we had known sooner. However, I don't feel guilty about having put my baby down to sleep on his stomach rather than his side or back. Like many other SIDS parents, I was just dutifully following the advice that doctors were giving at the time my son died in 1991. When the American Academy of Pediatrics first came out (in 1992) with its recommendation against sleeping prone, Dr. Benjamin Spock, author of the classic *Dr. Spock's Baby and Child Care*[7], was still advising that "It is preferable to accustom babies to sleeping on the stomach from the start if they are willing."

I don't believe that parents should feel guilty even if their babies died while sleeping prone *after* the new advice emerged. Decades of accepted practice cannot be changed overnight. Besides, researchers themselves have noted that millions of babies who sleep face down on soft mattresses in overheated rooms do not die of SIDS while many who sleep on their backs on hard mattresses in cool rooms die nonetheless. Infants have died in all positions, including back or side. Often, babies prefer to sleep prone, and it becomes nearly impossible, especially as they grow older, to keep them from rolling over onto their stomachs. Each of the three babies I had had before Christian slept on their stomachs and never had any problems because of it. I now try to keep my subsequent baby, Genevieve, on her back or side, but I find that she often rolls over onto her stomach. During her first six months of life, I used folded receiving blankets to maintain the side position, but after that she became so mobile even while sleeping that it was impossible to keep her in any position. Because the experience of SIDS has taught me that I cannot be in absolute control of everything all the time, I try not to let worry about her sleep position drive me crazy. I'm doing the best I can to follow the experts' current advice, and that's all any of us can do.

Rather than feeling guilty, I feel some anger when I read projections in the media that perhaps 2,000 American babies may be saved annually because of the campaign to advise mothers to place their babies on their sides or backs. American doctors, who normally lead the rest of the world in research and medical advances, seem to have lagged behind the rest of the world in research on this important issue. The United States campaign was launched in 1994 in reaction to epidemiologic studies conducted overseas since the mid-1980s. These studies showed that the rate of SIDS dropped by about 50% in countries where campaigns have been effective in promoting back or side sleeping among infants, according to the U.S. Department of Health and Human Services. Why wasn't the United States at the forefront of these studies and campaigns? My anger stems from the fact that my son died while sleeping on his belly and that this was his only known risk factor for SIDS besides being a boy. (Boys are more at risk for SIDS than girls, by as much as 60% to 40%.) Yet all my "should haves" and "if onlys" will not change the past, so I must make peace with myself on the sleep position issue on the basis that I followed the best advice I had at the time.

Another major guilt-raising question that SIDS parents often face involves suffocation: "How do I know that my baby didn't suffocate?"

Several studies have shown that babies do not suffocate in ordinary bedclothes. Autopsy findings in babies whose faces were covered in the crib are identical to those in babies whose faces were uncovered by bedding.

Longtime SIDS researcher J. Bruce Beckwith addresses the issue of suffocation vs. SIDS in a booklet copyrighted by the Colorado SIDS program.[8] Dr. Beckwith notes that one of the findings in SIDS babies is "little pinpoint hemorrhages (petachiae) found in the chest organs of 87% of the cases." These hemorrhages result from the instantaneous and complete closure of the upper respiratory tract at the end of a breath, Dr. Beckwith explains. "If I were to go out and attempt to strangle someone or put a plastic bag over their head, it would be almost impossible to produce the hemorrhages. The findings differ in SIDS and suffocations, with 95% confidence levels."

To resolve our guilt about any issue, we sometimes need someone to help us look at the situation from a new angle. For example, when I talked about regretting taking antibiotics and mild medication when I was pregnant, a friend told me, "But you were just taking care of yourself! Maybe if you hadn't taken anything you would have become sicker and more exhausted and maybe that would have hurt the baby." I was so preoccupied with self-recrimination that I had not done myself the favor of considering that my intentions had been good.

When you feel that "if only" you'd done one thing differently your child would still be alive, remind yourself of all the times you *did* do something differently and you probably were able to change the outcome of events. Think about the times you watched children at a swimming pool and, through your vigilance, may have kept them from drowning. Think about the time you grabbed someone's arm just when they were about to step off the curb in front of an oncoming car.

Also, consider the times you or someone you know were careless or negligent (and every human being is at times in his life). If no disastrous event results from such behavior, the behavior is normally forgotten. In other words, millions of people have done stupid things and gotten away with it! Human beings are imperfect. Accidents can happen. Only hindsight is 20/20.

When we get "stuck" in our grief process—on guilt, anger, or another issue—it is often because we do not want to give up our child. We believe that if we give up our emotions about a baby we'll give up the baby. In truth, we need to replace those negative emotions with positive feelings that rejoice in the baby's short life.

The "what ifs" and "if onlys" will kill you if you let them. There's nothing more self-destructive than guilt. The pastoral counselor I was seeing, Joanne Hill, helped me to see that I was holding on to my unfounded guilt as a way of punishing myself. Delores Charboneau, a good friend who is also a counselor in a psychiatric hospital, listened over and over to all my protestations of guilt and kept reassuring me that I was "grasping at straws" to blame myself. I had medical reassurances from my cousins Michele Walz Stegeman, a Minneapolis midwife, and Mary Guhin Whittaker, a Dallas obstetrician/gynecologist, and also from SIDS experts such as Dr. Beckwith, Dr. O'Brien, and Dr. Barbara Bruner.

All these people helped me to realize that guilt is for some reason a strong characteristic of mine. Those of us who have this trait torment ourselves with imagined or unrealistic guilt. (I only fully realized what a guilt trip I had been on when I told other SIDS parents that I would be writing this article in the chapter on guilt. "Oh," they said, "You're the perfect person to write that chapter!" I feel guilty when the dog hates its dog food. I feel guilty when the hamster dies of old age. I feel guilty for feeling guilty!)

I also believe I had, until my son died, an unrealistic belief that life was basically fair, that people usually get what they deserve. Except for the deaths of my father and brother, life had always been pretty fair to me. Therefore, when SIDS struck us, I thought I must have done something to deserve it.

In *When Your Child Is Gone: Learning To Live Again*,[9] Dr. Francine Toder includes a guilt inventory devised by Dr. Donald Mosher of the University of Connecticut. "If your guilt quotient is high, the discomfort that this sense of guilt creates may cause you to dwell on your possible transgressions continuously, looking for a way to absolve or to punish yourself," says Dr. Toder.

William Ermatinger, the facilitator of our local SIDS parent-support group, helped me to put my guilt into perspective by stating, "If you think you know what caused your baby's death then you think you're smarter than all the medical experts who have been studying SIDS for decades."

Dr. O'Brien also helped relieve my guilt feelings when he stated that it's actually surprising that more babies don't die of SIDS, considering what dramatic changes the central nervous system undergoes during the infancy period.

We must realize that whatever bad thoughts we had about the pregnancy or about the baby didn't kill him. Thoughts can't kill. We need to let go of our childhood "magical thinking," which may continue to lead us to believe that our thoughts control the world. Being mature means accepting that not everything is under our control.

It may help to write down all the things you think you should have done and all the things you think you should not have done. Then focus on accepting them. You cannot change them, so you might as well accept them and forgive yourself.

Also, make a list of all the good things you did for your baby. When we submerge ourselves in guilt, we often let ourselves forget about all the positive things we did. As my husband Gabe says, our baby was conceived in love, lived in love, and died in love. He was entertained, pampered, and spoiled. So what more should we or could we have done?

If you think you need to be tortured for your sins, inflict insults upon yourself during vigorous exercise! In the chapter "Strange and Novel Ways of Addressing Guilt" in the book *Living Beyond Loss*[10] , David Epston gives tongue-in-cheek suggestions for torturing and insulting yourself in order to demonstrate to yourself how exaggerated and even ridiculous your guilt feelings may be.

If you can, discuss your guilt feelings among peer contacts and in support groups. You may be surprised, but they really will not rise up and stone you! It's likely that they have many of the same doubts and fears that you have.

If possible, try to laugh about your guilt and lack of self-esteem. I saw a great cartoon by Bob Thaves in the first year of my bereavement that helped a lot. A therapist says to his client, "You must learn to like yourself." And the client responds, "I refuse to lower my standards that much."

Another saying that helped me is, "The biggest fool is one who worries about that which he cannot help." Feeling unjustifiably guilty is probably the biggest waste of time there is. What does it get you except despair?

With the help of many friends and SIDS experts, I finally came to realize that I would have found a way to blame myself no matter what I had done during pregnancy or when the baby was newly born. If I had taken birth control pills after he was born (and I did not do this even though some were prescribed to me), I would have thought he died because of that even though there is no known link between birth control pills and SIDS. If I had gotten a tubal ligation and taken medication during it, I would have thought the medication stayed in my milk and killed him later. If I had had any kind of genetic testing, I would have thought that killed him, even though there are no links between genetic testing and SIDS. I was out to blame myself no matter what.

However, in fact, I did the best I could. I nursed my baby around the clock. I took him to the doctor when he had a cold. During my pregnancy and thereafter, I didn't smoke, drink, or take any drugs besides a prescribed antibiotic and a mild cold medication. When I put him down to sleep that last time I truly thought he was okay. And even if I had done something "wrong," I never intended to. I would have jumped off a cliff if it could have saved him. So I have finally reached the verdict: I am not guilty.

Still, I must confess that occasionally, when I am tired, sick, or just feeling blue, the thought creeps back into my mind that maybe I could have done something differently and changed the outcome. When this happens, I try to dispel my feelings by rationally analyzing them. However, social workers tell me that SIDS survivors may always feel some degree of guilt and, rather than completely rid ourselves of guilt, we may just have to learn to live with it.

Even three years after Christian died, it still amazes me that a baby can just up and die for no apparent reason. My refusal for so long to believe that such a thing could actually happen is what kept me feeling guilty. I thought, "Nothing this awful could happen without someone doing something bad or stupid to make it happen, so I must have done something wrong." As I learned more about SIDS and read about risk factors, I—like many other parents—tried to place myself high or low on the risk ladder. But such an attempt is useless because researchers have found no risk evaluations that are clinically useful in determining who is at risk for SIDS.

Also, more than two-thirds of SIDS babies and mothers have no apparent risk factors. Dr. Marianne Bombaugh used to assume that

SIDS was caused by child abuse, child neglect, poor prenatal care, or maternal substance abuse during pregnancy. Then her second son, Teddy, died of SIDS after getting the best of care in utero and during the two months of his life. When an emergency responder gave Dr. Bombaugh the news, her first thought was that God was getting back at her for her previous belief that SIDS only happened to people who had done something to cause it.

Even if you did do something that is considered a risk factor for SIDS—such as smoking—there is no direct causal relationship between any risk factor and SIDS. Among babies in even the highest risk category—born to drug-abusing mothers with poor prenatal care—only about 1 in 100 die of SIDS. Moreover, the proportion of SIDS deaths has not increased over the past 15 years, even though the number of infants born to drug-abusing mothers has skyrocketed over the same period. (Some researchers have concluded that whereas use of cocaine and other drugs during pregnancy is not a cause of SIDS, babies of drug-abusing mothers are more likely to be born prematurely, which is one of the biggest risk factors for SIDS.) If it bothers you that you smoked or abused drugs during your pregnancy, forgive yourself and don't do it next time. Flogging yourself over and over doesn't do anyone any good.

No matter how guilty you feel you are, there is a well-traveled road to resolution. It involves confession, penance, absolution, and forgiving yourself. Admit your guilt, say you're sorry, do something you feel helps to make amends, and then stop punishing yourself.

In fact, many people find incredible solace in religion. According to prevailing doctrine, God will forgive anyone who says he's sorry. Although many SIDS parents rightfully get irritated when people say it was "God's will" that their babies died of SIDS, that belief actually comforted me for a while in the intensity of my guilt. It let me off the hook; it helped me to find some grand design in my suffering. Many Catholics and people of other religions will find comfort in the guilt chapter in the book *Mother Angelica's Answers, Not Promises.*[11] She says it is "not God's will that we become so strapped down with our guilt that we no longer accept His love, the love that forgives."

So stop being so hard on yourself!

Chapter 4

"Why My Baby? Why Me?"

In the early months of 1994, world champion figure skater Nancy Kerrigan was seen night after night on the television news holding her just-bashed knee and crying pathetically, "Why? Why me?" SIDS survivors know all too well that defeated battle cry. "Why me? Why my baby?" we ask again and again when we are stricken by this random, senseless killer.

Ms. Kerrigan's question, "Why me?" was answered clearly when it was discovered that the attack on her was planned by people affiliated with her chief United States competitor Tonya Harding. When blame was clearly established and guilt admitted, many of us breathed a sigh of relief. At least the randomness, the senselessness, was gone. Good old-fashioned greed had done in Nancy, not some unseen, indiscriminate force. We now had concrete characters at whom we could point a finger and shove our anger. It made us feel better, or at least less helpless. Tragedy is not as bewildering or frustrating when we can target the culprit. Unfortunately, we cannot yet target the culprit behind SIDS. It is vague and unseen. It creeps like a thief in the night into our peacefully sleeping babies' rooms and robs them of their very existence. It also steals from everyone who has loved the baby, robbing them of their sense of security, their image of order, their trust in what ought to be.

Questioning and protesting the "whys" of death is a natural thing to do. In fact, it is necessary in order to come to any resolution about the death. The best advice Joani got for dealing with the "why" question was from Gwen and Kevin Robinson, who lost their first child, Rachel, to SIDS. They told her, "Believe whatever makes you feel better. If you can find the answer in God, that's great. If religion gives you comfort, hope, and peace, go for it. But if a belief in reincarnation makes you feel better, believe in that." Also, don't be surprised if you find yourself jumping on and off any number of different horses on the carousel of "Why?" believing one thing this week and something different the next.

It is normal for a child's death to cause a parent to scrutinize and challenge his philosophy of life or faith in God. Joani was so baffled about why God would do this to her that she visited a pastoral counselor twice a month for more than a year. Her husband, especially, had always been very religious. Joani just could not understand how God could do this to such a faithful servant and his family. Delores Charboneau, a friend of Joani's who came to help shortly after Christian died, put it succinctly when she said, "I can't understand why God is rotten to His friends."

When Joani first tried to answer the question, "Why?" she theorized that God had taken Christian to somehow make her life more meaningful. But that belief just made her angry because she believes that nothing could have made her life more meaningful than to have been able to raise her baby boy. Now she usually finds it more comforting to believe that Christian's death was an accident of nature, but that God was there to accept Christian's soul after he died.

In parent-support groups, when SIDS parents discuss the "why" issue, some parents have shared the fact that they found it comforting to believe their baby was a mature spirit sent by God to learn just a few things and to teach a lot. Others theorized that maybe they could not have a baby in the next world without having one here. Some acknowledged a trust in God; He gave them the children they were supposed to have, and it was in His plan that this child not live beyond babyhood. Others agreed with Joani that their SIDS loss was an accident of nature, a random event in an imperfect world.

Many people have written about the "why" question. In the popular book, *When Bad Things Happen to Good People*[1], Harold S. Kushner says that "God does not cause the bad things that happen to us but rather stands ready to help us cope with our tragedies if we could only get beyond the feelings of guilt and anger that separate us from Him." Bad things happen in nature, and "laws of nature do not make exceptions for nice people." Rabbi Kushner does not find it comforting to believe in a God who plans tragedies: "I don't believe in a God who has a weekly quota of malignant tumors to distribute and consults His computer to find who deserves one most or who could handle it best." Rather than ask why we deserve bad things, Rabbi Kushner says we should ask, "If this happened to me, what do I do now and who is there to help me do it?"

Other writers disagree with Rabbi Kushner's picture of a God not in control, a God without a plan. "Who could find hope in a relationship with a God like this?" asks John Bramblett, a bereaved father who lost a two-year-old son to an accident and wrote *When Good-Bye Is Forever: Learning To Live Again After the Loss of a Child*[2]. Instead, Mr. Bramblett finds his hope in a God who is in control: "He is a God of eternal life, a God who defeated death itself." Belief in a God in control helped Mr. Bramblett achieve a spiritual awakening that "peacefully put to rest the fear of my own death and the emptiness over Christopher's death."

A more unconventional answer to "Why?" is contained in *Many Lives, Many Masters*[3] by Dr. Brian L. Weiss, chairman of psychiatry at Mount Sinai Medical Center in Florida. Dr. Weiss says that a patient to whom he was giving "past-life therapy" began channeling messages from "the space between lives," which contained remarkable revelations about Dr. Weiss's family and his son, who had died at age 23 days. Dr. Weiss was "very heartened" by the suggestions that his son had agreed to be born to him and his wife to "help us with our karmic debts and, in addition, to teach me about medicine and humankind (and) to nudge me back to psychiatry." Dr. Weiss's belief in this tie between science and metaphysics has given him "a strong feeling of oneness and connection with the heavens and earth."

The above-mentioned books have all been helpful to numerous SIDS survivors, yet some must find answers completely on their own. "It would be great if someone could give us all the answers," one SIDS mother said, "but unfortunately no one has them." Many SIDS parents say they come to a point where they finally stop asking, "Why me?" because it doesn't get them anywhere. Many parents stop beating themselves up psychologically for the death and simply conclude that life is not fair. Others simply trust that although they will never see the reason in this life, they will see it in an afterlife. Still others, as they attend parent-support group meetings and see people who face even greater burdens than they, finally conclude, "Why *not* me? When so many others suffer so greatly in life, why should I be spared?"

Whatever our resolution, we all in some measure come to the conclusion that we as human beings are simply not as "in control" as we would like to be. As Godwin wrote, "Like the tide...some things... arrive in their own mysterious hour, on their own terms and not yours, to be seized or relinquished forever." This lack of complete control is scary, but it can be accepted and we can make peace with it.

It is important to remember that even if you knew the reason your baby died, she would still be dead. Reasons have no power to change the past. And the unrelenting pursuit of reasons can not only make you miserable but also halt your grief process. To move beyond pain, we have to let go of our need for reasons and admit that we are human and that humans do not always, or even often, know why things are.

Footprints
Anonymous

One night I had a dream. I dreamed I was walking along the beach with God, and across the sky flashed scenes from my life. For each scene I noticed two sets of footprints in the sand. One belonged to me and the other to God. When the last scene of my life flashed before us, I looked back at the footprints in the sand. I noticed that at times along the path of life there was only one set of footprints. I also noticed that it happened at the very lowest and saddest times of my life. This really bothered me, and I questioned God about it.

"God, You said that once I decided to follow You, You would walk with me all the way, but I noticed that during the most troublesome times in my life there is only one set of footprints. I don't understand why in times when I needed You most You would leave me. God replied, "My precious, precious child, I love you and I would never, never leave you during your times of trial and suffering. When you see only one set of footprints, it was then that I carried you."

One Point of View
by Jay Lamb

Since grieving the loss of our son, Ben, my wife and I have read poems and letters that described the sadness others have felt at the loss of an infant. A few of these also seemed bitter and angry. Reading those, we felt special sympathy for the authors and wondered if there was anything that could possibly be said that might help soften their grief. It made us think of a spiritual philosophy that has helped us to cope with the loss of Ben.

Our belief is based on the assumption that there is a God and that all aspects of our lives have meaning. When we lose a dear one, sorrow is a normal and natural part of life and it is right to grieve. However, we should not allow ourselves to go on for years being consumed by that sadness. At one of our SIDS support meetings, someone wisely noted that the rest of our lives become a testimonial to the meaning of our baby's life. Will that testimony be one of purpose, love, and direction, or one of self-pity and grief? Wouldn't our son rather have us focus on the many good memories of his life rather than that single painful one? Shouldn't his birth into our family improve us rather than diminish us?

After Ben was born we decided not to have any more children. We had our perfect family, one wonderful girl, Sara, and then Ben. Thirteen months after Ben's death, another daughter, Rebecca, was born into our lives and has been an absolute delight. Would we do anything to bring Ben back if we could? Of course! Would we trade Rebecca, now one year, to have Ben back? Never! As parents who love each child immeasurably, we could never choose one's life over the other. It is impossible for us to add up the minuses and pluses of Ben's death and Rebecca's birth to arrive at a quantitative evaluation. We cannot, from our worldly perspective, calculate which direction would have been the "best" for us, if we could have chosen. We could not have been more thrilled than we were when we were given a son, yet Rebecca is a blessing to us beyond words. How would our lives have been enriched and changed if Ben had lived? This maddening question is eased by our believing and accepting that these events, however tragic at the time, are happening as they should and serve our higher good.

Quite simply, we believe that in this world, we do not have sufficient perspective to make judgments of this kind. All the events of our lives have meaning and fit into the mosaic of a larger picture, and each event that takes place has an ultimate relationship to what our purpose is in this world. We are unable to guess why our son was born to us only to leave so abruptly, but we do believe that one day, when we make the transition to the other world, we will understand this fully. From the broader view of the spiritual world, we will see the unfolding of our lives, and the reasons for what has taken place will become clear.

"Why? Why Me?"

by Richard A. Watson, M.D.

It was 6 am 10 years ago. I was kneeling on the floor, holding in my arms the dead body of my six-week-old baby boy, Mark Thomas. I was not thinking about God at the moment. Indeed, I was hardly able to think at all. Rational thought had given way to a log jam of emotions, a panicked sense of unrealness, disbelief, frustration, rage, and helplessness. An accusing voice within me challenged, "You are his daddy; you are a doctor. Do something! DO SOMETHING!"

But there was nothing that could be done; he had died some time in the night. They call it Sudden Infant Death Syndrome or "crib death." The body was cold, resuscitation impossible.

In the following hours, so many thoughts, so many emotions raced through my mind. I turned to God in both prayer and anger simultaneously. I never needed God's help more. I prayed for strength. And yet another force within me would lash out in anger. "Why me, God? Whatever I have done wrong in my life, I do not deserve this—not this. I want my baby back. Why are you doing this to me? Why? Why me?"

In the weeks that followed, many well-intentioned Christians offered my wife and me all sorts of speculation; second-guessing God's reasons and intent. None of their rationalizations were of any help to us. At last, a Christian missionary to Africa who had himself suffered extreme personal hardship shared a cogent point of view. She said that God fully realizes that in this world there can never be an adequate explanation for such intense and seemingly pointless pain and loss. Yet through this trial, God offers us, as a special grace, a challenging test of our love for Him. "Can you love Me enough to trust Me and love Me still; even though I cannot reveal, not while you are yet in the world, the reason for this harsh and unmerited suffering?"

Having experienced a tragedy of this magnitude, I found that I have become more intensely sensitive to the suffering of others, especially of other fathers. Some years back, a little girl fell into a deep dry well and lay there trapped for many hours. The impenetrable bedrock surrounding the well prevented rescuers from reaching the child. At first they were not certain whether the little girl had survived the fall. Finally they were able to lower a small microphone down into the well. What a relief it must have been for that father to hear his little girl singing a nursery rhyme and to know she was alive! Oh, but then to hear her suddenly cry out, "Daddy, it hurts me. Daddy, Daddy, where are you?"

"Oh, my little baby girl, don't you worry. Your Daddy's coming! If I have to claw through the granite with my bare, bleeding knuckles, your Daddy's coming!" But there was really nothing that her Daddy could do. All through the long hours of the night, as rescuers inched their painstaking way toward the goal, the unanswered cries of the little girl were recorded. "Daddy, Daddy, where is my Daddy?"

Another time, the newspapers carried the story of a father who watched his home burning down. His little boy was trapped in the flames. He and the firemen could hear the little boy's voice, but could not reach him through the flames. "Daddy, Daddy; it hurts. Daddy, where are you? Please, come help me!" How that father must have suffered; it took three men to hold him back!

God may not, in this world, justify to our human minds our seemingly senseless suffering, but Our Heavenly Father has lifted up as a comfort to us His own example in the suffering of His only begotten Son. He cannot yet say, "Let Me explain." What He has said for now is, "I and My Son will suffer first—for you."

It seems to me that the Church teaches us more (and there is no end to all we can learn) by focusing on Jesus, God the Son, and how He suffered for us on Calvary. However, it is not very often that our attention is turned to the pain that God the Father bore for each of us and for our salvation on Calvary Hill. For us fathers, there can be special understanding and insight: that the Father God, the Creator of all the universe, the heavens and the seas, would hold back and watch while mortal men nailed His only begotten Son to a tree. He watched His Son, His naked body racked with pain, search the black, uncaring sky, crying out across all history, "Abba, Abba. Eli, Eli, lamma sabachthani?" "Daddy, Daddy, where are you? I need you now. Why are You letting them do this to Me? Why?"

What power in all creation could hold back, like those firemen's arms, the immediate, wrathful intervention of Almighty God, our Father? Only one power, the power of God's love for you and for me.

But why was all this necessary? Why?

My wife and I take consolation in our belief that God has seen fit to share with us, mirrored in our mortal reliving, the brutal suffering that

He Himself endured in the death of His Son out of love for you and me. In that faith and hope, we look forward to the time when God invites us into His heavenly kingdom. On that day, I will bring along with me neither bitterness nor anger. Rather, a whole bagful of questions. And on top of the bag will be the big one, "Why? Why did my son have to die? And why did Yours? Why is there pain and suffering? And why sickness and death?"

Because God, in His goodness, has shared this one special insight now, there will be then, with all these questions, neither rancor nor remorse. Rather, as one imperfect, unworthy father to the Father Who is God, I will be free at least to ask, and free to understand, fully and joyfully, for all eternity: "Why? Why me?"

This article was first published in The Linacre Quarterly *of May 1991. It is reprinted with permission.*

A Jewish Perspective on "Why?"

By Marjorie Romanoff

"God wanted it that way." Or, even worse, "It was her time." Those were some of the most irritating words of comfort that were either spoken to my husband, Milford, and me or written by countless people, many of whom we did not even know.

Our daughter, Janet Beth, was killed in an automobile accident in December of 1969 when she was 15 and a half years old. Milford and I were coming from the other direction and saw the car plow into the Volkswagen in which Janet Beth was a passenger.

More than 600 people attended Janet Beth's funeral at our temple, and I had the task of writing almost 1,600 thank yous. The many messages were the result of two large newspaper articles telling of Janet Beth and her service to her friends as well as to the community. And she was only 15 and a half! We always felt that she was placed on earth just to spread her abounding love and enthusiasm, which was distributed to all around her, especially those in need.

Did God want her to die? Was it her time? Unequivocally, no! The accident was caused by too many commercial establishments located on a heavily traveled street that had too few traffic lights. In addition, the drivers of the two cars were each 16 years old and were unable to make the mature decisions that come with experience.

How can any thinking person say that God took my daughter? What chutzpah to claim that we know what God is thinking! That very assumption is an affront to our sensibilities because it assumes that we know what God is.

In Judaism, the Orthodox, who are primarily fundamentalists, believe that whatever is written in the Bible is correct. They believe in a God who gives rewards for good behavior and punishment for bad.

In Reform Judaism, we believe that God is a presence, an unexplainable presence. While there is not space to go into greater detail in this article, we believe in the message of the three major prophets and 12 minor prophets, which implores us to become a just and moral society where righteousness and brotherhood are the rule.

Many Holocaust survivors blame God for the hideous murders of every one of their relatives and friends. They have become atheists or are angry with God.

Having lost one of the most precious members of our family, neither our sons, who were so devoted to her, nor we, can blame God who is, after all, unexplainable. We mortals may live to be 120 years old, but God is billions of years old. He preceded everything. How is it possible for any person to explain or blame God?

Our hearts go out to everyone who loses a child. Parents weren't intended to bury children. Janet's presence is with us every waking minute that we aren't consumed with work, family or friends. Perhaps that is why Milford, at age 75, serves on 15 community boards and makes a real difference while continuing with his work as a general contractor. I know that is why I, at age 73, throw myself into my work supervising student teachers and teaching a class to international students. Without our work, we would be thinking of Janet and our loss constantly.

We bless our seven grandchildren, aged 12 to 23, who have learned about Janet from their fathers. Maybe that is why they try so hard to be a blessing to our family, and they are.

So, can we promise anyone who has lost a child that time heals all wounds? Certainly not. However, time does erase that initial, devastating grief that we think will never pass. And life goes on. Working hard at something we really enjoy has been the best medicine for us, but each person needs to move forward and solve that problem for himself. God cannot do it for you.

Although the author of the above article is not a SIDS parent, her story has been included to lend a Jewish perspective to the question of why bad things happen.

A Grandmother Asks, "Why?"

by Millie Lutz

I miss my grandson, I want him back so much.
My arms ache to hold him and feel his baby touch.
God has plans for all of us, the Bible does say;
Is this then the so-called "Wonder of His Way"?

I have grieved and wept for this lost one of mine,
Who only lived with us for a very short time.
Was it because Our Lord decreed that he should die?
I cannot accept; I can't stop asking, "Why?"

I'd never heard that abbreviation SIDS......
The unexplained, instant death which attacks young kids.
Once we called it crib death; but then they changed the name.
It matters not; the loss still remains the same!

You have an infant who is healthy, bright and bold,
Whom you expect will live 'til he is very old;
But while he's just a tiny babe you lay him down,
And, suddenly, he's gone when you turn around.

This poignant sorrow simply wouldn't go away.
It seemed to hurt me more with every passing day.
Though I have truly tried to bear all of this,
I long for him and to have his hand to kiss.

Pondering if I'd spent too much time at play,
I queried, "Did this happen to show me His way?"
Can the answer to "Why?" be really found in church?
Scientists say it shall be found in research!

Constantly I ask, "Can't anything be done
Which would keep this from happening to anyone?"
I agonize, "Must a child again have to die?"
How can I accept? Will I always ask, "Why?"

In nightmares it seemed that I slept in a pit!
Then one night I arose and declared, "This is it!"
None of this mourning nor the funeral fuss
Will succeed in bringing our child back to us.

Solace hasn't come from the tears which I have wept.
Yet I've remembered his memory can be kept,
And I feel that there may be help for you and I
If we will do more than cry and wonder, "Why?"

Now I look for sponsors to help PROJECT SIDS
In the hope that all small ones may become big kids;
And today I believe our boy was born to die
So that we'd aid this search for answers to "Why?"

When You Don't Believe in a God
by Ned Balzer

Much has been written about how faith in a god can sustain a parent
through the terrible time following the death of a baby. But what about
those parents who are unsure of their faith or who don't even believe
in a god?

I am such a person. My parents were Mennonites, but I grew up
attending a Congregational (United Church of Christ) church. After
high school I stopped going to church at all, and eventually I began to
actively disbelieve in any god. The idea of a god whose whims we
must obey on pain of eternal punishment didn't make any sense to me
and seemed instead to be an invention of a culture and political system
struggling to control dissent. I believed that there were mysteries to
life and the universe, but those mysteries either would eventually
reveal themselves to science, or else they were simply beyond the
natural limits of our comprehension. For me, belief in a god wasn't
necessary for the universe to be mysterious and complex.

When Margie and I married, having children wasn't at the top of the list of my life goals, but it was very important for her. If that's what my love wanted, it was fine with me. We didn't try to start a family for several years. The first time Margie got pregnant was more or less by accident, and I felt terrified and completely unprepared. A few weeks later, that pregnancy ended in miscarriage, and I found myself reassuring her that we would try again as soon as possible. But I was still doing this for her rather than for myself. Within three months Margie was pregnant again. She endured nearly eight months of nausea and fatigue, and a scary labor and delivery. Late in the afternoon of November 10, 1992, my world changed completely as I watched her push Willie out into the waiting hands of the doctor. He was alive, and I cried uncontrollably as I fell in love with my son.

After three months Margie returned to her work as a schoolteacher, and I to my graduate studies; Willie started in a family day-care situation. I was sitting in class, four months to the day after Willie's birth, when another student came to the door with a phone message: There was a family emergency, and I was instructed to call a social worker at Highland Hospital. The social worker told me only that Willie was in the hospital; she asked for my location and said that the police would soon be there to pick me up. I prayed to a god I didn't believe in that Willie would be okay. After a long wait, an unmarked police car pulled slowly up and I climbed in. A female officer in the back seat told me that the day-care provider had found Willie unresponsive in his crib. Efforts to revive him on the scene and at the hospital had not been successful. I couldn't understand what she was saying at first—if they hadn't succeeded in getting a response from him yet, why weren't they still trying? As the truth slowly dawned on me, I managed to croak out the question, "Is he dead?" The officer answered, "Yes," and then, "I'm sorry." It was the most terrible moment of my life.

The emotions I can remember most strongly in the days and weeks that followed were disbelief that he was really gone, and sadness, and anger: at him, at myself, at everyone, and at a god I didn't even believe in. I tried to drive the grief out of my head by concentrating on the many small tasks that came up in the aftermath of his death: putting away his clothes and things from the nursery, having duplicates of photographs made, writing letters to let distant friends know what had happened. I had been a first-time father and had just begun to get used to the full-time job of taking care of Willie. Suddenly that job was taken away from me, and I found myself clinging to every little task that I could equate with taking care of his memory. I tried to drag these little jobs out as long as possible because any time I finished something, it felt like another part of Willie died. Perhaps prayer serves to fulfill this need for people who believe in a god; for me it didn't help, although I tried.

It wasn't long before another emotion crept in: fear that I was being punished for my disbelief. I had led a charmed life, I felt, and nothing really bad had ever happened to me. I could just imagine a god waiting for a moment when I was happier than I had ever been before to deliver a blow like this, punishing not only me but my innocent baby boy as well.

In the months following Willie's death, we attended meetings of a SIDS support group in our area. There were several openly religious couples who also attended the group. I was dwelling more and more on my disbelief in a god, and I felt both jealous and resentful of these people who had their faith to support them, as if somehow they were having an easier time of it than I was. A couple of times I went to churches in the area, without really knowing what it was that I was hoping to find there: an understanding of what had happened; relief from the pain; faith in a god; or at least the comfort of knowing that I hadn't been wrong all along not to believe? Whatever it was I was looking for, I didn't find it.

But a couple of experiences in those early months brought the beginnings of a sense of acceptance. One was a hike that Margie and I took along California's Big Sur coast. As we drove to the trail head, along a road that hugged the cliff above rocks and crashing waves, I realized that I was no longer afraid to die. I wasn't feeling suicidal, but rather in awe of my little boy, who had gone before me across that threshold. The hike took us through coastal chaparral at the peak of the spring wildflower bloom, and a calmness grew in me. We stopped in a clearing for lunch and sat quietly. Suddenly a bobcat stepped out of the brush onto the trail. He gazed at us for a brief moment, and then trotted unconcernedly away. The look in his eyes seemed to convey that none of us is on this earth for long, and why we are here must remain forever unknown.

For me, at the heart of religious or spiritual belief is a desire for answers to questions such as what the purposes of life and death are. I have struggled to find a purpose in Willie's death, a struggle made more difficult by the suddenness of SIDS and the absence of explanations for it. As an atheist, I have also struggled with the question of why I need his death to have a purpose in the first place. I haven't found any all-encompassing answers to these questions. Perhaps if I were a different person, a believer in a god, I would have found these answers, and they might even have brought me relief from the pain of grief. But maybe, for me, this relief would have been premature. I think the pain I have been through has been necessary, in order for me to accept the truth of what happened.

Willie's death has neither strengthened nor weakened my disbelief in a god, but it has helped me find a more peaceful and accepting relationship with the world. An acceptance of who I am and what I believe has led to a greater acceptance of other people, no matter what they believe or don't believe, and a deeper connection with them. Despite my atheism, an abiding desire someday to be reunited with my little boy is never far from the surface. Even if it is irreconcilable with my disbelief in a god, this desire is what keeps Willie alive.

How Faith Helps Us

by Jeannie Nelson

It was love at first sight! We were young and invincible. I was 18 and heading off to college soon. He was 22, a free spirit, and just living life one day at a time. One year later, we were married, working full-time, and eager to assume the responsibilities of our impending parenthood! We were blessed with a beautiful baby girl. We chose a special name, Kelsay Deanne, for her—my maternal grandparents' name and my own middle name. Even then, as young as we were, we knew how important our families were and will always be to us. What a bash we had to celebrate Kelsay's first birthday. It was more a celebration of success for us as parents than anything. We were scared being parents and wanted to do everything just right.

Five years followed; I had returned to school part-time hoping to pursue my lifelong dream of joining the professional medical commu-

nity. My husband, Donny, had proven all those people wrong who
thought he was incapable of responsibility—including himself. He
began a career in computer technology and continued to spend time
being the best Daddy in the world. Were we growing up or what?
We decided we couldn't wait any longer to have another child. We were
blessed again with another beautiful girl. She arrived on Thanksgiving
in 1993. She was absolutely angelic and had us totally mesmerized
from the start. We chose another family name, Victoria Louise—after
my paternal Grandpa Vic and Donny's paternal Grandma Louise. I
never really understood about the extent of love until I had two children
to shower it upon. By the time her first birthday arrived, we felt like old
pros. We had many people tell us how beautiful our girls were and how
lucky we were to have such good, healthy kids. Every time we heard of
tragedy, we would remind ourselves how lucky we were.

We weren't sure when or if we would be ready for more children.
We wanted to give our children the best of everything we could. There
would always be enough love to go around, but love doesn't pay medical bills or mortgage payments. We could only do our best.

I unexpectedly turned up pregnant in February 1996. We had been
so busy. My first thought was, "Did I even see my husband that month?
It must have been that damn snow day." Snow is almost unheard of in
Dallas, Texas, so it was easy to pinpoint. Oh well, so much for me
thinking that I am in charge of my life. I remember saying to Donny,
"I sure hope God knows what He's doing!" After the initial shock and
deciding that things would take care of themselves, Donny and I were
very excited. The girls were thrilled. October was a long way away,
and none of us was patient. Kelsay's activities, as well as our own,
and Tori's "wildness" kept us very busy and kept me stressed.

I was not a very nice person during this pregnancy, and I knew it. I
didn't feel like I could control myself or my emotions. I often thought,
"I'll be glad when I finally have this baby and things can get back to
normal." Normal chaos, that is.

Finally, on October 18, 1996, at 3:58 am, he arrived! Donny and my
sister and my best friend, Jen, were with me during the delivery. I had
had natural childbirth with my previous children and had a relatively
easy time. We expected this one to be quick, too. My pregnancy was
"pretty much ideal" according to my doctor, and delivery time would

probably be cut in half from my last birth. It wasn't. My labors aren't "pretty much ideal."

After two hours of labor and the nurses not seeing much progress, I was frustrated. I started praying intensely to God to help me. Within one half hour, Tyler James Nelson was born. After delivery, while talking to Jen, she told me how proud she was of me and asked how I could handle the pain of childbirth so gracefully. I told her it was divine assistance and that I was literally praying to God to help me. We decided then that prayers were amazingly powerful. We were raised Catholic and attended parochial school for nine years. We had strong religious convictions, but were not zealots. Jen and her husband, Rusty (both family and dear friends), were asked to be Tyler's godparents. Jen and Rusty don't have their own children yet, and we were all looking forward to them "practicing" on Tyler.

The next days, weeks, and month all seem to be a blur now. Tyler had been very strong from the beginning, often forcing me to stop and take notice of him during pregnancy. (He had me scared he was twins for a long time because he would simultaneously kick me in the ribs on my right side and under my hip on my left side.) During my one-day stay in the hospital, the nurses all commented on how strong he was, lifting his head up off my chest most of the time. Donny and I were stunned that he was a boy. We didn't feel that we had to have a boy; we just wanted a healthy baby to add to our family. I didn't even know I wanted a boy, and now I was totally wrapped up in him. What an incredible feeling—a son. I now understood the saying about little boys "belonging" to their mothers. He was my own miniature version of my husband, dark hair…sparkling eyes…complete love. I told all my friends how funny it was that Donny was so enthralled by his son and that for someone who didn't care if he had a son or not he sure was a proud Daddy! The girls wanted to touch Tyler, to hold him, and to be near him constantly. Kelsay was a "little mother" to him. They were both proud of him—to them, he was "theirs." And do you know what? They actually shared him. Totally amazing! I was returning to work at my Dad's lab the Monday after Thanksgiving weekend. Actually, I never really took a break from work. Because of the nature of my work, I couldn't do a lot of my job duties while I was pregnant. I always felt guilty for the strain that extra work put on my Dad, and I was eager to help him in any way possible. My parents have done everything for me; it was the least I could do.

After spending the first week at home, under house arrest by my husband, I began taking Tyler to the lab with me to do office work. My Mom had started helping at the lab during my pregnancy. I was nursing Tyler and still couldn't be around the chemicals. Mostly, our time at the lab was spent visiting with his grandparents. (Thank you, God, for that time with them.) My Dad was eager for me to come back full-time, and I was anxious to get back too. I really enjoy the relationship working together has helped us build. It was time for me to get back to work.

I am lucky enough to have the best sitter in the world. Her name is Ruth Ann, and she is a gift from above. Everyone should be so lucky to have a Ruth Ann. But I'm afraid Ruth doesn't feel that way. Tyler was at her house on December 5, 1996. One day short of being seven weeks of age, Tyler died unexpectedly. She found him and had to immediately deal with the reality of the situation. She's been keeping children for about two decades, sickly children as well as wild, healthy ones. Never before had she encountered anything like this.

I'll never forget the page I received and the call I placed to her home only to find out that my precious child was not breathing. The events that made it possible for her to even find me that afternoon are bewildering. (Thank you, God, for allowing her to reach me.) I had Kelsay with me; Tori was at Ruth's house with a member of Ruth's family and the other kids Ruth kept. Donny had been paged to go to the hospital.

Kels and I beat the ambulance there. We didn't even know what was going on. Had he choked or something? Had he suffocated in a blanket or something? How could he just stop breathing? I called Jen at work, and she was there almost instantly. My Dad was on his way too. A nurse named Kathy, I think, and a hospital patient support person, whose name escapes me now, but her memory is burned in my heart, took us to a family room, and the nurse kept us informed about what was going on. Before anyone arrived, this wonderful woman stayed at our sides to lend us strength, support, comfort, and words. Specifically, she said a prayer out loud for me. I wanted to pray, but all I could get out was, "Oh God!" (Thank you, God, for helping her lend me words.)

The following hours at the hospital are scrambled in my brain. My mind no longer had the boundaries of time, and I felt like I was venturing through uncharted waters. We had our families with us, and many friends and complete strangers were offering support as well. When Donny arrived, the nurse told us what they were doing for Tyler. Apparently, the paramedics had gotten a weak pulse on him, but he wasn't breathing on his own. She took us back to see him and I will never forget that scene. It looked like something out of the show "ER." The whole room was packed with people trying to save my baby's life. I looked at Tyler and begged him to breathe, to not go away, to hang on, to live! I encouraged him, "You can do it." He didn't. I asked the nurse if they had any idea how long he had been down, and the room seemed to freeze. A paramedic told me they had worked on him for about 15–20 minutes before they got a pulse. I felt my body go limp. I had enough education to know that it would take a miracle to bring him back. The nurse took us to the family room, where we spent a while trying to contact people. Then the nurse came back and asked Jen to go out in the hall with her. I knew why, and I could hear her as she told my sister that Tyler was not going to make it. Jen had asked for them to contact a priest when she first arrived—just in case, she thought, so Tyler could be baptized. (Thank you, God, for giving her that insight!) The nurse told Jen that a priest was on the way and that they would continue to do CPR until Tyler was baptized.

Tori had been brought to the hospital. Kelsay was being occupied by some friends who had come to be with us. Donny and I took Kelsay to a private room and explained what was going on and that Tyler was going to die. It was an unthinkable thing to tell an 8-year-old that her world had just been shattered. She decided that she didn't want to see Ty in the hospital and that she would remember him the way she had last seen him—in her arms.

When Donny, Jen, and I went back to see Ty again, the scene was completely different. There was not a sea of activity going on around him anymore, just two people gently performing CPR to keep this child with us long enough to be baptized while, technically, alive. After he was baptized, they stopped CPR and let me hold him. He died in my arms. I can remember how peaceful he looked and thinking that he must not have suffered. He looked like he was sleeping and like he would wake up at any minute. If only love could have brought him back! We all took turns holding him and weeping. My Dad had gone to pick up my Mom, and when she came in to see Tyler I was afraid for her. She had just lost her Dad, and I was afraid it would be more than she could handle. She, on the other hand, could only think of me, her baby, Donny, and all the pain we were enduring. I've never felt more connected to my Mom. (Thank you, God, for Mom and Dad!)

Our families were given the opportunity to spend these last moments with Ty before the medical examiner's office was called to pick him up. An autopsy would have to be performed. Ty was perfectly healthy, except for a mild cold that had just been checked out by his pediatrician two days before. We signed a consent form for Ty to be a soft tissue donor. We still had no idea why he died.

I later found out that the police had been there to conduct an investigation. I vaguely recall seeing them in the family room. They questioned Ruth Ann, who welcomed this because she too wanted to know why Tyler had died, and she felt that she had nothing to hide. They questioned my husband about Ruth and the quality of care. He said he was uncomfortable with the insinuation that Ruth could be at fault. As far as we are concerned, Ruth and her family are an extension of our family. (Thank you, God, for not letting them question me!)

A nurse told us a little about SIDS and gave us a number of a support group. I remember telling someone, "I hope they find something that was wrong with him so I'll have an answer to why he died. Please, God, don't let it be SIDS. Don't let it be something I can't understand."

We went to my parents' house and were surrounded by a huge network of loving family and friends. (Thank you, God, for our "life support system.")

The autopsy was inconclusive with a cause of death "pending further analysis." I remember thinking, "We're never going to really know." We went through the process of planning a rosary, funeral, and graveside service. The services were beautiful and were attended by a lot of people. We stayed at my parents' house for about a week, going back and forth to our house only to get what we had to have. The holidays were upon us, but no one wanted to do anything. Our children were looking for us to set an example of how to deal with this, and we didn't know how. I was afraid that our entire family was going to be ripped apart.

We talk to the girls a lot about Tyler dying and how we feel. They are encouraged to talk themselves, but not pressured. Kelsay is a silent griever and tries to shelter us from her pain. She is much too mature for eight. Tori woke up every night for the first four weeks after "Ty-Ty" died. She'd crawl into bed with us and just want to snuggle. She couldn't get enough love and comfort. Kelsay attends a private, Catholic school and seems to be satisfied with the fact that Tyler is in heaven with God. (Thank you, God, for her faith! I need to borrow it now and then.)

Donny and I are just beginning to allow reality to set in. We've been on autopilot for all this time. Things and people act as distractions, but Tyler's death is always on our minds. We just miss him! We cling to each other, not sure of what tomorrow will bring, and we pray that God knows what He is doing. The holidays are over, and things are calming down some. Is this the calm before the storm? I pray to God for strength. I beg Tyler to help guide me and watch over all of us.

We have begun collecting angels now that we know one personally. We've joined a local support group and spend hours reading information on the SIDS Network Web Site. Don and I have also stayed up for hours reading *The SIDS Survival Guide*. The book is powerful; it is strength; it is just what I needed. We are scheduled to join a grief support center for children called The Warm Place. (Thank you, God, for all those who support us through loving thoughts and prayers!)

It has been only one month and three days since my sweet baby boy left this world. We know he will never leave us.

For Anyone Who Has Lost a Child

by Margaret Lee Dove-Hedges

I lost my son Michael to SIDS on March 4, 1991. He was two months and one day old. At first, all through the ride to the hospital, I kept on thinking that everything would be all right. But it wasn't. At 4:55 pm, the doctors told me that they had done all they could. I felt as if my world had stopped and nothing would ever be right again. I had to go in and tell my son good-bye and that I loved him very much.

My son has been gone for two years, and I still miss him as much as I did the day he passed away. My husband says, "We are all put on this earth for a purpose, and when we have served our purpose we pass on." I don't understand why my son was called so soon, but I know he is happy and safe.

Michael, we all love and miss you very much.

SIDS

by Désirée Spencer Stamps

Shock
Unnerved
Death
Denial
Extreme
Numb

Impossible
Needless
Fault
Anger
Neglect
Throb

Despair
Empty
Accept
Tearful
Hope

Search
Yearn
Nightmare
Desire
Remember
Outrage
Misery
Endure

Chapter 5

Fathers:
The "Second-Class" Grievers

T he most common question asked of a SIDS father is, "How is your wife?" Each time it is asked, society's assumption that fathers must grieve less than mothers is reinforced. Of course, husbands do ache for their wives and fear for their well-being. Nonetheless, a father cannot help feeling that inquiries about his wife's status alone insinuate that his ties to the baby were not as deep or as significant as his wife's.

From the time a father discovers his baby dead, or more often learns second-hand of his baby's death, great demands are placed on him. Often the tragic news that is tenderly broken to a mother is given to a father "straight," with everyone assuming he will "take it like a man." In addition, it is often assumed that fathers are more able to handle such things as the needs of the baby's siblings, keeping up with the bills, and handling the details of funeral arrangements.

The Horchler family's experience was typical: While Joani lay in bed being comforted by friends and relatives, Gabe and a male friend transported Christian's little casket from the funeral home to the church and prepared the family van to take his body to Philadelphia for burial. Yet was Gabe really less devastated than Joani? Did his son not touch his heart as deeply, just because he is a man? Being a "fix-it" type by nature, it was heartbreaking to Gabe to feel so useless and out of control. Here was the thing Gabe most wanted to fix—for himself and his heartbroken family—and yet the thing that most defied fixing.

It is not that wives seek to burden their husbands or assume a strength that may or may not be there. But in her hour of chaos, a mother is not expected to see the unfair expectations being heaped on her spouse. A mother is often far too disoriented to look out for anyone else's interests, and unless the circumstances demand it (such as with a single parent), little is usually asked of her.

It is not unusual, and in fact should be expected, that a father begins to feel resentful about this. It seems absurd to him that he should be considered the "problem solver" any more than his wife is, as if his ability to fix the car, sink, and toilet will automatically enable him to fix the grief that accompanies death. Yet some men, not knowing anything else, take these burdens on willingly, desperate for something to do. To a businessman, taking care of the business of death may be a comfort. What is important is that it be an option, and not an expectation, whenever possible.

Are Fathers and Mothers the Same Type of Grievers?

To say that a man deserves the same degree of comforting as a woman after a baby's loss is *not* to say that men and women grieve in the same way. Psychologists observe that men do grieve differently from women when they lose infants. In general, men are more likely to feel and express greater anger about the death, just as women are more likely to feel and express greater guilt. Men are more likely to keep busy after the death, whereas women are more likely to carve out time and space to grieve. Men are more likely to be private in their grief and to hold back tears and other emotions, whereas women (again, in general) have an easier time talking and crying about the death. Fathers also tend to have a tougher time than mothers on the anniversary of the baby's death, whereas most mothers seem to have it worse on the baby's birthday.

A 1980 study by F. Mandell, E. McAnulty, and R. M. Reece in *Pediatrics* looked at 28 fathers in 46 SIDS families and found patterns of behavior peculiar to men.[1] These behaviors included attempts to deny the reality of the child's death and to avoid the pain of grief work; the assumption of a manager-like role immediately after the baby's death; the intellectualizing of grief and blame; an increased involvement outside the home; a concern to have a subsequent child; and an avoidance of professional support. Most fathers did not want to talk about death and their feelings. Those who did typically expressed a decreased sense of self-esteem and remorse over lack of involvement in their infant's care.

By contrast, mothers in this study were tearful, frequently incoherent, self-absorbed in grief, and seemingly unaware of much around them. They needed to verbalize and express feelings, displayed a tendency to withdraw, and expressed a fear of subsequent pregnancy. In general, fathers seemed angrier and more aggressive than mothers, who appeared more depressed and withdrawn.

One of the greatest sources of conflict between a husband and wife who have lost a baby is this very subject. One assumes the other must not be grieving, or grieving "right," which in turn indicates either inadequacy or a lack of love for the baby. Recognizing that men and women grieve differently, and giving a spouse permission to grieve as he or she wants and needs to, is a great gift each spouse can give to the marriage.

Going Back to Work

Also handled with less compassion for fathers than mothers is the issue of going back to work. Often, but not always, the father earns the lion's share of income for the family. Thus, a father may be required to return to work before he is ready to leave the haven of home. He is required to smile at clients and co-workers as if nothing significant has happened. He must find a way to care about ledgers and budgets and his subordinates' trivial differences. If in the line of sales or freelance work, he must also somehow muster a self-start. In the end, the pressure of grief combined with the pressures of work can be overwhelming.

On the other hand, for some fathers, the workplace *is* the haven: a place to immerse oneself, a place away from death and mourning. Many fathers prefer a pressure-filled job: It allows for the avoidance of the even more uncomfortable pressure of grief. In both cases, whether the demands of work come too soon or not soon enough, numerous fathers have found that professional counseling and parent-support groups can be invaluable. Even if a father wants to or must mask his feelings on the job, he has a healthy outlet for his emotions and time for his grief work to progress after hours.

Like the rest of the world, a SIDS father's boss may expect him to grieve in a certain way. If his boss is a workaholic, he may think more work is just what the father needs. He may also assume that some arbitrary length of time, such as three days or three weeks, is long enough to give special consideration to his employee. Unfortunately, grief has its own timetable. A father may be 50% more productive in a matter of days, or below par for more than a year. Being aware of grief issues is the best thing an employer can do for his employee. Providing him or her with a copy of this book may be the best way to begin his or her grief education.

The Hazards of Suppressed or Delayed Grieving

Unfortunately, many fathers avoid working through the emotions of grief. Yet, invariably, years later those emotions are still bubbling below the surface. One father suppressed grief over his daughter's death for more than 12 years. Throwing himself into his busy career was his personal method of pain relief.

"I functioned and even got promotions," he said, "but I was not happy and my marriage broke up three years after the death." When he finally "brought everything to the surface," he was hospitalized for two weeks for serious depression and suicidal tendencies. Yet, he says, "It was the best thing that ever happened to me because I found a good therapist and got involved in a support group called Compassionate Friends. It took me over a year to let out all my feelings, especially those of guilt. But once I did, I really started to heal. I felt so much better after three years that I was able to start leading support groups. I've learned that it's never too late to start the grieving and healing processes."

A Father's Anger and Guilt

Though a more egalitarian society has emerged over the past few decades, our society still expects that a mother will spend more time with a child than a father. Even in dual careers, mothers most often arrange child care, shop for clothes, and stay up with new and sick babies. Whereas parental leave may now be available for both men and women, studies have shown that men are less likely to feel comfortable about taking it, both for financial and career-goal reasons.

Whatever social ramifications this has is not important here. What is important is the personal issue of a father having spent less time with his lost baby. The lesser amount of time that a father has spent with his baby may cause him enormous regret. As Gabe lamented, "I thought I had the rest of my life to spend with him." Instead, Gabe spent much of Christian's few short weeks constructing a new deck.

Sometimes feelings of guilt bring up anger at everyone involved, even the mother, who may have had that precious time with their child.

Many times a father's anger is centered around the loss of his hopes and dreams for the child's future. The night Christian died, Gabe said, "I had already planned the schools he'd attend, the things he'd help me with around the house." Yet there was no one and nothing at which Gabe could direct his anger, and he was left feeling frustrated and vulnerable. At the same time, Joani felt angry and frustrated about Gabe's loss of his only son, with whom he had so closely identified. The similar emotions they shared brought them closer together, but feelings of anger can also divide couples. When such emotions come to the surface, it's necessary to acknowledge them as healthy and try to vent them openly in the presence of those who will understand.

Tears

Tears are important. Yet they cannot be coaxed or yanked or threatened out. For many men, tears take time and privacy. That is not to say that a father needs to be alone to cry. But he needs the safety of those who love and accept him. This may mean his family and close friends or just his wife and other children.

Many fathers are concerned about crying in front of their children, especially the boys. They fear that they are not setting a manly enough example. Yet child psychologists agree that it's not only okay, but very important, for a father to cry in front of his children. Many years after his brother's death, one SIDS sibling commented on how touched he had been to see his father cry about the loss. Because his father cried so seldom, it spoke of how deeply his father had loved the baby. The sibling also concluded then and there that his father must also love the rest of the family.

Finding Support

As stated earlier, fathers are less likely to attend support groups than mothers. This is in keeping with their tendency to hide their feelings just as our society expects them to do. They are also less likely to seek support and understanding from professional counselors. However, those who do use these resources often find it enormously beneficial to be in a situation where they can openly express their feelings with others who are going through the same thing. For those who do not prefer these options of support, groups like the Maryland SIDS

Information and Counseling Program or SIDS Alliance chapters offer
one-on-one contact with another bereaved father who is further along
in his grief process. Finally, there are also several good books to consult. One is *Men and Grief: A Guide for Men Surviving the Death
of a Loved One*[2] by Carol Staudacher. Others are those written by
bereaved fathers, such as John Bramblett's *When Good-Bye Is Forever:
Learning To Live Again After the Loss of a Child*[3] and David Biebel's
Jonathan, You Left Too Soon[4] (which deals extensively with the subject
of paternal guilt).

The Unique Burden of Fathers
by Bob Shaw

SIDS fathers, hit with what will probably be the worst crisis of their
lives, often hear from well-meaning counselors that everyone grieves
differently. Some folks weep, while some are stone-faced. Some folks
talk, and others just "work it out on their own" and don't say a word
to anyone. It's just a matter of personal preference, they are told, and
there's no right or wrong way to grieve.

I say baloney.

There *is* a way to do it wrong, and SIDS fathers seem to suffer the
consequences of it far too often. It's because fathers face a uniquely
confusing burden in SIDS deaths. Too often, men don't instinctively
know how to grieve. They are plunged into loneliness and anger that
can turn well-adjusted, hard-working men into emotional cripples.
Handling grief wrong can mean constant, gnawing unhappiness that
lasts a lifetime, as opposed to just a year or so.

It's a lesson I began learning the day my son died, April 29, 1991.
Benjamin was my first child, and my wife Stephanie and I often called
this healthy, handsome baby a gift straight from God.

I don't have to tell any SIDS parent what the first months after a
child's death are like. They know the horror of feeling like you're on a
roller coaster that has just fallen off the track. They know all about the
rage, the emptiness, the anger at God, the loss of a will to live, and the
feeling of losing your whole future.

Like most men, I was always taught that in times of crisis, you must find solutions to your problem, to be strong and useful. I was also taught that it was a more feminine quality to weep, talk about feelings, and grieve openly. Due to this teaching and my own personality, my instincts were to withdraw and not talk much.

Meanwhile, I noticed how my wife talked with friends and family in a deep, personal way. I saw that my own typically male, strong and silent Clint Eastwood approach wasn't working. There was no "bad guy" to be angry with. There was no solution. There was nothing that this SIDS father could do for other people, or even for himself.

These male-vs.-female expectations were reinforced by the often-repeated question, "How's your wife?" Not, "How are you?" Not, "My God, I am so sorry you are hurting." People were more concerned about my wife, in large part because they expect a mother to be closer to her children than a father. They don't really expect a father to grieve much at all.

Fortunately, we had an effective local support group and a good grief counselor. I was encouraged to talk about this disaster, write diary entries, and face reality, no matter how painful. By actively grieving, we were able to resume normal lives—including feeling happy to be alive—as quickly as anyone.

But in my years of attending and leading support groups, there have been accounts of many men who were not so lucky. In our meetings, many SIDS mothers arrived by themselves. No one ever asked the obvious question—"Why isn't your husband here?"—but the women typically volunteered the answer anyway.

"He doesn't believe in this. He never says a word about it. He just sits there. I think he blames me, but I don't really know."

We heard about husbands who, years after a SIDS death, still had not talked with their wives about the death. In this, the most awful and important event in their married lives, some men were unable to communicate on any level. Relationships had been strained. Some marriages broke up, heaping tragedy upon tragedy.

Sometimes, men need an excuse to grieve and to tell their experiences and emotions to others, be it a spouse, support group, or counselor. Some will take a practical approach. No man would break a leg, then "tough it out" and keep on walking for months, when doctors were available. Likewise, they see SIDS grief as something broken inside them, something they admit they need help in mending.

Some take a spiritual approach. What does God want me to do? Does God want me to become an emotional cripple, destroy my marriage, and shatter my family or hopes of a future family? Does God want me to respond to this tragedy with another?

Some fathers focus on the needs of their families. Dealing with grief in a direct way is the fastest and best way to get back on track with other children who need a father.

How a man actively grieves doesn't really matter. What does matter is that he communicates his grief in some way that is meaningful to him and his loved ones.

Do it right, guys. The stakes are high.

Editor's note: Bob Shaw is president of the Iowa SIDS Alliance.

The Missing Person
An Interview with Pete Petit of Healthdyne
by Joani Nelson Horchler

As he witnesses his living children growing into adulthood, Pete Petit has rejoiced over the years. He remembers the football games, the gymnastics and cheerleading competitions, and the graduations. But through so many of these special times, he is reminded that there is always a person missing. At times like these, "I still feel the pain," says Pete, who is founder, chief executive officer, and chairman of the board of Healthdyne Technologies.

It has been 24 years, but Pete vividly remembers the day Michael Brett Petit, his six-month-old son, died. It was a Sunday evening at about 7 pm in June 1970. "I had been mowing the lawn and was on the porch drinking some water when I heard my wife scream," Pete recalls. He ran up the stairs to his son's room and took Brett from his wife's arms to begin CPR. Brett was not breathing, but he was rushed to the hospital with Pete continuing resuscitation efforts. Brett did not survive.

Like many SIDS parents, especially at that time, Pete did not realize that an apparently healthy baby could suddenly die for no known reason. "I was extremely frustrated when I found out what it was. I thought, 'I'm a well-educated person; why didn't I know this could happen?'"

Within a week of his death, Pete had conceived the idea of a small and portable physiological monitor that could be used on infants. He took the idea to Dr. Scott James, Brett's pediatrician, and asked whether such a product would be valuable if used in the home. Fortunately, Dr. James had enough insight to advise Pete that this would be useful on infants who were having episodes of apnea. He told Pete that he needed better devices for use in the hospital nursery and also that it was his personal opinion that SIDS was simply a result of infants having episodes of apnea at home as they often did in his hospital neonatal nursery.

"Fortunately, Dr. James was a very forward-thinking doctor who gave me a great deal of support and encouragement," Pete says. Dr. James worked with Pete on the development of the world's first home apnea monitor, which they called the "Infant Monitor." Within eight months of Brett's death, Mr. Petit quit his job as a product-development manager at Lockheed and formed Healthdyne, which today is the world's largest manufacturer of home apnea monitors and employs more than 2,500 people in several areas of high-technology home care.

Grief counselors often say that SIDS fathers are too quick to throw themselves back into the workaday world and often do not take the time to deal with their grief. But Pete's work became his therapy. "I was extremely confused by Brett's death, and I wanted and needed to do what I could to prevent this from happening to other babies and their families. I basically lost myself in the development and design of the Infant Monitor, and this had a great deal to do with my healing."

Pete says he did not feel any guilt about Brett's death. "I remember feeling angry, but I don't allow myself to stay angry very long. Anger is not a productive human emotion. You have to have faith and forgive. You have to channel your anger into something positive. For me, designing the Infant Monitor meant I would be helping others, and this was positive."

In fact, Pete says, "We all have a role to play in situations like these. Each parent has to find his or her own particular role. It might be helping others in a parent-support group, or raising funds for more SIDS research, or educating the public about the tragedy of SIDS."

What if Brett had not died? Would Pete still have invented the Infant Monitor? What about the 2,500 people who work for Healthdyne? Would these people have jobs elsewhere? How much time would have passed before someone else invented the monitor? What about all the SIDS parents who use monitors?

To all these questions, Pete has basically one answer: "I believe there is a reason for the things that happen to us and that each person has to come to grips with what those things mean for him." His own role, he believes, was to develop an international home health-care company as a result of his own personal tragedy.

"I know the Lord could have accomplished everything we have achieved even if we had not lost our son. But the fact that we lost our son has resulted in good things happening to a great number of people. Somehow, knowing this has made my loss worthwhile."

Pete says that his company has received many letters, poems, and articles from people who believe that their babies' lives were saved because a monitor alerted them to their babies' distress. "I think that there have been thousands of babies saved by our monitor and those of our competitors," asserts Pete.

"It's been a long time now, but I still have strong feelings about Brett's death," says Pete. Part of his emotions arise from his belief that his son might have been saved if he had been on a monitor. "I frankly believe that the odds are certainly with the parents who have their babies on monitors," he says.

Pete put his own daughter, born three years after Brett's death, on one of his company's earlier monitors. "Fortunately, she had no alarms that were considered significant, and today she is a healthy and beautiful young woman," says Pete.

Pete has served for many years as chairman of the SIDS Alliance, an organization dedicated to eliminating SIDS by supporting medical research and increased public awareness and understanding.

89 Days of Sunshine
In Loving Memory of Rachel Lorraine Andell: 7/13/94–10/10/94

by Jonathon L. Andell

You were mine eighty-nine fleeting days.
    Your mother had you eleven months.
    She wept with joy the day she knew you were coming.
        I missed my chance to share that extra time.

When you were in the womb I didn't think I was up to the job.

    When you left me—

I can't even begin to describe the loss,
        the hole in my heart,
            the shattered hopes and dreams.

I've lost jobs before.
    Add up all those hurts and multiply them by a thousand.
    It doesn't come close to how it hurts not to have you.

I was good at my job of loving you and caring for you.
    It came to me naturally
        to my surprise and delight.

How I loved that job.
    How I want it back.

For eighty-nine precious days, I had the best job in the world.
    Because, anxieties and troubles and all,
    You were pure sunshine, beaming right on my heart.

Never in this world will I know why you had to leave me behind.
    And never will I leave behind the pain and sorrow of losing you.

But I hope and pray that somehow you know this, too:

Never will I forget the
    bright,
        beautiful,
            joyous
                SUNSHINE that you were.

St. Louis Community College

Current Check-Outs summary for STOFFEY,
    Wed Nov 12 12:42:36 CST 2008

BARCODE: 300080004481766
TITLE: SIDS : a parent's guide to unders
DUE DATE: Dec 03 2008
STATUS:

BARCODE: 300080004482818
TITLE: The SIDS survival guide : informa
DUE DATE: Dec 03 2008
STATUS:

An Awesome Dream

by Chuck Dohrman

I was on a business trip in New Jersey when I got the call that would change my life forever. It was February 5, 1991. I was told that my two-and-a-half-month-old son, Zachary, had been taken to a hospital near our home in Upper Marlboro, Maryland. I was not told that he had already died. I was told only to come to the hospital. In retrospect, I think the only way they got me there was by not telling me that it was all over. I don't know what I would have done had they told me right away, but I don't think I could have made that trip home. They got me back with the hope that something was being done to save Zach. I bargained with God all the way home.

With the benefit of more than two years' hindsight, I now see that the tragedy could not have been handled better—from the time the ambulance was called to a day later, when the Maryland SIDS Information and Counseling Program called to tell us that Zach had died of SIDS.

Still, nothing could take away the feeling of total devastation that enveloped my wife, Terre, and me and our families. The biggest, most important thing that had ever happened to us was having Zach. He was our first child. Terre comes from a family of three girls, and her two sisters have three girls. So Zach was put on a pedestal when he was born. To us, he's still special, just because he existed. He's still our first-born son and always will be. His death will never change that.

Our second son, Luke Jackson Dohrman, was born 13 months after Zach passed away. Having Luke has brought back the joy of being a parent, and while different, Luke is just as special as Zach. Luke is Zach's little brother and Zach is Luke's big brother. However, part of us will always be committed just to Zach.

I spend the time that I would be spending with Zach, if he were still here, on SIDS work in his memory. And what helps is that Luke seems to know; he seems to realize that he's a special kid and that his parents love him very much...even more than we would have if we had never lost a child. I also realize that we would probably not have had our special and unique son Luke if we had not lost Zach, because we probably would not have conceived again so soon.

I've never felt guilty about Zach's death. I think we always did our best for him and that nothing we could have done could have saved him. And I never blamed anyone—not me, not Terre, not the babysitter who was caring for him when he died. However, I did feel extremely angry, initially at God, and I vented my anger at anybody and everybody, and mostly at the people who loved me. I soon realized that because of my type A, very action-oriented personality, I had to channel my anger into doing something...anything. I either had to go hell's bells in a positive direction or hell's bells in a negative direction. I chose positive.

My way of surviving my overwhelming grief was to throw myself, just two months after Zach passed away, into fund-raising for the Maryland SIDS Information and Counseling Program. I wanted a way to let everyone know I'd lost a child to SIDS and to help find out what killed my son. I looked for a way to tie my business involvement in with my need to help other parents stricken by the tragedy of SIDS. With Bell Atlantic Mobile as the title sponsor, I started an annual golf tournament and dinner at Turf Valley that raised $5,100 the first year; $22,000 the second year; and $30,000 the third year. Many people cautioned me not to get so involved with my work that I would end up repressing my grief, but I think what I did helped me deal with Zach's death head-on. I didn't have time to shut down. It hit me every day when I woke up and threw myself into another day of volunteer work.

I also went with Terre every month to a parent-support group meeting of the SIDS Information and Counseling Program. I tried to help other SIDS dads feel more comfortable there because I think that most men have problems coming to meetings. For many, it's easier and more important to work than to sit around commiserating.

I had a hard time going to church, even around the holidays, for one and a half years after Zach's death, mostly because of my anger at God. But now I don't believe God did this to me. When it came time to have Luke baptized, we had a nice talk with our pastor about birth, baptism, life, and finally death. He said something that I took to heart: "Death took Zachary, and God was waiting there ready to receive him." I truly believe it now.

Today, I believe Terre and I are pretty much through the grief process. We can look at our pictures of Zach and actually feel happiness when we see that certain gleam in his eyes, instead of only pain because he's not around.

Zach made a lot of positive changes in our lives. It took me more than a year after his death to realize how much pain there is in this world, but I feel that awareness has turned me into a more sensitive, caring, and giving person to people in general. My faith has strengthened. I understand now what's important and what's not really important.

The worst thing a person can go through is the death of his or her child. But going through it helped me to help my family when my dad died 11 months later. I believe Zach's death also helped my father accept his own impending death. He felt like he could look forward to seeing his grandson in heaven. I'm only in my mid-30s, but like my father, I'm not afraid to die. I believe in God, and I know there's a heaven. I want to be there to see Zach again.

I had an awesome dream several months after my father died. It took place at my grandparents' house, and everyone of significance in my life was there. Even though my grandfather is dead, he was alive in the dream. It was a happy time. Walking through the city, I saw my father, strong and tan. I asked him what he was up to, and he said he was building skyscrapers. He had always enjoyed constructing things. He told me, "You'll have to come to dinner and meet the mayor." When we all went to dinner, my Dad proudly announced, "Here's the mayor!" The mayor was Zach.

My Would-Be Perfect Family
by Robert Lopez

This is the story of a would-be perfect family. That is my wife, my son, my daughter, and me. Going back to 1989, I remembered how my wife labored about 18 hours to deliver my son Daniel. The doctor was so tired from the ordeal that when she delivered him she said Daniel was a girl, but a second later reversed her opinion. We were happy either way because it was over—or was it? Six months of colic proved us wrong and gave us an experience we will never forget.

Going forward to June of 1992, we were again expecting a baby at the end of the month. As time approached my wife would ask me to feel the baby kick. We both thought it was going to be another boy, but we didn't care as long as he was healthy and didn't have colic! When the day of June 27 arrived, we were surprised that it was a baby girl! She was born with no complications.

I named her Angelique. I still remember that day: The deep blue sky was full of sunshine. That day I went home in a daze and couldn't get over the fact that we had a girl!

For the next two weeks, I stayed home, helping my wife at night with the baby. I really enjoyed being with Angelique, especially because she did not have colic. Soon I had to go back to work, and I felt sad that I could not be with her as much. Nevertheless, I looked forward to coming home and being greeted by my wife, my son, and my baby daughter. As soon as I would come in the door, I would hold my little girl and kiss her. I would lie on the sofa with her and put her on my chest, close to my heart. In addition to choosing her name, I also nicknamed her, "Our Mamanina."

As the summer went by, she grew to be a healthy and big baby. When my wife went back to work, we worked out an arrangement. She was to drop Daniel and Angelique at the sitter's house in the mornings, and I was to pick them up in the afternoons. The first day my wife went to work, it went smoothly. The next day, September 10, was also a normal day until I arrived at the sitter's house. As I was getting closer to the house, I saw fire trucks and police cars parked in front. I was getting worried, thinking there was some kind of fire. I got out of the car nervously and started walking toward the house when I was approached by three firemen and two policemen. One of them asked me if I was Mr. Lopez. They all looked scared and worried. I said that I was and asked why. They told me that they had some bad news concerning Angelique. They said that between 3:30 and 4 pm, the babysitter went to wake her up from her nap but found her not breathing. The babysitter immediately gave her CPR but had no success. Then she called 911, and the medics came. They also tried to give her CPR but were unable to resuscitate her. So they took her immediately to Holy Cross Hospital.

At this terrible news, I thought that my world was suddenly collapsing in front of me. When I arrived at the sitter's house, I remembered the sun being out, but now the sky was dark and gray. I felt weak and numb. I didn't know what to say. They told me that my wife was on her way to the hospital and asked whether I knew how to get there. They also offered to take Daniel to the hospital, but I told them that I could. They said that they were deeply sorry for what had happened and said that they would be investigating the matter more thoroughly. For a brief moment or two, I saw the babysitter coming out of the house in tears, but she was unable to talk to me.

On the way to the hospital, I felt much anxiety. I wanted to cry, but I didn't want to upset Daniel. He didn't know what was going on, or did he? I remember rubbing my fingers on the steering wheel so much that I developed a big blister on one of my fingers. I asked God to help us in this hour of darkness and hoped that everything was going to be fine. I thought about my wife, wondering how she was doing.

I finally arrived at the hospital after what seemed an eternity. As soon as I entered through the emergency room, I met a doctor, a nurse, and a chaplain. They would soon tell me that Angelique had died from SIDS. I broke down and cried bitterly and requested to see my wife. They took me to an area covered with curtains, and I saw the most devastating sight. My wife was sitting on a chair with Angelique's body in her arms. I cried so much that I couldn't stop. I could not believe "Our Mamanina" was dead.

After hours of being with Angelique, my wife and I reluctantly left her on the bed as we were told to do. On the way home, it was unbelievable how much it was raining, and at the same time I was crying so much that I could barely see the road. Somehow, I managed to get us home.

After the wake, mass, and burial, I was numbed with so much pain and tried so hard to find answers to why this had to happen. But I didn't find any straight answers. I thought that I had not been such a good person and that God was punishing me for the sins I had committed. I felt guilty, and so I decided to talk to our priest. He told us that God was not punishing us for our sins. And yet, he didn't know why it had happened either. He suggested that we should read the chapter on Job from the Bible and a book called *When Bad Things Happen to Good People.* I read both books and learned that God was not to blame nor was this tragedy His doing.

How did I survive this awful experience? By praying to God and reading books on SIDS, the death of children, and grief. I've also talked to other parents who have lost their babies from SIDS and to SIDS counselors.

It has been only four months since "Our Mamanina" died, and the hardest part is letting her go, knowing that she won't come back. But she will always be in my heart. Now I see the world through different eyes. No longer do I enjoy this world the way I did. For I know now that my goal in life is to walk in the footsteps of the Lord Jesus Christ and to serve and love Him for the rest of my life, for only in Him and the Virgin Mary can I hope to find true peace and joy. Only in them can I hope to see our Angelique once again.

I know that Angelique came into our lives for a purpose. And although I don't know what it is, I know it will be something good. I feel that Angelique was an angel sent from heaven and that, through her, I'm now more bonded to heaven than to earth. After all, a part of me is there and always will be.

I love you, my Mamanina, my sweet angel Angelique.

Surviving a Bereaved Wife

by Gabriel F. Horchler

The knock on the door jarred me out of a deep sleep, and I sensed at once that something terrible must have happened. Why else would I be roused at this hour and this place, a secluded conference retreat designed to shield attenders from external distractions? My room didn't even have a phone; the voice that followed the knock told me to call a neighbor back in Cheverly from the phone down the hall. I was jolted by the memory of a similar message, years before in Philadelphia, asking me to call a kind neighbor whose sad task it had been to inform me that my father had collapsed and died on the street. The Cheverly neighbor told me to call my wife Joani at the hospital, which I immediately did, and learned from her that Christian, our two-month-old son, was dead. This solid little boy—who had seemed so robust from the moment he greeted us with a strong, masculine clarion call right after birth—had died in his sleep of no apparent cause.

Joani's voice over the phone was surprisingly calm, and she appeared in control of her emotions when I arrived at the hospital about an hour and a half later. She was, as I soon discovered, in a state of numb disbelief, one that would soon be followed by bouts of anger and despair. Our emotional roller-coaster ride had started, and it would lunge us about for the next two years.

Little Christian looked so peaceful and beatific on that large hospital bed; this was no mortician's handiwork. Life must have slipped from him quietly and without trauma, so unlike the deaths I had witnessed in Vietnam. This was a great consolation to me, even though his death remained incomprehensible.

Given today's culture and attitudes concerning childbearing, some might wonder how a family could be elated at the birth of a fourth child, yet that was how we greeted Christian. His mother especially was ecstatic. Joani finally had a son, and her entire being radiated joy. The pains of a natural delivery were soon forgotten as she cradled and nursed Christian moments after birth, and the nurses were amazed at her cheerfulness and energy. The two months of his short life were blissful. The burdens of running a large household while caring for an infant did not seem to weigh on Joani; neither was she upset about end-ing—at least temporarily—a successful career as a journalist. She was content to be a career mom and to revel in our son's presence, a luxury she had not been able to indulge with our three daughters.

Suddenly, all this unraveled, and it was as if part of Joani died along with Christian. I found myself in fact grieving more for her than for our son. He was at peace, but she was anguished. Because Christian had been a hearty nurser, Joani's breasts remained engorged for several days after his death, a painful reminder of the intimacy they had so recently shared.

The next two years were very difficult. At times, Joani would appear reconciled to our loss, only to be engulfed soon afterward by a wave of grief. There was also an overwhelming urge to have another son as soon as possible, and she used her investigative-reporter skills to research how this could be ensured. We received much help from family, friends, members of the clergy, and various support groups during this time, and the periods of acceptance gradually dominated those of despair.

Nevertheless, it was Genevieve's birth that finally halted our emotional roller coaster. Because of Joani's determination to have another son, I became very concerned upon learning that we would have another daughter, but from the moment of her arrival, Genevieve totally disarmed us, and the residual pain evaporated. She has truly been our healing baby, a splendid affirmation of life over death, a beautiful incarnation of God's power to renew.

Always in My Heart

by Marta Brown

…"to love and cherish 'til death do us part"…As Bob and I exchanged our wedding vows, I reveled in that romantic language. I remember looking at my husband—the strong, handsome, loving man I had chosen—and thanking God for bringing us together. Cherish?

Yes, I wanted to make that promise. But at that moment, I had only a superficial idea of what that promise meant. The sudden, unexpected death of our son, Rob, seven years later, made me appreciate the warmth of being cherished. Bob's love and concern for me, at a time when his own heart was "torn in half," is something I will never forget.

When Bob arrived in the emergency room, a doctor told him that our four-month-old son had been a victim of SIDS. As Bob entered my room, I fell against him and cried, "Oh, Bob, what are we going to do?" Our seven years of marriage had taught me to trust him completely. Distraught as he was, he still managed to comfort me. I believe that God used our love to sustain us in our grief. When the nurse asked, "What can I do for you, Mr. Brown?" he replied, "Just help me take care of my wife." That's what it means to be cherished.

Later that evening, I again felt his unselfish love pouring forth. Lying down in a vain attempt to sleep, I heard sounds in the kitchen. There I found my husband painfully emptying the pantry of baby food, bottles, and other reminders. He told me he wanted to put away the baby things so I wouldn't become upset by seeing them. I believe that I began to cherish him at that moment.

Throughout the weeks and months after Rob died, I continued to rely on Bob for support. We prayed, cried, and talked with each other. In my contact with other SIDS mothers, I've found that many husbands could not give them support. I'm thankful that my husband was able to muster the strength to be able to console me during those nightmarish days, and that he cherished me enough to try.

Even now—many years later—the memory of my husband's caring and concern is always in my heart.

…"to love and cherish"…We found God's promise in that vow.

Editor's note: Marta Brown is immediate past chairman of SIDS International and its 1996 conference chairman.

Chapter 6

Children Grieving Children

"**M**ommy, Christian's throwing water down from the sky! He's having a water fight with us!" This positive response to rain came from Joani's third daughter, five-year-old Julianna. The innocent remark would have torn Joani's heart out, had it come any earlier in her grief process. But after two and a half years, Joani could actually laugh and respond, "Yes, Julianna, isn't Christian a funny boy?"

"It's not that we've denied Christian's death," explains Joani. "We just believe that Christian's spirit is alive and that he will always be with us as we move through life, making even ordinary things like rain more special and fun. We talk about him a lot, and these days the peace and joy his memory brings us usually outweigh the pain."

Getting to this point in the grieving process—where the mere mention of the baby does not burn blisters into everyone's hearts—takes most people (children *and* adults) quite a while. For children, it involves allowing them to experience the pain of the grief process, rather than yielding to a parent's natural instinct to protect a child from sorrow.

In earlier generations, it was common to avoid talking about death to children. Today we know this only makes it more difficult for them. They may show behavior problems, such as appetite and sleep disturbances, withdrawal from family and friends, concentration difficulties, increased dependency, regression to infant-like behavior, restlessness, and learning difficulties. In addition, eating, sleeping, bowel, and bladder problems are seen in children age five or younger, and school-age children may show phobic or hypochondriacal behavior. They may either withdraw or become excessive in their care-giving for family and friends, and some may replace sadness with aggression.

The booklet *Sibling Grief* [1], which is published by the Pregnancy and Infant Loss Center of Wayzata, Minnesota, considers age quite specifically when describing the impact of death on a child. It describes children of 8–12 years as having an adult concept of death and concern about their own death. They may carry on as if nothing happened but be inwardly frightened and show anger and irritability. A child of 5–8 years sees death as a natural process that could happen to him or her. According to the authors, "There's an increased sense of guilt, egocentricity, and 'magical thinking'—wondering how his actions could have caused or prevented the death." At 18 months–5 years, death is seen as an altered and permanent state, but still bewildering. Behaviors may include withdrawal, irritability, confusion, clinging, and being overly demanding. These, of course, are broad generalizations, and no child will perfectly adhere to any particular grieving style.

If there is no discussion or attempt to explain the death, children often imagine the worst, including that they did something to cause it. It's terribly scary and unsettling to lose the family unit as it has been known. But, handled openly, the death can actually open a door for families to grow together in a positive direction.

Joani found that her children felt different from other children because they didn't know anyone else who had experienced a SIDS loss. "I'm the only one in my school it happened to," lamented her eight-year-old daughter. To show them they weren't alone, Joani and Gabe took their children to family potluck dinners sponsored by SIDS support groups. They also took their children to a grief workshop led by Helen Fitzgerald, author of the excellent book, *The Grieving Child* [2]. At the workshop, the kids—all SIDS siblings—drew pictures, told stories, and wrote about their brothers and sisters. At the two schools attended by Joani's daughters, kind teachers had their students write sympathy notes to the Horchler children and helped them understand the girls' need for special support.

Many children have guilt feelings over the death, especially if they have been jealous of the baby and wished that he or she would just go away. Psychologists say that it is best to acknowledge children's guilt feelings by saying something like, "I know that you sometimes got angry at the baby and wished that he would go away from us, but your wishing had nothing to do with the baby's death. No one is to blame for the baby's death." Because parents also have some difficulty believing this, it is helpful for everyone to keep repeating over and over that SIDS is not predictable and not preventable.

The most helpful book Joani found to explain death in a comforting way to children is the lesser known book *Summerland: A Story About Death and Hope*[3] by Eyvind Skeie, a Norwegian pastor. In this spiritual story, the experience of death is portrayed through the image of an innocent child walking through a dark valley toward the source of all hope, "The One Who Is Waiting—the one who bids us welcome when all others must say good-bye." Joani's children found it comforting to think of their baby brother being picked up by "The One Who Is Waiting" and carried into a summer meadow where there is joy everlasting.

Children often ask, "Isn't the baby unhappy without us?" *Summerland* has a response: Those in the meadow "have somehow left all tears...behind them. But the One Who Is Waiting...weeps with us while he dries the child's tears and makes it smile again."

Explaining death to children depends a great deal on the child and the one doing the explaining. But two things are considered standard: First, keep your explanations simple and truthful. Explain what you know about SIDS, especially that this kind of death happens only to babies. Don't say things like the baby "will sleep in peace forever" lest you cause a child to fear sleep. Second, don't pretend you have all the answers. Be candid and say that although SIDS has a name, no one really understands it. You might say, "Some things in life don't make sense to me, either, and some things in life are not fair."

As difficult as it may be, children need to participate in the rituals surrounding death—the viewing, wake, funeral, and burial—to acknowledge that the person has really died and to start the mourning process. These rituals provide special times and places to remember and honor the baby and to begin the natural human quest for the meaning of the death. Jennifer Wilkinson has not regretted allowing her then four-year-old daughter Claire to see her baby sister shortly after she died and before the ambulance took her away from their home. "The issue of body and soul becomes so much clearer once you've laid eyes on the dead body of a loved one," says Jennifer. Seeing the "empty vehicle" that remained after the baby's life had been snuffed out helped her daughter realize that Larkin was clearly gone.

Likewise, Joani and Gabe have never regretted taking their three daughters with them to see Christian at the funeral home. "Touching him helped them to realize that he was really dead and could not come back as a person. But we explained that his spirit could stay with us always," says Joani. The family touched the hair that curled out from Christian's hooded sweater and cut a lock to keep in his baby album. They rubbed his icy hands to try to warm them and put farewell notes, a rosary, his teddy bear, and a copy of one of the kids' favorite books, *The Velveteen Rabbit*, in his casket. At home, each child chose some items (toys or clothes) to keep as mementos of their brother. All these rituals helped the kids say good-bye to Christian's body and helped them feel that they were doing things to honor their brother.

Amy, Amy
by Michael Purcell, age 5

Amy, Amy
I love you, love you.
I wish you could be here
But I know you can't.
I wish you could kiss me,
But I know you can't.

Missing Someone I Never Knew
by Lindsey Hosford, age 11

Most people believe that you can't miss someone you never knew, but I think a lot about my sister Susanna, who died of SIDS before I was born. I think she would have helped me with homework and tests. We would have planned parties and activities and other fun things together. She would have known about some of the problems I might have as I grow older.

I have an older brother, and he's great, but Susanna was a girl like me and I know I would have loved her very much.

A Spring Death

by Ilona Horchler, age 14

The house felt cold on that warm spring day of May more than five years ago. There was a great emptiness inside of me. I lay in my bed under the soft, cuddly sheets, and I clutched them in astonishment. This day was starting out as my worst nightmare. My father had left my room just two seconds ago after telling me that my baby brother had died. He had said only two words: "Christian died." He was trying to be sympathetic but left in fear that he would begin to cry. I saw my seven-year-old sister running by the door of my room crying.

All I could do was lie there. I didn't understand anything—I couldn't. I couldn't think, hear, or see anything. I slid shakily out of bed and walked to my dresser. All of a sudden I began to cry. Tears rolled down my cheeks one after the other as I thought about what had happened. How could it happen, and why?

I remembered when, on her birthday while holding Christian loving-ly in her arms, my mother had said, "This is the best birthday that I have ever had." I also remembered first hearing of my brother coming into the world from my second cousin Sylvia, who was to be Christian's godmother, after my Hungarian Scouts meeting on March 8, 1991. She stood at the top of the basement stairs and said to my two sisters and me, "You have a new baby brother." The house felt cozy and warm when she said this.

Now everything had turned upside down. By now my head hurt and, from trying not to cry out loud, my throat felt like someone had shoved a baseball down it. Questions flowed through my head. I want-ed to wake up from a horrible dream and to hold my brother close to me again—but no matter how hard I pinched myself, I would not be revived into this happiness. I dressed myself and stood in front of the mirror trying to dry my tears so as not to let anyone know I had been crying. I walked down the steps into a living room of sadness and confusion. Everyone was trying to figure out how a big, healthy baby could have just stopped breathing during a peaceful sleep. The doctors have a name for this crazy thing that they don't yet understand. The name is both matter of fact and chilling to the bone: Sudden Infant Death Syndrome.

Five and a half years later, I still find myself sobbing into a pillow. The pain will never go away. Through all of this I have greatly matured. I think more of the importance of life and try to excel in everything I do. I have been brought closer to God because He is my brother's caretaker now, but I also question Him. I am very much afraid of another death in the family and think of how I could not live with it. I know, though, that everyone's life was planned carefully and some lives must end earlier than others. I pray to my brother every night and will always love him with all my heart, for now he is not only a brother to me but a guardian angel as well.

Sister

In Memory of Meg Mihalko (9/15/89–10/23/89)

by Jon Mihalko, age 11

There once was a young boy
Who had a baby doll toy.

He wished and wished some more
For a sister and a whole lot more.

And when she came he was happy.
And one night when she took a nappy,

She died that very night.
He had an inner fight.

But when he thought of happy thoughts
Then he was winning the war he fought.

And do you know who that be?
He is no other than me.

(I was five years old when my sister died of SIDS. If anyone else wants to talk about his or her brother or sister dying of SIDS, please e-mail me. You can find my address in the appendix of this book under SIDS Network.)

He Should Have Been My Best Man
An Interview with Curtis Schweitzer

by Joani Nelson Horchler

For 24 of his 29 years, Curtis Schweitzer has lived with anguish over SIDS and a grief he is only beginning to resolve. When Curtis was a kindergartner, five-month-old Chad—the brother he had wanted so badly (and, as it turned out, the only brother he would ever have)— died of SIDS in a crib in the room he and Curtis shared.

As Curtis remembers it, his father had come in as usual before work to check on Chad and say good-bye to his two sons. "I went back to sleep, and the next thing I remember is Mom gasping and running out of the room. I reached into Chad's crib and he was cold and clammy. Mom came in after calling the ambulance and took me across the street to a neighbor's house. We had tomato soup for lunch, and to this day I still have trouble eating it."

Curtis was taken to school in the afternoon. When he came home afterward, he knew from all the cars and people that Chad had died. "I broke down and cried and it didn't seem like I could ever quit. I was in Chad's room when he died and I felt I should have heard him gasping for air; I thought he had suffered, and I blamed myself. I thought I should have saved him. After that, I tried to block it out and never talked to Mom and Dad about it. They never discussed it with me, either."

When Curtis went back to school the next day, his friends asked him troublesome questions such as, "What's it like to be in the same room with a dead person?" Curtis was as silent with them as he was with his family.

No family support groups were available at that time, and Curtis has always felt that "I was on the sidelines, having to keep everything to myself and deal with it on my own."

However, Curtis does not blame his parents. "In those days, everyone was expected to deal with their feelings as best as they could on their own and not bother anyone else. I felt bad for my parents because they didn't know how to deal with the pain so they just tried to shelter us from it by going about life as normally as they could."

But no matter how hard his parents tried to repress them, their emotions always managed to come through. "I remember my parents feeling sad quite a bit, and I always thought, 'Shoot, they're thinking about Chad again and how he could be here with us'—but we all left everything unsaid because that's what everyone expected us to do."

Within the past few years, the family has finally begun to open up about Chad as a result of a CBS movie made about Curtis's mother's life. The movie portrayed how dramatically the SIDS death affected Arlette's decision to become a surrogate mother for her own daughter Christa, who was born without a uterus. Arlette bore twins, a boy and a girl. When Christa named the boy after Chad, Uncle Curtis at first had a hard time even saying his nephew's name.

"I realized then that I'd been trying to run away from the pain, but it never went away. Part of the problem was that I never got to say goodbye to Chad. The last time I saw him was that morning when I reached into the crib and felt him dead."

People can learn from other animals about the necessity of saying good-bye, Curtis notes. "If one of a litter of puppies dies, the others realize that life is gone and won't dwell on it if they can see, smell, and feel the puppy. But if the dead puppy is taken away without that chance, you see the others whining and yelping at the gate. They're uncontrollable for a long time."

Besides never having said good-bye to Chad, Curtis also never resolved his guilt over having been in the same room with Chad when he died. The festering guilt made him overprotective of his own three sons. Each of them as babies slept in a bassinet next to their father, and, with the first, Curtis always kept his arm in the bassinet. If he rolled over and his arm fell out, he'd awaken with a start and, with the always-present fear that the baby had died, would slowly put it back in.

However, it took being electrocuted on a job to jolt Curtis into seeing a therapist. With his insides ready to explode, Curtis felt a hand reaching out to pull him to safety. At that moment, Curtis felt sure it was the hand of his guardian angel, Chad. Then he noticed the hand had his own wedding ring on it.

"I realized then that I had always thought of Chad as a god—that whenever anything good happened to me, it was always because Chad was helping me. My life revolves around Chad—I always tell all my problems to Chad, and I always think he answers me."

During therapy, it helped Curtis a lot to write a good-bye letter to Chad and, in effect, to "let him go." In it he told Chad how much he had blamed himself over the years for his brother's death. "It helped me because I realized that if it was him writing the same letter to me I wouldn't blame him. Now I know he doesn't blame me. I also told him that it was time for me to get on with my life and that I'd be with him again someday."

Besides getting therapy, Curtis has also been learning more about SIDS. "It wasn't terribly long ago that I found out that SIDS babies don't suffer, and that in and of itself has helped me."

Because his grief process was delayed and is not yet resolved, Curtis still can't think of Chad without feeling hurt. And he believes he will always feel cheated out of having a brother. "I was so excited when he came along, and when I was feeding him I'd tell him how much fun we were going to have together—how I was going to teach him how to build forts and go bike-riding and sledding on the dirt hill in the new subdivision. We'd roll around on the floor together, and he'd laugh and I'd tell him how I couldn't wait to wrestle with him."

When Curtis got married, he couldn't help thinking, "He should have been standing here beside me as my best man. A big part of my life is always missing."

In therapy, Curtis is finding it helpful simply to talk about Chad for the first time in more than 20 years. "The hurt never goes away, but I've finally learned I can talk about it. I can break down." However, because of all the mental roadblocks that were set up over the years, Curtis still has an easier time talking with strangers than with his family about Chad.

As a result of having his own three sons, Curtis isn't surprised at the enormous impact losing his baby brother has had on his entire life. "As soon as they're born, you love the youngest just as much as the oldest. You'd have more memories if you lost an older child, but the love and the pain are the same."

However, Curtis believes that if he had been encouraged to talk about his lost sibling earlier in his life, he could have dealt with the grief in a healthier way.

For children who lose brothers and sisters to SIDS, Curtis has some advice: "Don't hold anything in. Let out all of your good and bad emotions. Talk to your parents, family members, priests, and teachers. Don't be as hard on yourself as I've been on myself. Don't live inside yourself for as long as I have."

Editor's note: After telling their stories for this book, Curtis and his mother Arlette (whose article is featured in Chapter 17) had long talks about how they handled Chad's death. Arlette now says she realizes it was "foolish" to try to protect Curtis from the pain of Chad's death. "My husband and I come from very stoic German and Irish parents, and we always thought we had to keep our emotions in. We also didn't realize that a six-year-old could be so sensitive and perceptive, and we mistakenly thought that if we didn't talk about death it wouldn't affect him so badly," Arlette now says. "The mother in me thought 'being strong' was a valuable protection for my children, but now, too late, I've learned a valuable lesson—that it's better to confront the issues head on." Actually, it's never too late to make amends. Arlette and Danny are much more talkative with their grandchildren about Chad's death.

Helping Siblings Cope with Death

by Kee Schuth Marshall

I have a four-year-old son, Sam, who lost his three-month-old sister Margaret to SIDS on January 14, 1992, and then his father to a sudden heart attack just two months later. I would like to share how we dealt with our losses in hopes of providing assistance to others who have experienced similar losses and must help their young children understand and cope with death. Please keep in mind that I am not a professional counselor. We did, however, seek professional advice at the time from our children's pediatrician and grief counselors. In addition, following Margaret's death in particular, I tried to read as much as I could about how to help children deal with death, including several pamphlets provided by our local SIDS Information and Counseling group.

I was working when Margaret died. Sam normally attended a full-time day-care facility, but I had left him home with Margaret's new babysitter that day because he had a bad cold. The babysitter took both children for a stroll to the park and then to the Science Center at Sam's request. It was here that Margaret died in her stroller. Sam was there with her, and it is difficult for me to know exactly what he did or did not see. Almost immediately upon hearing the babysitter's screams, an off-duty paramedic began CPR on Margaret. Most people's attention— and apparently Sam's—was focused more on the distressed babysitter than the baby. Subsequently, both Margaret and the babysitter were taken to the hospital in separate emergency vehicles. Sam was left at the Science Center by himself until someone could determine who his parents were and how to reach us.

I was not in my office at the time. However, several of my colleagues went to pick up Sam and returned to my office while my husband was contacted. Jim went directly to the hospital. By the time I had arrived back at the office, many people already knew of Margaret's death. I did not know in the police car riding to the hospital with Sam and a co-worker; but once I arrived and saw everyone's faces I knew the worst had happened. While Jim and I spoke with the doctors, friends and hospital staff took care of Sam.

Jim's death was different in that Sam did not witness the events surrounding his death. Jim had left home to run to the athletic club to work out and then to run back. This was a normal workout for him and it was his first serious training effort for the 1992 triathlon season. As I was just finishing putting Sam to bed, the phone rang. Jim had passed out at the club, and I needed to go to the hospital. I called my next door neighbors to stay with Sam and drive me to the hospital. I learned shortly thereafter that Jim had died of a massive heart attack.

One of the first pieces of advice we received about Sam after Margaret died was that we should have him as involved with the funeral service as possible. We were told not to shield him from conversations about death and that talking about it openly in front of, and with, him would be helpful for him as he tried to understand what had happened. We were also told that children at his age (then three) take things very literally. Thus, we were advised to stay away from phrases such as "Margaret died in her sleep" or "she's resting peaceful-ly now" or "she's up in the sky in heaven." This was because Sam might then be afraid to go to sleep or fear that Margaret might be harmed by big birds in the sky.

Sam was involved with the funeral service. One excellent suggestion was to let Sam pick out flowers to take to her at the funeral home. I thought it most appropriate that he selected an entire bucket of baby's breath along with a few spring flowers sprinkled in. After leaving the funeral home, we took these flowers back to our house. He kept pointing them out to visitors with pride that they were his flowers for Margaret.

Jim and I had debated about whether or not to have the casket open at the funeral home. We decided that we would try because we wanted Sam to see that she was "all right" and that he need not be afraid for her. In addition, many people had never seen Margaret, and this would give them a chance to do that. We left the initial decision to the funeral director, who dressed her with the clothes I had provided. He said that Margaret looked surprisingly well. Jim and I went to the funeral home before the viewing to be with her in private first and to make the final decision about an open casket. We decided to do it, and for us, in hindsight, it was definitely the best decision.

We went home and picked up Sam and got ready to meet our visitors at the funeral home. The 20- to 30-minute drive from home to the viewing was spent prepping Sam on what to expect and what we were doing. Specifically, we told him that we were going to say good-bye to Margaret and that he would not see her again. We explained that Margaret was going to be with God and that He would take very good care of her so Sam would not have to worry about her. We said it was okay to cry, to miss her, to be sad sometimes, to talk about her, and to ask us any questions about her any time. During this discussion, Sam often repeated what we had said and was very interested in the conversation. I was amazed at Sam's memory, and I realized what an impact it had when, a week later, we were driving almost the same route as the one to the funeral home and he began to strike up the same conversation almost verbatim.

I had arranged ahead of time for someone to take Sam home from the viewing early: he was not there long (20–30 minutes). Sam was very comfortable with the person who took him home, which was one less thing for us to worry about.

Sam also attended both Margaret's and Jim's funeral and graveside services. I gave short eulogies for Margaret and for Jim at both funerals, during which Sam was by my side. After both of their services, I arranged for Sam to get out of the house while we received friends and relatives. This was such an emotional time that it was probably good for Sam to have some relief and for me not to have to worry about him while I greeted everyone.

Sam had nightmares the week following Margaret's funeral. He woke up crying hysterically but could not verbalize exactly what his dreams were about. Jim went in, lay down next to Sam, consoled him, and fell asleep with him. We later learned that this was a bad habit to start, but fortunately it seemed to help and only lasted a week.

When Jim died, Sam and I went through everything all over again. One important thing stands out, though, and it occurred during Jim's service. We had Communion at his service, so it was a long service for Sam to sit through. He wanted to leave me to sit with relatives behind us. The more I said "No" and "Be quiet," the louder and more deter- mined he was to do the opposite (as three-year-olds are apt to do). But I couldn't exactly get up and take him out of the church. I finally decided to let him have his way.

He took with him the visitor's card from our pew. The next thing I knew, Sam had started going to every pew to collect the visitor's cards. By the end of the service, Sam had collected several hundred of these cards from the entire church. This was like a much-needed comic relief, and many people expressed their appreciation to me later that I did not prevent him from doing this because it was like a member of the imme- diate family greeting them almost individually during the service. Quite frankly I was nervous about this and had really wanted to resist Sam. In the end it was like God reaching out to everyone who was grieving in this double tragedy—and it certainly kept Sam occupied during the service for me!

I guess all in all what I am saying is that sometimes you have to go with the flow. There are things you can plan and prepare for and there are things that will happen that you cannot anticipate. In hindsight I am glad Sam went to the viewing and the funeral service, and that I did not insist on "proper" behavior which—in addition to everything else— would have brought more attention to my already puffy, tired, and tear- stained face! Kids will be kids, even in the most horrible of situations.

Bless His Soul

In Memory of Her Cousin, Kyle Austin Koen
(Written on the day Kyle died of SIDS)

by Jennifer Wingfield, age 13

Almost three months old and he's six feet under
What's God trying to prove, I wonder?
It's just not fair, for he was so small,
He was so small he couldn't even crawl.
Too young to understand how good life can be
Dear God, could you not have let him see?

I just can't believe it, this feels like a dream
A dream, that's it! It's only a dream.
God wouldn't take the life of something so innocent and pure
Is he really dead? Are you absolutely sure?
Oh, it must be some mistake, this cannot be true
No, no mistake, his soul already withdrew.

I can remember holding this tiny child of whom I speak
His dark blue eyes and his rosy red cheeks.
Peacefully he left us all and went to a better place
Yes, he is really gone—reality I must face.
There was no mistake
It was just—bless his soul—his chosen fate.

Sadness in May

by Gabrielle Christine Horchler, age 9

My name is Gabrielle Christine Horchler, and I once had a brother
called "Christian Gabriel Horchler." We were both named after our
father Gabriel. Christian was born on the 8th day of March. He was one
of the cutest baby boys in the whole universe until May 9, 1991, when
he died of SIDS when he was two months and a day old. When he died,
we went to the funeral home to see him and stood around in sadness on
a day of May. Since then, we have been missing him every day and

wondering what he would be like now. But now we are starting a new life because we have a new sister called "Genevieve Désirée Horchler," who is the fourth girl in our family. But we will always remember Christian on that sad day in May and every day of our lives. And when I grow up, I would like to be a scientist so I can find a cause of and cure for SIDS and also a book writer about SIDS.

***

How We Helped Our Children... and How They Helped Us
by Joani Nelson Horchler

People occasionally comment to my husband and me that our children seem to have handled their baby brother's death in a remarkably healthy manner, and they ask us what we did to make it so.

Believe me, there were and are no magic maps to follow, and the road was often dark and stormy. During the first year, my then-nine-year-old daughter Ilona said several times, "The thing I want most in the world I can never have, and that is to have Christian back." My then-seven-year-old daughter said, "God kidnapped our baby." And our five-year-old daughter once said, "Big people don't die. Only babies die."

All of these statements vent bewilderment, frustration, and anger. They are simplistic but profound ways of expressing the feelings that we adults have, too. How did we deal with such statements? Simply by listening and by letting the kids be honest and open in showing their emotions about the death. And we let them see that it is normal for both adults and children to feel confusion and rage about an unexplained death like SIDS.

Because I was so angry about the death myself, I sometimes ranted and raved in front of my kids, and I often let them see me cry. But, in retrospect, I think—and psychologists confirm—that it's really healthy to cry in front of the children and even to let them see you're angry. After all, something truly devastating has happened. Why wouldn't you be angry and why wouldn't you cry? If you didn't cry in front of them, they might think you didn't love and miss the baby. Also, anger is a very natural part of the grief process, and I think it's healthy to let your children see that you're angry about what has happened. As they see you resolve your grief, they too will learn to resolve their angry feelings.

Our eight-year-old and six-year-old both expressed their anger, not overtly but rather by acting out (occasionally getting angry at everybody and everything in sight). I told them that it was okay to get angry as long as they didn't hurt anyone. I told them that feelings of anger are normal and that those feelings would begin to go away over time.

From talking with literally hundreds of SIDS parents, I have found it very common for SIDS parents to be impatient and often annoyed by their other children at times like these. I remember taking the kids to my husband's office for a visit about four months after Christian died. What I had intended to be a fun, relaxed family outing turned into a tense time because I was so irritable. To put it bluntly, I was hopping mad that Christian wasn't riding the Metro with us, and I couldn't help recalling the happy, carefree visit we'd made only five months earlier to show off what we had thought was our extremely healthy baby. When we picnicked on the lawn of the office building, we talked about how I was angry because we didn't have Christian with us. Talking about it openly seemed at least to help the children know that I was not angry with them, and I told them that, like me, they could help relieve the stress of their anger by swimming or hitting a tennis ball, or even by breaking something they'd been given permission to break. Our kids are swim team champions, and I think much of their anger was safely channeled into smacking the water.

Don't forget guilt. I expressed some of my guilt feelings—over not having checked the baby sooner the night he died, over having taken an antibiotic and a cold medicine when I was pregnant, and so on—in front of my oldest child when I didn't think she was listening. She asked, "Mom, is that what really caused Christian to die?" And I replied, "No, but we all feel guilty when someone dies, and we all need to talk about what we think we might have done wrong in order to realize that we really didn't do anything wrong." Guilt is a normal reaction when anyone dies, and I feel that coming out into the open and expressing some of my own misgivings may have helped her deal with her own sense of guilt. She had actually said several times, "Mom, did I do something that caused Christian to die?" And I would respond, "No. I always saw how wonderfully you treated the baby; you didn't do anything wrong." I responded that way because it was the truth. If I had ever sensed that she had wished the baby would go away forever, I would have responded, "I know that you got angry with the baby sometimes and wished that he would go away forever, but it's normal to feel that way about a new baby, and nothing you or anyone wishes can make a baby die."

My husband is a much calmer person than I am, and he didn't show his emotions nearly as much as I did. But I think that worked out fine because he provided stability and kept them going about their normal routines as much as possible—by continuing to take them to their piano and ballet lessons, Hungarian Scout classes, and their many other activities. He and I both felt that life should go on as normally as possible, even though we did not ignore the horrible thing that had happened to us.

My oldest daughter once expressed regret that I hadn't woken her up after I discovered Christian dead so that she could have seen him in a more natural state than when she later saw him at the funeral home. I replied, "I'm really sorry if you think I didn't do the right thing, but I did what I thought was best for you at the time and I can't change that now." I don't know whether this response was "right" from a psychologist's point of view, but it seemed to work.

To a large extent, just following your own parental instincts will work. Just be loving, tender, and truthful. And roll with the punches. As difficult as it may be, you may have to try to have a sense of humor about some of the embarrassing comments that just naturally pop out of the mouths of babes. About six months after Christian died, some of our neighbors were asked if they were planning to have a second child. Our then-three-year-old daughter Julianna piped in and said, "They'll have another baby when (their first child) dies!" As intense as our grief still was, this provided a sort of comic relief. We all couldn't help cracking up at this morbid, yet totally innocent comment from the mouth of a babe.

What has perhaps helped our children most is our new baby Genevieve. She has not replaced Christian—simply because he was totally irreplaceable in all of our hearts. However, she has brought all the joys of babyhood and having a baby sibling back into our home. One of the main reasons I wanted my children to have another sister or brother is that I didn't want a baby sibling's death to be their last memory of having a baby. Too, I wanted them to experience the fact that most babies live and thrive. I was surprised at how quickly they adapted to the heart and respiratory monitor, and how they viewed it as a friend that would help alert them to any problems their baby might have rather than as a threat that this new baby would die. We tried to be forthright and candid in dealing with their questions about whether this new baby could die: "Yes, she could, but it's not at all likely, and we are taking all the precautions we can to make sure it doesn't happen." Again, the keys are listening; being honest; answering questions to the best of your ability; and letting kids vent any confusion, frustration, and anger.

What Mister Rogers Has To Say
An Interview with Hedda Sharapan

by Robin Rice Morris

Fred Rogers, the long-time, caring host of *Mister Rogers' Neighborhood*, and his associate producer, Hedda Sharapan, have been helping children deal with the emotional issues of life for more than 25 years. As a natural part of life, death has been addressed by the pair on the television program and through conferences around the country.

"Fred Rogers believes that 'Anything human is mentionable, and anything mentionable can be manageable.'" Hedda says. "This is especially true when dealing with the issues that surround death."

Incorporating this belief with those that are always the building blocks of his show—including the importance of encouraging children to feel good about themselves; helping children learn the skills needed for growing up; and encouraging appreciation and respect for others—Fred Rogers made a program about the death of a fish and the death of a dog he had when he was a boy. In a newer program, in the week about Then & Now, a dead bird is found in the neighborhood, and Mister Rogers talks about the recent death of his cat. (This program repeats annually.) These programs, which Hedda has taken to many SIDS conferences over the years, have been a helpful resource to children and adults alike.

In her talks, Hedda stresses the following things to those who are dealing with a grieving child:

■ There is no recipe book for how to deal with children and death, but honesty—which children can intuitively sense—is essential.

- Often what helps children helps us. This would include such things as talking about the baby by name, remembering out loud with others, and being close to someone you love.

- Remember that each person has his or her own timetable for grieving, and when one member of a family is up, another might be down. This includes children and is both normal and to be expected.

- Every child is different, with his or her own pace and methods of expressing grief. As Mister Rogers often says, "There is only one person in the world like you." This is hard when a child's way is not the way of his or her mother or father. But the freedom to grieve in his or her own way and pace is critical to a child's healing.

- It is important to understand how children feel about baby siblings. Jealousy is a normal and natural reaction to the arrival of a new baby. Often, a new sibling is accepted with mixed feelings, and there may have been a time when a child has "wished away" his baby brother or sister. Parents or other adults need to acknowledge that this may have happened, and that, as Mister Rogers sings, "Scary Mad Wishes Can't Make Things Come True." Emphasize that there are angry times in loving families.

- Keep in mind, and tell your grieving child, that "The Very Same People Who Are Sad Sometimes Are the Very Same People Who Are Mad Sometimes." (You guessed it, another truly brilliant Mister Rogers song.) The heavy sadness won't last forever. We all have a full range of feelings—times of sadness and times of fun. We can't assume that a child who is off playing is no longer grieving, nor that laughter—from any griever—is out of place in the early days after a death.

- Admit to a grieving child, as this Mister Rogers song does, that "Some Things I Don't Understand Why, Why, Why." Especially with SIDS, where there are no answers to why, it's okay to admit that you don't know.

- It may be difficult for children to see a parent cry, but seeing parents cry is more healthy than seeing them hold back the tears. Terribly sad occasions without tears are confusing to a child, and he or she may wonder if the baby was really loved or is missed.

- Mister Rogers ends each program by singing, "It's Such a Good Feeling To Know You're Alive." That theme is especially helpful on the programs about death. It helps to balance the sad talk with hopefulness.

- Everyone needs closure after a death. Children need to react to, and come to accept, the baby's death as much as any adult does. For that reason, children's attendance at funeral services are encouraged. Funerals help survivors believe that the death has really happened and allow them to be with people who care about them. Of course, this does not have to be an "all or nothing" attendance. Often attending just a portion of the viewing, funeral, or burial is enough for a child. In addition, Fred Rogers and Hedda have created an excellent activity book for children to use during visitation or at home. Entitled *So Much To Think About: When Someone You Care About Has Died*, it is usually available from your funeral director through the National Funeral Directors Association. It can also be obtained from Fred Rogers' production company, Family Communications Inc., 4802 Fifth Avenue, Pittsburgh, PA 15213. Also available from the same address is a booklet for adults called "Talking with Young Children About Death."

- Many parents worry about what is "normal" in a grieving child. Hedda believes that if your child is in real emotional trouble over the loss, "you'll know. Children give us clues, and you can trust your instincts." Through SIDS and other support groups, parents can feel reassured when they hear how other children are reacting. There are caring professionals in almost every community who can help parents deal with their children's needs.

- Every child has the right to be sad. Quite naturally, it pains adults to watch a child grieve. They wish for their children a happy childhood. As one of Hedda's friends told her son, "Let's just be sad until we're not sad anymore."

- Realize that for children, play is the most natural way for them to deal with their feelings. Though it disturbs many adults, it is perfectly natural for a child to be "playing funeral," running up and down the stairs and screaming with a baby doll in arms (a reenactment of the SIDS discovery), or lying in front of the coffin to see what it feels like to not move. Adults don't need to analyze the play—just respect it. Play helps children work through the issues and come to some peace about the death.

■ Most of all, help your grieving child again and again, as Mister Rogers does, by letting them know "You are special." Children need to know that the people who are important to them care about them no matter what they're feeling. We all do.

For My Baby Sister Stephanie

by Tony Paik, age 5

She made me so happy when
*   She came home from the hospital.*
She was so cute and pretty.
I always picked her up,
Even though Mommy thought I was too small
to hold her the right way.
I would sing "Itsy Bitsy Spider" to her
And she would smile at me.

Then I remember Mommy telling me
*   She was gone!*
I cried when I saw her grave.
I wanted to dig her out,
*   And hold her again.*
I wanted to be with her more than anything!

I miss her right now.
I wish she was still home with me.
I will never forget her.
I will see her one day and
Until then
She will never leave my heart.

I never thought it could end like this,
*   My baby sister dying.*

Chapter 7

Grandparents: A Grief Doubled

There is an old Swedish proverb, "Grief shared is grief halved." But for a grandparent sharing in a SIDS grief, the pain is doubled. There is first the pain of losing the grandchild, and second the pain of watching helplessly as one's own child—the baby's father or mother—is tortured with grief.

One common reaction for grandparents is, "Why not me? I'm old and have lived my life. He was just a baby—just beginning his." This is not a wish for death, but for a trade in the tragedy if there must have been one. People of all ages feel that God had His rule book all wrong, or was at the very least not paying attention. But this anger is especially poignant for those looking on toward the end of their lives anyway.

Another pain is that of never having seen the grandchild, which is common in our industrialized society. Perhaps a trip was planned for the summer, but the death came first. The peek into a casket may be the only time a grandparent sees his or her beloved grandchild. The sadness can be overwhelming.

On the other side of the coin is the grandparent who lived very close and took an active role in his or her grandchild's daily life. The grandparent may have been the Saturday night sitter, or even the full-time weekday child-care provider. These grandparents feel a day-to-day emptiness and face many physical reminders. (The last time she was here she took a bath in this very sink!)

There may also be feelings of jealousy or previously built-up animosity between sets of grandparents, especially if one set has been much closer to the grandchild than the other. For the parents' sake, this is the time to build bridges, not burn them.

Sometimes grandparents may try to mask their grief in order to "be strong" for their children and other grandchildren. But this can actually lead to a feeling of resentment by the bereaved, or wondering if the grandparent really cared. Family relationships can be strengthened through shared weakness, and a grandparent has every right to be weak in the face of a SIDS tragedy.

Many bereaved grandparents work through their grief by plunging themselves into SIDS-related charity work or other socially productive activities. Christine Fackler Salemi, who writes about her grandson in this chapter, worked tirelessly keying in this book's outside contributions and also spearheaded a quilt-making project for SIDS. Beverly Powell, who also shares her thoughts about losing a grandson, found relief by serving as chairperson of the board of advisors to the University of Maryland SIDS Institute. Both women believe that their grief process has been helped along by "giving back" through SIDS-related activities.

Oh, for the Purely Material Losses
by Dora Nagy Horchler

He was born during bombardments and homeless at age three months. Too, my youngest son Gabriel almost starved to death when I could no longer nurse him as we fled Hungary on evacuation trains during World War II. At age three, Gabe's burst appendix was operated upon by a young, inexperienced surgeon in an Austrian hospital that did not have any penicillin. A warning of tuberculosis followed. Many years later, my son—by then a completely healthy young American man—fulfilled an agonizing year of combat duty in Vietnam.

Yet when I look back at my family's exodus from Hungary through artillery fire, I don't feel any regret. We had been wealthy in our native land and lost our home, our money, and even our jewelry (when the suitcases that held it fell off a crowded evacuation train). But our losses were purely material. And in exchange for them we got the chance to become closer to God and to feel the gratitude due Him for leading us to safety. We ended up here in Philadelphia six years later with four happy, healthy children who had relished their poor but cheerful transitory home in the scenic western Alps.

Yes, our losses in those days were only material.

Forty-some years later, on May 10, 1991, the phone rang at 5 am. Awakened suddenly, I thought at first that it must be one of those annoying anonymous calls. But there was also a vague feeling of fear, like the premonition of a catastrophe. And, when I recognized the cracked voice of my youngest son, I knew it was something very bad.

"Christian died last night," he said.

"Crib death?" I asked at once. This frightful, unexplainable menace to infants' lives—about which I had often heard and read—had hit friends and acquaintances, but never us. Not until now.

The evening before I had thought intensely of little Christian Gabriel—my twelfth grandchild, my son's only son, the precious little brother of Gabe's three little daughters, the boy my darling daughter-in-law Joani had long hoped for. I saw Christian shortly after his birth and then again at Easter for the first of what I thought would be many visits. He was a sturdy, healthy baby, and I longed to see him again, to hold him and hug him. It was with plans for a visit to his home that I went to bed. And now this awakening...

My son could hardly talk. He was physically and emotionally exhausted by the horrible shock of his loss. He asked me to notify his sisters and brothers, and I promised to come to him as soon as I could. I waited an hour and then called my eldest son and my younger daughter who live close to me, and then my son in Maine. I could not reach the big sister of all the others; she was away on vacation with her husband. Her mother-in-law promised to tell them when they arrived home. Bebe, my youngest daughter, could free herself for the day, and by 9 am we were already on our way to Cheverly, Maryland.

We found a seemingly empty house. Kind friends had taken the three little girls for the day. The parents moved and looked like ghosts. Ken, Joani's good-looking, stalwart young brother, was there, too, exhausted and devastated. Soon friends and neighbors came; their sympathy was touchingly sincere. They helped us to persuade Joani and Gabe to lie down and sleep. They had many more things to face and needed strength. Ken, too, needed a rest and wanted to go home, but before leaving told us what happened. We would hear it over and over again, re-opening the wound, re-enhancing the cruelty of the loss, and—in a way—reliving the pain. As Joani often lamented, it was so ironic that Gabe had suffered yet survived so many trials in his life when his chubby-cheeked, sturdy little son could not even endure a peaceful nap.

That day was followed by more days, weeks, months of sadness, intensified by the fact that the previous two months had been perfectly happy. Little Christian's birth brought so much joy, fulfilling so many dreams and desires. This should have been a warning: Perfect happiness, so rarely experienced, cannot last long in our earthly lives. Why? We do not know. We do not know God's plans, and we cannot question them. It hurts to think of past happiness when tragedy strikes, but later the memory of it does comfort us.

The loss of a child, even of a very small one, causes a wound that never heals. The thoughts, "How old would he be? What would he be doing now?" accompany us through life. But at the same time, we have to be thankful for the others, whom God gave and saved and whose growth and development we can follow and enjoy. We value and appreciate them more because we suffered that loss.

All in all, a catastrophe is like a thunderstorm: It causes hurt and damage, but it also cleanses the air and throws a revealing light on many things. Little Christian's death made us aware of the kindness of neighbors, the sincere devotion of friends, and the strong ties of the family. To me, it was a special comfort to see how all my children hastened to their brother's side and shared his grief.

AGAST: An Alliance for Grandparents
by Sandra R. Graben

Our second child, Catherine Ann, had been married six years. While I did not bug her (says I), they were not in as big a hurry as I was for children (grandchildren). Finally, they announced that a baby was due January 17, 1989. Not only was the 17th of each month a birthday in the family, but this would be my parents' first great-grandchild and our first grandchild. Excitement reigned.

Timothy David Hulme (T.J.) was born as promised on January 17, 1989, in Phoenix, Arizona. He was a wonderful baby. At that time we lived in Texas, and I made a point of seeing T.J. at least once a month. On July 29, 1989, I headed to Phoenix and played with T.J. on Saturday and Sunday. He had a new tooth, and on Monday he pulled himself up on the TV stand. Leaving that day was hard, but a teenager waited in Texas.

While changing clothes after my return home, I received a phone call that changed my life. Catherine was holding T.J. He was dead! Preliminary diagnosis was Sudden Infant Death Syndrome. But he was too old, we had thought—6 1/2 months! I remembered thinking, "Thank you, God!" as his fifth month passed. So, how dare He? This beautiful, healthy, loved, wanted child? Why my kids? Why my family?

My anger gave me strength. Action was called for. I knew of two friends who about 20 years before had had children die of SIDS; both babies were girls aged 3–4 months. I called them. They had received no support from family, friends, or church. At least my children (the parents) received peer contact immediately, and group counseling was available. Texas had some support available, but I lived an hour from a large city, so my self-appointed job was to visit each doctor, each clinic, and the one hospital in our county with information on SIDS.

What made me angriest was the lack of knowledge, the awareness beforehand of SIDS. In Texas, I contacted the state health department, worked health fairs, and spoke on SIDS to civic groups. My daughter, her mother-in-law, and I attended the National SIDS Alliance meeting that year in Houston.

On Cathy's return home, friends, including professional golfer Mark Calcavicchio and his wife Sheryl, offered to put on a fund-raiser. In January 1990, the first professional–amateur golf game for SIDS research was held. It raised $40,000 for the T.J. Hulme Research Fund. Mark won the Phoenix Open that year, held the pro–am the following Monday, and announced that he wanted to give Cathy and Tim money from his winnings to attend the International SIDS Conference in Australia!

By 1992, Cathy and I and my subsequent grandchild (Jason Lee Hulme, born September 11, 1990) had attended most national and many state conferences. More grandparents were attending. In 1993 a breakout session for grandparents was held. Afterward, seven grandparents from several states formed a support group called AGAST (Alliance of Grandparents Against SIDS Tragedy). The chance to talk to other grandparents who had a grandchild die was a relief. The anguish of being unable to help your child or yourself through the turbulent stages of grief is overwhelming. A talk with a person who has walked the same walk frees the inner knots and gives one the ability to speak freely.

In November 1994, AGAST was recognized as a 501(c)(3) charity, allowing all donations to be tax-deductible. I became the coordinator rather by default, but I have felt it to be worthwhile. The mailing list now numbers about 600 grandparents across the United States. More health professionals know of AGAST and recommend it to grieving grandparents, whether the grandchild died of SIDS or other causes. There are AGAST peer contacts in 27 states. Internationally, 10 countries have grandparent contacts. A newsletter is mailed four times a year. AGAST sustains itself on donations and grants, is run by volunteers, and works with the national SIDS Alliance and its 50 state affiliates.

Every time I, as coordinator of AGAST, talk with a newly bereaved grandparent or a grandparent whose grief has surfaced again, I am reconfirmed in my commitment that before I die, at least I shall have done everything that I can to give parents and grandparents foreknowledge of SIDS. If this devastation strikes their families, they will know where to turn for help and be able to receive support. This is all I can do for my grandson, T.J. Hulme (January 17, 1989, to July 31, 1989).

The Double Hurt of Grandparents

by Beverly Powell

As mothers, we try to protect our children from pain. When our child's child dies, we suffer a double hurt in seeing them suffer and not being able to shelter them. I felt so frustrated and upset that I could do or say so very little to ease my only son John's and his wife Alice's pain at losing their only son Christopher to SIDS in April 1988.

As grandparents, we also wish—in many cases—that we could take the baby's place. The first thing my mother, the great-grandma, said when she heard of Christopher's death was, "I wish it could have been me."

The anger and frustration are penetrating. I remember two incidents that made me extremely angry after Christopher died. One was an aborted fetus left on an aircraft and another was a baby left in a trash-bag. I was just furious that my grandchild had been so loved and yet had to die, and here were babies being mistreated and left to die.

I'd heard about SIDS, but that was something that happened to somebody else, not my own children and not my own grandchild.

I have friends who lost three of their four children in an auto accident 20 years ago. Neighbors would cross the street so they didn't have to say anything to them. It was left to my bereaved friends to break the ice. It was so ironic that they had to make others feel better. I thought such a tragedy could never strike me, and then when Christopher died I said to her, "I know now what you went through." I've had some bitter feelings toward people who have refused to deal with Christopher's death. I have friends who have never, ever mentioned Christopher's name to me, and I have reluctantly learned to accept that.

Whether I mention that I have three grandchildren, including one who died of SIDS, depends on the occasion and the setting. If I don't feel like explaining, I say I have two granddaughters. But with someone like an old high school friend, I'll say, "I have two granddaughters and a grandson who passed away."

I've tried to channel my anger about losing Christopher into constructive things. For example, I served as chairperson of the SIDS Institute's board of advisors for several years.

I also cherish my granddaughters, who were born to Alice and John after Christopher's death. Kelly is five and Shelby is two. Alice was in the doctor's office with them four times last week, but I try never to question anything she does. I have to respect the fact that I've never walked in her shoes, and I don't know what anxieties I'd have. When people say she's overprotective, I tell them, "You've never lost a child and neither have I."

Since there is so very little I can do to shield my son and daughter-in-law from the pain, I just try hard to be understanding. I view my role as supporting them in that way.

A Letter from Grandma Nelson

by Doris Guhin Nelson

Dear Joani, Gabe, Ilona, Gabrielle, and Julianna:

It will soon be the first year anniversary of Christian's birth. You can always be proud of having made Christian's too-short life such a happy time. I feel blessed to have had a month to be with him. I feel that now he is a special angel—up there with my son, his Uncle Brad—and wants his family to think of him happily. It is difficult to accept his death, but we will always remember him with happiness.

Love,
Grandma Nelson

Sweet Memories of Jacob Barlow Kruse

by Christine Fackler Salemi

your birth,

first day home,

helping your Mommy and Daddy,

watching you sleep,

watching you play with your mobile,

listening to you coo and sing,

Christmas Eve,

seeing you in your new crib,

watching Mommy while she bundled you in your snowsuit,

when you blinked your eyes real fast

after Mommy kissed you all over your face,

watching Daddy bounce you on his knees to help you to fall asleep,

nursing sounds,

holding you,

touching your soft skin,

seeing how much you were looking like your Daddy,

your christening day,

Mommy and Daddy coming to my house carrying you.

These are the memories that I hold very dear

and try to focus on.

Forgive Me, My Daughter

by Jean Andre

I want you to be the little girl
  who tore her many-layered petticoats
  on the parallel bars or in school,
  and once even chipped a tooth.
I want you too, to be the child with
  bloody knees who had matching holes in
  her new leotards.
Or maybe the one who fell from a swing
  and needed a half dozen stitches beneath her eye.

Oh, I could hold you then
  there was magic in my kisses that
  stemmed the pain and a doctor nearby
  for more tangible aid.

But what do I do now, now that you
  are a woman, and your sorrows are
  commensurate with your age?
I stand immobile as your wan face
  leans over the broken turf
  where your infant son, your only child,
  will soon be interred.

I clench my fists knowing
  there is no solace any longer in my
  arms for agony of this magnitude
You are deaf, too, to my murmurings:
  you hear only the echoes of his
  laughter and his cries.
Of course,
  I am here when you need me.
But I can only pretend I am a strong
  and wise grandmother when, in truth,
I remain a mother, heart-broken twice.

Chapter 8

When a Baby Dies
at the Child-Care Provider's

Child-care providers play a special role in the lives of children and their parents. It is likely that parents have scrutinized the provider's background, looked for signs that he or she will provide abundant hugs and kisses, and left their child only after safety and nurturing seem ensured. Yet as all survivors know, there is no way to ensure against a SIDS death. And as the child-care provider learns, the cost of lending your heart for a daily wage can be tremendously high.

For parents, there are overwhelming feelings of guilt when their baby dies at the child-care provider. Why wasn't I with him? Why did I go to work that day? Why did I have a career at all? Would it have happened if I had been there? Can I forgive my provider, even though I know there is nothing to forgive? And for child-care providers, there is another kind of guilt and even more questions: I was responsible for the baby, so am I responsible for the baby's death? Did I miss something I should have seen? Do the parents blame me? Am I welcome to attend the funeral? Can I also have some "good-bye time" with the baby? Will I lose my license? Can I handle caring for an infant again?

The three things child-care providers must do if a baby dies while in their care are (1) notify the paramedics, (2) notify the child's parents, and (3) notify their licensing agency. As Jodi Shaefer, director of the Maryland SIDS Information and Counseling Program, says, "While they may hear accusations or ignorant comments, no provider has lost a license due to having a SIDS death occur in her home." Even so, child-care providers are concerned that parents of other children in their care "may fear SIDS as their fault or contagious," notes Ms. Shaefer. "That's why we need to give them much of the same information and support we give the parents."

Several child-care providers say that they were not provided with any information about SIDS when they went into the business. The shock and horror of finding a previously well baby not breathing or even obviously dead are tremendous blows. Yet because the baby was not their own, most people question what the big deal is. As child-care provider Donna Shelton notes later in this chapter, family and friends are not hesitant to say things such as, "Why are you so upset? He wasn't yours!" They expect the baby's death to be treated as a very bad day at work that is now over. Even child-care providers themselves may wonder why they can't get over it. Yet the reality is that grief and anxiety can continue for many months and even years.

An excellent video, "Caregivers Hurt, Too," describes the emotional trauma providers experience and includes information on support and resources. Emergency procedures, the investigative process, and strategies to reduce the risk of SIDS are presented. The video is available for $30, including shipping and handling, from the Maryland SIDS Program, 630 West Fayette Street, Room 5-684, Baltimore, MD 21201-1585.

Parents who lose babies in a child-care setting have different issues to deal with than parents who lose babies in their own homes. These questions and unique concerns are addressed at length by SIDS mother Jennifer McBride in her article in this chapter.

Many SIDS parents have additional difficulty in understanding and accepting a baby's death when the infant was not in the usual location or with the usual caretaker when the death occurs.

"If only I'd been home with her, she wouldn't have died," is a fairly typical comment heard in SIDS support groups. However, "no data exist to suggest that infants are more vulnerable to SIDS because of a change in location or caretaker," says Dr. Carl E. Hunt, chairman of the department of pediatrics at the Medical College of Ohio. It is common for infants at the vulnerable age for SIDS to experience changes in locations and caretakers, and there is no evidence to suggest that avoidance of the change would lead to prevention of the death, Dr. Hunt states.

As Child-Care Providers, It's Our Baby, Too

by Donna Shelton

It is often said that SIDS is every parent's nightmare. Well, SIDS is also every child-care provider's worst dream. And I, as a day-care provider, lived through it.

Little Edward was seven weeks old when his parents, Mark and Nancy, brought him to me for day care. During the two months I cared for him, he continued to smile and started laughing and loving playtime. The fateful day arrived when he was three and a half months old.

It was a fairly normal day at first. He woke up from his morning nap early, and I spent some extra time playing with him. At about 4:30 pm, he got fussy, so I laid him down as usual in a crib in my bedroom. At 5:15 pm, I noticed he was lying face down. "You silly boy," I thought while casually reaching into his crib to turn his head. I can't describe the feeling of total horror I had when I felt him and realized right away that something was terribly wrong. Though it hadn't been very long since he had died, his muscles were like empty sponges with no tone whatsoever. When I flipped him over he was blue in the face. My husband Bill was home and called 911. We followed the resuscitation instructions given to us, but nothing could be done.

Because they chose me to care for and love him when they could not, I couldn't help but feel I had let Mark and Nancy down. The guilt was enormous. Yet, right from the start, they were wonderfully understanding. Not only did they not blame me, they made me feel like a part of their family. I had a private viewing with just Mark and my husband alongside. We were relieved and honored that Edward's family felt close enough to us to ask us to be with them at such a tragic time in their lives. I think it was because they realized that we also had grown to love Edward very deeply and we felt his loss as if he had been our own child. The four of us also went together to a support-group meeting for parents. Not too long after that, Nancy and Mark moved to a town too far away for them to keep attending the meetings. But I continued to go religiously. For me, the group was the only outlet I had for my grief and feelings of loneliness.

The implicit message I got from most of my family members was, "He wasn't yours. Why are you so upset?" People who haven't experienced it can't understand the devastating impact of finding a precious baby dead and trying frantically to breathe life back into him. In my own life, I had already learned how much life is to be cherished. My husband and I had tried for many years to have a baby and were finally able to adopt a son whom we treasure as our own. Two and a half years later, I gave birth to a son. I went into the business of child care because I adore children, especially babies. I continue to care for children even now, seven years after Edward's death and despite my fears, because I need babies and they need me. I always strive to give them the same care and nurturing their mother would give.

I also continue to spend many hours each month on volunteer activities for the Virginia SIDS Alliance. I currently serve as chairperson of the Family Services Committee, and in that role I try to include child-care providers as much as possible in support programs. For several years, the group's SIDS hot line was in my home, and I answered it. Thus, I was very often a parent's or child-care provider's first point of contact with other SIDS survivors after a SIDS death. I find it strange that many people, and often even SIDS parents, don't realize that child-care providers feel much the same anguish that they do.

My advice to parents and child-care providers is to reach out to a support group and share your feelings openly. True understanding is the most comforting thing you can find. We as child-care providers feel much of the same guilt that parents feel about not having been able to prevent a SIDS death, and talking to others who have been through SIDS deaths helps us realize that we did nothing to cause it.

I also plead with parents to reach out to their child-care providers. I know how very much I needed to hear from Nancy and Mark that they didn't blame me. Because we talked and cried and looked at Edward's pictures together during those first few unbelievable months, we developed a strong bond. Even though we don't get to see each other very often anymore, I rejoice in the two subsequent children they have and in their mended lives. I can't imagine how I could have lived through a situation in which the parents wouldn't talk to me, or even blamed me. The death would have been even harder on all of us.

A Parent's Perspective

by Jennifer McBride

All my life, I knew that I wanted to be a mother. When I was 31, I finally got the chance. I'd heard of SIDS and the risk factors associated with it. While pregnant friends ignored these risks factors, I paid attention to every one and did nothing during or after my pregnancy that would have put my infant son at a higher risk. He was a strapping, serious, wise-looking child, and I loved him as I knew I would from the moment he was conceived. Then, on December 9, 1992, six weeks after I brought him home from the hospital, three days after I'd started back to work, my son, Maxwell Aronson McBride, died during a mid-morning nap at the day-care provider's house.

I didn't have the choice of staying home with my child. Neither did I have relatives close by. So, when my allotted maternity leave was over, I was forced to find someone else to care for my child. I asked friends for day-care references, I consulted local newspapers and day-care associations, I interviewed several at-home day-care providers, checking their references and their histories through the state offices.

Finally, I found one—Michelle—whom I thought would be qualified to take care of my son. We worked out a schedule that allowed me to have a "lunch date" with Max. On Monday I went home for a quick bite to eat. When Michelle had wakened Max from his morning nap, she called me at home and told me to come over. I stopped by her house on my way back to work and nursed Max. While nursing, I talked to Michelle about Max's morning. I was surprised when she indicated that he'd slept for more than two hours because he rarely slept longer than 20 minutes for me while on his back, unless I slept beside him. It turns out that she was placing him on his tummy to sleep. I asked her if she'd heard that the American Academy of Pediatrics was now recommending side or back sleeping to reduce the risk of SIDS. She said that she had not. We discussed it for a bit and, in the end, I bowed to her eight years of experience in taking care of infants—of course, she knew more than this first-time mom. Because he almost always fell back to sleep after eating, I laid him down—on his back—in the playpen she had set up for him. I breathed a sigh of relief when

Max (and I) survived his first day away from me. Tuesday passed in the same way.

On Wednesday, Michelle called, right on time, for my "lunch date," but, before I could get out the words, "I'm on my way," she said "No, don't. I couldn't wake Max up. The paramedics are here and they want you to meet them at the hospital."

"Please, God, don't take my son," was all I said and thought as I tried to contact my husband, who was at lunch. "Please, God, don't take my son," was all I said and thought as I drove myself to the emergency room. "Please, God, don't take my son," was all I thought as I discussed insurance details with the emergency room clerk. Although I asked repeatedly for any details about my son's condition, they were unable to tell me anything. Instead they led me to an isolated "Community Room," where I could continue to try to reach my husband and family. My husband, Max, Michelle, and her father all arrived at the hospital at about the same time—at least one hour after I had arrived. My husband came into the room with me, and by 2:00 our pediatrician came in for the third time. The first time, he said that the ER doctors were working on Max, the second time he said that it wasn't looking good and that they would have to stop resuscitation efforts soon. The third time it was over.

Our pediatrician encouraged us to see Max one last time. Through our tears, Michelle and I saw each other in the hallway on my way to hold my son. I think I hugged her; I know I asked her about Max's sleeping position when she found him. When I held Max, and for some time afterward, I was only conscious of the fact that he didn't look like my child and that he was dreadfully cold and heavy.

We all suffer in similar ways when we lose a child to SIDS. But when a child dies while at a day-care provider's, the parents feel a different sense of guilt. I remember hearing one side of a conversation my mother was having at my home immediately following Max's death. She said, "Jenny interviewed at least seven people, and this one came highly recommended." To the next caller she said, "Jenny interviewed at least a dozen people, and this one came highly recommended." In truth, I don't know how many I interviewed, but why did my mother feel compelled to lie on my behalf? Why were the callers immediately convinced that either the day-care provider was negligent or that I was negligent in choosing her? Was I? There's my guilt. Max was fine when he was with me. I should have insisted that he nap on his back. I should have…

I spent the Christmas holidays at my parents' house and walked for hours in the woods gathering fallen tree limbs and making "nesting birds" (it's supposed to be good luck to have one in your house) to give as thank yous to all those who had been kind to me during this difficult time. When I returned home, I went to Michelle's house to take her one. Part of me wanted to reach out to her, even though she only took care of my son for two and a half days; she was the only other one to have taken care of him. I thought that because she had known him, she would share my grief. She was very uncomfortable seeing me. I told her about the SIDS support group in the area; she wasn't interested. She had plans to go out that night, so I gave her the bird (the nesting one) and left. I haven't seen her since.

Two and a half years have passed since Max died. A lot has happened in that time. I became active in the North Texas SIDS Alliance. I became pregnant again right away. I'd always wanted more children. There was nothing I could do to bring Max back, I would never be allowed to raise him. I wasn't getting any younger. Why wait? It was the best decision I ever made.

My son, J.B. (Jacob Blanding), was born five weeks early—only nine months after his big brother died. By the time J.B. was born, President Clinton had signed the Family Medical and Leave Act, which, when coupled with a great employer, allowed me to take 15 weeks off as maternity leave. (I never did understand the six-week rule. They don't wean puppies from their mothers until eight weeks!)

Monitoring J.B. seemed the way to go for me. Because most health professionals agree that there will undoubtedly be more than one cause of SIDS, it makes sense to me that some children currently dying of SIDS may be able to be resuscitated. Therefore, monitoring him would enable his caregiver to begin resuscitation efforts immediately, ensuring that every effort had been made on his behalf. My mom and J.B.'s Aunt Koko took turns staying with him for the first month after I went back to work. During this time, my husband decided that family life wasn't for him. So, on my own, I had to face my worst fear: securing day care for my second son.

This turned out to be harder than I thought. By the time I found Noel, I had been referred all the way to the Easter Seals Nursery for Special Needs Children on the other side of town. No one wanted to take a perfectly healthy baby on a monitor. Most of the day-care providers I consulted were totally ignorant about SIDS. Of course they weren't as motivated as I was to learn about it...yet. One provider was taking care of an infant my son's age who wasn't on a monitor and wouldn't take on the risk of my son. She couldn't accept the fact that my son was at no greater risk than the other child and that, at least in my son's case, she'd be notified if he was in distress. It was a very frustrating time for me. Anyway, I found Noel, and she was a godsend to both J.B. and me. Life was finally smoothing out again.

Then, on December 14, 1994, I had my second brush with a SIDS death at day care. A new child, Kyle Koen, died at Noel's during his mid-morning nap. Talk about deja vu! It was his mother's third day back at work. This time I saw, as a third party, what both sides go through when a child dies at the day-care provider's. The parents immediately look for the reason. Why did their son die? How was he being cared for? Was the sitter to blame? She didn't pay as much attention to him as I would have. Would he have died if he'd been with me?

Of course these questions when directed at the day-care provider often elicit a defensive response: "I checked on him every 10 minutes during his nap. I began CPR right away and didn't miss a beat when calling 911." What each person can't really admit or share with the other is the enormous amount of guilt, helplessness, and self-doubt that they're feeling. My own experience of wanting to reach out to the provider was re-enacted by Kyle's parents, Tracy and Karl. What I understood this time around, though, is that the day-care provider can't feel the same loss as the parent. In fact, no one can. Even each parent's loss is unique. Noel was certainly affected and devastated by Kyle's death, but she didn't have the same experience with him as Tracy and Karl did. She didn't anticipate his birth and life. Kyle wasn't a part of her and her husband. He was a child that she was paid to take care of during the day, and she did that job admirably. It was very important to Noel to hold day care the next day. For her, life went on. For Karl and Tracy, it stopped...temporarily, then moved on forever changed in a different direction.

Now, two and a half years into my recovery, there are some things that I've learned and would like to pass on. For the parents who suffer the loss of a child to SIDS: Eventually you need to move to a place where you understand that nothing the day-care provider did or did not do caused the death of your child. No, she didn't love your baby as you did. Yes, she had her own way of doing things that may not have been to your liking. But she did not do anything that caused the death of your child. The autopsy ruled that out. By understanding and accepting this fact, you can begin to release your own guilt. If she didn't cause the death of your child, you weren't remiss in hiring her.

For day-care providers, now that the American Academy of Pediatrics has taken a firm stand in supporting the National "Back to Sleep" campaign, you should support it too. Over the years, the one thing that we can count on is that children will die of SIDS, one in 1,000 each year. With more mothers working these days, it's only a matter of time before you will experience a SIDS death in your home. Protect yourself and the children in your care by being educated about how to reduce the risk. Always remember that the child you are caring for is the most important thing in someone's life.

Only the Sitter?

by Donna Allen

I was babysitting for a two-month-old baby and his two sisters and one brother when the baby died.

I picked him up out of his playpen, carried him over to the bed, and tried to give him CPR. But it didn't work, and the air rushing out of him sounded so awful that I didn't know what to do.

His parents held nothing against me, thank heavens. They included me in every part of their lives for the next couple of weeks. I told them that I'd like to attend the funeral if it wouldn't upset them, and they said that they wanted me there. They said that I was a part of their family (even though we were really just friends) and that they wouldn't have it any other way.

At the funeral, the mother and I looked at the baby together. She took my hand in hers and began to cry—again. Then we hugged each other for a long time and sobbed out our anguish and sadness together. Other guests there, people I'd never seen before, came up to me and said they had known how much those children loved me and offered their condolences to me. Who was I? I had never met any of them. I really wasn't one of the family, although I felt, and still do feel, like one. I don't know how they knew who I was.

Needless to say, the way this whole family treated me was wonderful and unbelievable, and it helped a lot. When it first happened, I was shocked when the police and firemen treated me so well and with such respect.

After all, I was only the sitter. I felt like the bottom of the totem pole, the very last person people would worry about. Thank you, my friends. I'll be eternally grateful.

This article was reprinted with permission from Children's Hospital of Wisconsin.

Chapter 9

How To Be a Friend to a SIDS Survivor

"The road to a friend's house is never long," the saying goes. But it is incredibly long when your friend has just lost a baby to SIDS. What do you say? What do you do? What can you offer that could make even the least bit of difference? There is none more able to answer these questions than SIDS survivors and the friends who saw them through their nightmare of loss.

Joani remembers her first reactions to friends and neighbors who visited to express their sorrow and offer help. "I actually felt resentful of people who tried to help. I wanted to send them away. I thought 'How can they just waltz in here, view my tragedy as if it were a Shakespearean drama, and then waltz home to their mundane worries like what color to paint the bathroom—their lives going happily along while mine was mired in utter disaster?'"

Joani fought the urge she occasionally had to send everyone away and leave her alone in her suffering. "I'm now glad I didn't because relatives and friends were, all in all, a real help and comfort to me and my family. And many of them had suffered losses in their lives that, even if they weren't SIDS losses, made them understanding, sympathetic, and helpful."

The most helpful, Joani found, were the people who didn't ask what they could do but just went ahead and did useful things, like taking phone calls and messages, running errands, and providing meals. Many of the neighbors in her close-knit community of Cheverly, Maryland, organized to bring nutritious meals each night for three weeks after Christian's death. "It was tough enough to force ourselves to eat, let alone to have to find our way around a grocery store." Other things that helped to ease the burden of daily life included some friends taking the girls to their neighborhood swimming pool, a friend of a friend who lent the family a beach house for an entire week, and yet other friends babysitting for a weekend so Gabe and Joani could get away to the Eastern Shore and bicycle together. In addition, Joani's sister in Albuquerque gave Joani her credit card number and said to call any time she needed to talk—a true lifesaver one night at 2 am when Joani was feeling suicidal. Joani's mother also allowed her to call collect any time she needed to talk in addition to paying for Joani to meet with a pastoral counselor for more than a year after Christian's death.

The Dos and Don'ts of Helping a SIDS Survivor

by Joani Nelson Horchler

What to do and say:

- Be there. Come to the house or call to say, "I care and I want to help."

- Listen! Even when talk about the baby or circumstances of death make you uncomfortable. This is not about your comfort. Not now. Take the attitude that the griever is the leader, and any topic of discussion he or she chooses is okay, for as long as he or she wants and even if the conversation seems repetitive or as if it is going nowhere.

- Remember that it is usually the simple, little things that mean so much.

- Freely recall the lost baby by his or her name. Although it may seem a little taboo to you, to a SIDS survivor it is a way of acknowledging the baby's existence and importance.

- If you have organizational skills, take the initiative and be an organizer. Put together a list of friends and relatives willing to bring meals to the bereaved family for several weeks after the death. Be sure to give the list to the grieving parents so they know what to expect, and keep in mind that the family needs nutritious food, not just cakes and pies.

- Answer the phone. Ask for an address book, and take charge of informing those who still have not heard the tragic news.

- Be available to run errands, clean the house, babysit, write an obituary for the newspaper (example on page 166) and call it in, or anything else the parents may be too emotionally drained to do (or even remember that it needs doing).

- If you know them to be the kind of people who like personal touch, then give a hug, caress a hand, put an arm around their shoulders. Afraid they will fall apart in your arms? Perhaps they will, but what better place than in the strength of a friend? Again, try to follow the griever's lead, and adjust your physical contact to their level of comfort.

- Seek and write down the names of any SIDS or bereavement support groups available to the grievers. Photocopy them, and make them available to anyone who might need them.

- If the mother has been breastfeeding, offer to run to the store to get whatever she needs to ease the pain of stopping. Someone must first talk to her obstetrician/gynecologist to see whether medication or cold compresses are best.

- Assist the parents in planning the funeral. This may include finding a funeral home or church; helping select a singer, pianist, or guitarist; or many other tasks.

- Help set up a memorial to the child. When the obituary is called in to the newspaper, include in the last paragraph where donations can be sent.

- Investigate places the family can get away to after the funeral if they want. (Friends, relatives, and sometimes even kind strangers may be willing to lend them a beach house or cabin for a few days or weeks.)

- If you would like to give the survivors a gift (sometimes given instead of flowers, but by no means socially expected), consider a locket for the baby's picture, a special box in which to keep mementos of the baby, picture frames (especially for siblings), or framed poetry.

- Assist any family members in finding—or purchasing—appropriate clothes to wear to the funeral. (Lynette Charboneau, a long-time friend of mine who is also a busy lawyer, took time off work to buy the material for a black hat with a veil that would cover my face.)

- Consider the needs of any siblings. A toddler will be distraught that his or her mother and father are acting so strangely and seem so unavailable. A five-year-old might love a game of checkers, while a tender teen might need the same listening that his or her mom and dad needs. Think of both the practical needs (How long has it been since Jason ate anything?) and the emotional (Does Sarah need someone to cuddle with?).

- Feed or walk the poor dog! Grievers are likely to forget about the needs of their pets at such a tragic time.

- If the casket will not be open, the parents may want to have photos of their baby on it or near it. Bring over a collage photo frame and ask the parents if they would like you to help them select and arrange pictures of the baby in it.

- Consider how long you think it should take for a survivor to "get over it," and then forget it! There is no time limit, and grieving is tough work that takes much longer than most people expect. Give the survivor all the time he or she needs, and be prepared to wait months and even years for your friend to be anything like his or her "old self."

- Remember important days such as birthdays and the death anniversary. A call, visit, or card means a great deal to the survivors, who are wondering if anyone else still remembers.

- If you have a baby of similar age, be sensitive to the pain of the survivor. Assume your visits should be without your baby at first, and even as much as 6–12 months later, ask how the survivor feels about being around your little one.

- Do feel free to say any of these things:
  —"I'm sorry."
  —"I can't begin to imagine your pain."
  —"I feel so sad that you have to go through this."
  —"This must be extremely difficult for you."
  —"I want to do whatever I can to help you. What can I do?"
  —"Talk for as long as you want. I have plenty of time to listen."
  —"You were good parents." (Or say how wonderful the baby was.) Say anything you know to be true and good about the care they gave.

What not to do and say:

- Don't visit for too long unless you are close friends or doing something specific to help.

- Don't expect anything—from a cup of tea to your definition of "dignified" grieving.

- Don't be afraid of reminding the parents about the baby; they will never forget the baby and find it comforting to remember with someone.

- Don't be afraid to cry or even laugh. Both provide comfort in addition to giving the survivor permission to do the same.

- Don't expect them—and for goodness sakes do not admonish them—to "be strong." If there is ever a time to allow oneself to be weak and needy, it is after a SIDS loss. Survivors need to be able to break down; and as hard as it is to witness, they need to suffer through the pain to move through the grieving process.

- Taking initiative is encouraged, but do not pack, move, or even handle the baby's things unless asked to by both parents.

- If at first your offers to help or attempts at comforting are rejected by a survivor, don't take it personally. The survivor won't even be likely to remember the incident in the future, and neither should you. Give them a few days, or even weeks, and try again.

- Don't wait until you know the perfect thing to say—there are no perfect or magic words. Just go, say what is in your heart, or be silent and cry.

- If you have lent the parents baby items or clothes, don't ask for them back unless it's absolutely necessary, and even then try to wait until they are offered. The survivors may not be ready to sort through baby things for some time, and feeling pushed to do this before they are ready can cause a tremendous strain.

- Don't blame anyone for the death—not the doctors or the babysitter or anyone. In a survivor's mind, the possibility of blame opens the window to all of their personal self-doubts. If someone is to blame, it could be them. What they need to hear repeatedly is that the only culprit was a mysterious killer called SIDS.

■ Don't impose your religious views on them. Now is not the time to sermonize or spiritualize. And whatever else, NEVER call the loss "God's will" (even if that is your true opinion).

■ Don't give pat answers. There is no way to wrap up a baby's death philosophically in a neat and tidy package. Pat answers are most often used by the ignorant, as opposed to the ill-meaning, but that is no excuse. The following are pat answers and what you don't want to say. (While these may seem obvious, all of them have actually been heard by a SIDS survivor.)

—"You'll be a better person because of this."

—"Calm seas do not a sailor make."

—"I understand."

—"It was all for the best."

—"It will all work out for the best."

—"You're young. You can have other babies."

—"At least you have other children."

—"It's good the baby wasn't older. You'd miss him more."

—"You should feel..."

—"Now you'll have an angel in heaven."

—"It was meant to be."

—"You're fortunate that you didn't lose your whole family."

—"Some people have it much worse than you. Just look at all the starving kids in..."

—"Maybe your baby would have been on drugs as a teenager, so it's better that he and you avoided all that."

—"Your baby is in a better place now."

—"I know exactly how you feel. My dog died last year."

—"You have to forget about this, put it behind you, and get on with your life."

—"God picked you for this because He knew you were strong enough to take it." (Then, God, make me weak!)

—"I don't know how you can stand this. Why, if my child died, I'd die, too." (Implies you love your child more than the SIDS survivor loved hers. Also suggests suicide.)

—"God must have really loved you to have chosen you for this special burden." (Grand Prize Jerk's Award #1)

—"Well, that was a waste of nine months." (Grand Prize Jerk's Award #2)

—"At least you don't have to pay for his college education." (Grand Prize Jerk's Award #3)

A Friend's Memory of William Kendal Herrera

by Renee Scolaro

In November 1989, I sat in the restaurant where I work, enjoying lunch and talking to friends. I looked up and saw my friend and employer, Bill, walking briskly out of the restaurant. Someone asked him where he was going. "The baby's sick," he said and disappeared out the door. We returned to our lunch, thinking nothing was unusual about a baby getting sick.

A few hours later, I realized Bill had not come back. I soon learned that Bill's and Deneena's beautiful son, Kendal, had died that afternoon. No one knew why yet.

I thought back to a few days before, when Bill had brought Kendal to the restaurant so he could do paperwork in the office. Bill had put Kendal in a high chair pushed up to the desk, where he could play with some toys. I had walked up to the office door, which was open, to say hi and had "oohed" and "ahhed" as usual at Kendal's big round eyes, looking up at me beneath unusually long lashes. He was smiling and laughing as he played. And that was the last time I saw him.

The night he died, I went to an unrelated church service. The congregation was singing songs about the power of God. I remember thinking, "God, why don't you prove how powerful you are and bring Kendal back to life, like you did some people in the Bible?" But I knew such a prayer would go unanswered. I ran out of the church in tears.

It has been nearly three years since Kendal died. I'm much closer to Bill and Deneena now, but it's only been in the past few months that I've spoken to Deneena about Kendal. I've listened to her talk, and I've asked her questions, and we've both cried.

Bill and Deneena have a second child now, a beautiful ten-month-old girl named Devon. Three or four days a week, I take care of her. As she plays and learns to crawl and talk, I look up to see the walls adorned with pictures of her big brother. She never got to meet him, but there are people who loved Kendal who will tell her all about him.

William Kendal Herrera died of Sudden Infant Death Syndrome. The night of his death was the first time his parents had heard of this mysterious killer. I've said to Deneena that reading the articles and seeing what she and Bill have gone through have made me afraid to have my own children. Deneena said to me, "There are risks in life, Renee. Don't let fear rob you of joy. The seven months we had with Kendal were the happiest of our lives."

Letter from a Friend
by Cheryl Lambson

Dear Margaret & Lee,

Words don't come easy for me at this time, as I try to express my sincere and deep sympathy. I am trying very, very hard to understand why such things happen.

Please know that you and your family are constantly in my prayers and thoughts. If you need me for anything, I am at your disposal.

Although Michael was here a very short time, remember the good, good times you had and shared with him. Cherish those memories. Rejoice in the fact that for a time he was on this earth, and that while here he was truly loved.

I believe that Michael has gone to a safer and better place, and that his spirit will live on forever. I also believe that he is in the hands of God now and that he will be all right.

Take care, my friends, and I will be in contact with you as we all try to overcome this loss. Although I only knew him for a while, I loved him too!

Your friend,
Cheryl

Untitled
by Oscar Wilde

If a friend of mine gave a feast,
and did not invite me to it, I should not mind a bit,
But if a friend of mine had a sorrow and refused to allow me
to share it, I should feel it most bitterly.
If he shut the doors of the house of mourning against me,
I would move back again and again and beg to be admitted,
so that I might share in what I was entitled to share.

If he thought me unworthy, unfit to weep with him, I should
feel it as the most poignant humiliation, as the most terrible
mode by which disgrace could be inflicted on me.
He who can look on the loveliness of the world and share
its sorrow, and realize something of the wonder of both, is in
immediate contact with divine things, and has got as near
to God's secret as anyone can get.

A Comforting Note from Friends in England
by Philip, Diana, and Patrick Beddows

Dear Joani and Gabe,

We were all devastated to hear news of Christian and send you our
deepest condolences and love, particularly as we have always been
very fond of you all and always looked towards you as "family."

We know that Christian has begun a new and everlasting life
and thank God for bringing him into our world so that he could
enter the new.

With all our love and best wishes,
Philip, Diana, and Patrick

Befriending the Grieving

by Robin Rice Morris

The first time I heard the name Joani Horchler, I was in the kitchen of a mutual friend. She was making a dinner to take to Joani and her family, all of whom were still reeling from the reality that Christian, Joani's fourth child and first son, had died in his sleep.

Though I did not know this fellow community member, my heart sank, and I quieted. Like anyone, I wanted details—how, when, how did her three daughters react, how did Joani react? I wanted some way to wrap my hands around this impossibility and understand it. My friend told me what she knew, and I remembered Joani from time to time as my life went on.

It was in our local park more than a year later that I first met Joani. I had forgotten her name but certainly not the incident. When she told me her story my heart sank again. So this is the woman who had her heart ripped out, I thought. This is the mother every mother dreads becoming.

Why did she tell me her story? Mostly because she still needed to talk, and someone—anyone—everyone to listen. Yes, more than a year later, she still needed to speculate and hypothesize and generally unload out loud. I could tell she was afraid I'd judge her because she often seemed to need to justify her actions. I let her know that I trusted her judgment as a mother, and that if anything could have been done, she would have gone to the ends of the earth to do it. She was like a lost soul in the desert, finding just enough water to go on another day.

Joani later told me that she shared her story with me because I seemed comfortable hearing it. That unlike others she had encountered, I didn't feel the need to rush her, or tell her how to fix her pain, or change the subject. After 45 minutes I could tell she was torn between feeling guilty for monopolizing the conversation and feeling relieved to have gotten to tell her story yet another time.

Since becoming a partner on this book (really, her book, and her labor of love for Christian's memory), I have gotten to know Joani much better. Still, almost three years since Christian's death and after another daughter was born, Joani needs to talk. We talk about the dreams she had for her son that now will never be. We talk about how she thinks about Christian every day. We talk about how she may be a better person for all of this, but she'd happily be her "old rotten self" for one more look at Christian alive. And we talk a lot about me now, too.

I am not a trained psychologist, but I have learned a few key things to keep in mind when being a friend to the grieving. 1) Listen, over and over. 2) It's more important to be "sad with" than "strong for." 3) Eliminate the words "you ought" and "you should" (as well as "I ought" and "I should") from your vocabulary. 4) Remember that you don't have to identify to be understanding. And 5) above all, use the baby's name often.

They say that a crisis will show you who your friends are. I also believe it will show you who you want your friends to be, and that any investment in a grieving friend pays off many times over.

Just Say, "I'm Sorry"
by Gail Fasolo

You don't know how I feel—please don't tell me that you do.
There's just one way to know—have you lost a child too?
"You'll have another child"—must I hear this each day?
Can I get another mother, too, if mine should pass away?

Don't say it was "God's will"—that's not the God I know.
Would God on purpose break my heart, then watch as my tears flow?
"You have an angel in heaven—a precious child above."
But, tell me, to whom here on earth shall I give this love?

"Aren't you better yet?" Is that what I heard you say?
No! A part of my heart aches—I'll always feel some pain.
You think that silence is kind, but it hurts me even more.
I want to talk about my child who has gone through death's door.

Don't say these things to me, although you do mean well.
They do not take my pain away; I must go through the hell.
I will get better slow but sure—and it helps to have you near,
But a simple "I'm sorry you lost your child" is all I need to hear.

Chapter 10

Planning a Funeral and the Role of the Clergy

After every SIDS death, there are arrangements for services and either burial or cremation to be made. Many people who read this book will have such arrangements still ahead of them. Others, however, will be long past them. This time is a blur for almost all survivors, but we hope there will be an overall feeling of peacefulness and comfort to accompany what memories you do have.

Unfortunately, some people take advantage of the survivor's "blur." He or she may later have feelings that range from an unidentified ambivalence to outright anger. The first part of this chapter, which includes two transcripts from uplifting funeral services, can help show what treatment a survivor should have received and thus help a survivor sift through the negative feelings of his or her own experience. The latter part of this chapter features two articles on how to plan a child's funeral and how to avoid potential pitfalls in dealing with funeral homes.

Within a few days, and sometimes a few hours, most SIDS survivors will have some type of contact with a member of the clergy. If a family is not already connected with someone, often the funeral home director will make a suggestion from the contacts he or she has on file. Whatever the circumstances, the good minister will meet the survivors wherever they are on their spiritual journey, even if, up to that point, there has not been one.

Of course, not all ministers graduated at the top of their classes. According to Rev. Byron Brought, who worked with SIDS parents Amy and Gary Maynard after the death of their baby, "Unfortunately, there are as many quacks in the ministry as in any other profession." It should not happen, but there are times when bad ministers do little more than add insult to injury. Tragically, many SIDS survivors have experienced eulogies that rarely—if ever—mentioned their lost baby, that were too theological to understand, or that screamed of hellfire and damnation. When this happens, the event forever taints the survivors' memories, when it could have—and should have—offered comfort and reassurance.

Rev. Brought offers a few guidelines he follows when addressing a tragic loss such as SIDS. Most importantly, he avoids saying anything that would imply the death was "God's will." He calls it a tragedy, stressing that sad things happen: "It would be nice if it all fit into a neat pattern, with the bad things happening to just bad people and good things to good people, but it does not work that way." Rev. Brought also stresses that any child is a gift from God, and not our own. "We let go *not* into nothingness, but back into the hands of God."

In cases where Rev. Brought does not know the family, he calls ahead of any services he will perform to meet them and learn specifics about the child. Regardless of whether the family members are professed believers, he tries to "lift the hope of the gospel as powerfully as I can." After all, this is what he believes, and offering this message is precisely his life's work. "But not in a judgmental way at all. I stress the mercy and grace of God." In addition, Rev. Brought looks to see that the family is attending to their grieving, including helping them to be angry in a "proper, not destructive, way." He also will make self-help referrals, such as to survivors groups or organizations. Unless it is expressly desired, he will not make a follow-up call in person after the services of those he did not previously know.

A Christian Celebration of Christian

by Father John J. Hurley, Jr.

We come here this morning asking, "Why did this happen?" Why did God allow wonderful, sweet Christian Gabriel Horchler to die of SIDS, the Sudden Infant Death Syndrome? How could God allow this to happen? I cannot answer. I do not know. But, like you all, we have come together today to struggle to find the answer.

And, as we consider this short but very rich and eventful life, we see God's plan. His divine Providence unfolds over nearly a year. Yes, we recall that it was nearly a year since Christian was first conceived in his mother's womb, just as the psalm we heard today reminds us.

Then, two months ago, Christian came into the world. He saw the end of Lent and the joyful celebration of Easter. And, he lived through it all, right up to the end on Ascension Thursday, when he followed in the wake of Christ into heaven.

At the beginning of the Book of Acts, St. Luke describes Christ's ascension for us. The two angels (one of whom was probably the same Gabriel who announced Christ's coming and is also the middle name of Christian) were there addressing the disciples and saying, "Why are you standing here looking? Jesus, who has been taken from you into heaven…will come back in the same way as you see him go there."

And, just afterwards, Luke describes the selection of the disciple to replace Judas, whose feast we celebrate today. The disciples did not stop their lives, but saw they had to carry on, just as baby Christian's brave family has done in the past several days.

His youngest sister Julianna is happy that her baby brother is flying around in heaven now. Oh, that we could share in the faith of the little children, as we are called to. Instead, as we grow older, this childlike but so profound faith slips away.

Christian's mom and dad are so comforted that all three of the other children (Ilona, Gabrielle, and Julianna) were so kind and loving to their baby brother. They were never jealous of him, and they always helped their mother with him. Christian's big sister, Ilona, wrote a lovely letter to her brother, which is in his casket. She shares her mother's gift for lovely writing. Ilona wrote: "I wish you did not have to die, but you are probably having a good time up in heaven." She added, "I know you would help us all get into heaven by saying a good word for us." She enjoyed being with her brother even more than going on a school field trip!

Then, of course, sister Gabrielle had a very special relationship with Christian. They shared the same names, in reverse. His name was Christian Gabriel, and her name is Gabrielle Christine. She was always good to her baby brother. She even gave Christian a lovely soft cloth book to keep with him in his coffin: *Pat-A-Cake*. Gabrielle and the other children also gave Christian a stuffed bear to keep in his coffin.

All the family are going to write a little bit in a journal every day to Christian. They are writing in the same book that several of you have already signed your names in. Christian's family is going to keep him a part of their everyday life. They are counting on him to be our guardian angel. This is how it should be, of course. Just as Christ is with us always, so are those close and dear, like Christian. It is part of the belief we profess in the communion of saints.

Joani knows this. She had a brother who died when he was 28. Joani always felt that Brad's spirit was looking out for her from above. After he died, Joani was afraid, but then Brad's spirit came to her in the night and gave her a feeling of peace and tranquillity. I know that Christian will bestow the same sense of peace upon his family.

Christian had a short but full and wonderful life on earth. His father loved him very much. One of Gabe's fondest memories was the time he took Christian to the Library of Congress, where Gabe works, and showed him off in his little tuxedo. Christian was also very special to his two loving grandmothers, who enjoyed him very much as they cared for him.

But Christian was one who was also very important to other friends and relatives, and also in the parish. Too bad everyone doesn't get to church as regularly as he did, sitting over there, even if he might get in a bit late. His was a life that many could emulate. The British poet Cecil Alexander once wrote: "Christian children all must be/Mild, obedient, good as He." Christian was every bit that type of child, following the example of Jesus.

So, we are here today to honor a special person, one who accomplished so much during his life on earth. There are sad thoughts here. But we need to remember that Jesus is with us, the Lord Who loves us is merciful, and suffered Himself, and knows what sorrow is like.

God loves us. He is here with us, today. True peace we can only hope to find one day in heaven, like Christian we trust already has. Yet, even here on earth, in our pain and suffering, we can receive from the Lord a little taste of that peace which the world cannot give. God loves us very much and is with us today in our sorrow.

William David Waugh

by Fern Stanley

We have gathered here today to commit to the earth the physical body of William David Waugh, born January 20, 1992, died August 31, 1992. As Sean O'Casey wrote, "A few brief moments in the garden of life, going where the primroses go, and then the night came, and we lost him."

The sorrow and grief felt by all those who had the chance of knowing Baby William, as some of his little friends called him, is immense and unavoidable.

It has been said that only human beings grieve. That we are the only creatures who know that to love deeply is to open ourselves to the pain we must feel when those we love are lost to us. But the only way to avoid such pain in life is to avoid the love, and love is that which makes the life worth living.

Regardless of circumstances, we are never prepared for death, nor can we be. We are always shocked when it comes. But, in a case such as this, where life vanished so suddenly from one so young, the shock and the attendant pain and grief seem unsurmountable. Out of anguish, we inevitably question, "Why? Why death? Why now?" And there are no answers that satisfy the questions. No answers that can bridge the irreparable loss.

We can only meet such questions with our grief, that uncontrived mixture of sadness, anger, denial, loss, pain, and so many other emotions, knowing that the heart that accepts and fully experiences such grief is the heart that is open. And the open heart never grows bitter, or if it does, it cannot remain so. In time, there will come a gentleness, a returning quietness, a restoring stillness.

To aid in this process, I've always encouraged the bereaved not only to grieve the death of their loved ones but also to celebrate their lives. I first thought that this would not be possible with William's loss because of the brevity of his time here. As if the sturdiness of the tree that lives a hundred years somehow could outweigh the fragile and precious beauty of the flower that lives only a day. I was wrong.

I realized just how wrong I was when talking with Steve and Shawna. Clearly, this life that they were privileged to cherish for these months has shaped and molded their own lives in ways not yet even recognized. They learned to set their priorities according to the needs of another. They dreamed dreams of William's becoming, and the growth they would all enjoy, nurtured by the warm and supportive family they were in the process of building. Though the pain they feel at his loss will never completely vanish, its harshness will be softened in time. And the joy they shared in their time with him will remain a part of their lives forever. He turned their lives upside down, caused them sleepless nights and some stressful days. During Shawna's recovery from surgery, Steve shared more of the primary care-giving than many fathers have the opportunity to do.

But this beautiful boy, William, was also their delight—friendly, playful, smiling, happy to be with people, never saw a stranger. It seemed to them that a hug and a smile from Baby William made the whole world worthwhile, no matter what else was going wrong.

They had planned to teach him as he grew, but found that already he was teaching them about life. One of the more important lessons they felt they were learning from him had to do with living in the moment. Sure, William cried when he was hungry or took a fall, but as soon as real needs were met, or the first shock of pain had passed, he went wholeheartedly into whatever came next, never looking back, living in the moment.

This lesson will be very hard to put into effect after such a loss, not only for Steve and Shawna, but for all those who loved William. He was, after all, grandson, nephew, cousin, and friend, as well as beloved son. And perhaps, for a time, a part of living in the moment should be to remember William, and to feel at the greatest depths the pain of his loss. For this is a part of the work of grief. To facilitate grief's work, there must be tears, many tears, to wash away pain and sorrow. And there must be talk, lots of talk that brings forth healing memories.

The birth announcement that went out last January included this piece called "Ode to Baby Waugh" by Steve and Shawna. They wanted it read in this service.

Happiness for me is loving
and sharing daily joys
With the special kind of closeness
between a father and his baby boy.
Learning from each other—
we will pamper you
And watch as you discover
and share the world with you.
Happiness for me, is loving
and sharing daily joys
With the special kind of closeness
between a mother and her baby boy.
Steve and I are lovers,
best friends, and partners, too—
And more and more each day;
joy for us is sharing this
special time with you.

For a moment of silence now, may we hold tenderly in our minds and hearts Baby William David Waugh.

PRAYER: Spirit of Life, Source of Love, which is everlasting and before which our generations pass as shadows, we have come together and have remembered and honored this much-beloved child.

We mourn his loss and yet celebrate his life. We express sorrow and yet affirm the power of love. Even in the midst of grief, may each be granted the knowledge that a steadfast heart and a quiet mind will return in time, and that each will once more be able to receive the blessings of peace—the peace that passes all understanding, that peace which the world can neither give nor take away.

May this peace be with us and abide with us.

A Funeral Director's Personal Experience with SIDS
by Sondra L. Held, MSW

As director of bereavement for the A. W. Bennett Funeral Home in Richmond, Virginia, I work daily with family members struggling to survive the death of a loved one. Mine is a profession that is becoming more common as society in general and the funeral industry in particular realize that people need help to cope and move forward.

Unfortunately, I know of the need for my profession from personal experience. Our son, Douglas E. Held, was a corporal in the United States Marine Corps stationed with the peacekeeping force in Beirut, Lebanon. He was killed that fateful Sunday when a Shiite Muslim drove a Mercedes truck loaded with explosives under the building that housed him and other Marines. Douglas, who was only 21, had been scheduled to come home in only three weeks. His wife, who was pregnant when he died, delivered a bouncing baby boy four months later. Her beautiful baby boy—my grandson—died of SIDS at 15 weeks.

Thus, I have "been there." I have had the typical experiences of not feeling normal; of wondering what is wrong with me; of feeling out of control; of feeling unable to cope with what used to be daily routine; of being unable to maintain existing relationships. I have asked myself the questions that bereaved people most often ask: "Why? Why my son? Why my grandchild?" I felt that I must have done something horrible to make God so angry with me that He took away one of our sons. God and I had some very one-sided conversations because His will was not mine. I yelled, I cursed, and I learned that God has very wide shoulders.

In the beginning, a cloak of shock enables us to get through the funeral. This is a time when funeral homes should help parents by giving them gentle suggestions on how to make this almost unbearable time more manageable and more meaningful. At Bennett, we advise parents to consider obtaining a heart or charm that breaks apart and can be worn by both the baby and the parent. If parents would rather have a religious symbol, they might want to buy doubles of a star of David or of a cross. (These may be purchased from jewelry stores, as I believe it is a conflict of interest for funeral homes to sell them.) If parents want to help dress their babies, we encourage that. Parents can write notes or draw pictures and put them in the casket along with a favorite toy or doll. Funeral homes should provide rocking chairs so that parents can spend time holding and rocking their babies. One mother whose baby's service we held did not want to see her daughter in a casket. Thus, we invited her to place her daughter in her own baby carriage for the visitation and service. A bassinet or cradle are other alternatives to consider.

Funeral homes can aid in the long healing process. At Bennett, we host a holiday season remembrance service with a priest and a rabbi in attendance. We hang bronze ornaments (shaped in angels for the babies who are remembered) on a tree. Afterward, we have a catered fellowship session.

On anniversaries—your own day of need—it often helps to do something for someone else. On the first anniversary of my son's death, I organized a friend's retirement party. I was so busy with the party that it made the day more tolerable for me. On your child's birthday anniversary, you might want to arrange a party for some needy children and bring in a clown. You might want to donate things to a facility for the mentally handicapped or buy a gift for someone in your baby's name. Lighting candles in your home on special days is a nice way to remember your baby.

You must seek out people who have also lost a child. The Compassionate Friends, based in Oakbrook, Illinois, with chapters nationwide, is wonderful. Many cities now have groups within Compassionate Friends that offer assistance to parents whose children have died of SIDS. Your funeral home may have a counselor with whom you can meet. We do not walk this way alone, and, when life is darkest, help is just a phone call away. Please take advantage of whatever is available to you, and God bless you.

Sondra Held facilitates a Richmond-area SIDS support group and the Mechanicsville, Virginia, chapter of Compassionate Friends.

Planning a Special Funeral

by Joani Nelson Horchler

Looking back, many of us who went through those bone-numbing first few weeks of shock can hardly imagine how we made it through the funeral at all. We were walking ghosts, merely shadows of ourselves. It was hard to decide what to wear or eat, let alone to plan a special funeral.

That's why it's so important that funeral directors have brochures available that can help. When we were planning our son's funeral, I wish we'd had an excellent pamphlet called "Have You Considered?... Planning Your Child's Service." [1] This pamphlet, prepared by the SIDS Foundation of Washington, offers dozens of gentle suggestions for planning a child's funeral. (For information on how to obtain copies, see bibliography.)

When my husband and I went to the funeral home for the first time to pick out an infant casket, we were appalled by the fact that only two were available, both in fiberglass. Gabe was shattered that he did not have time to build his son a nice, simple wooden casket and that the funeral home did not have one. In fact, some families have made their own caskets. Jennifer Wilkinson tells how a woodworking friend designed a casket, which he and her daughter's godfather made together.

We instinctively put notes to our baby and mementos—a rosary and special toys and books—in the casket, but nowhere was it suggested that we do so. We also used our own van rather than a hearse to transport the casket. However, we did not receive any information from the funeral home on these and other options available for making a child's service special. In fact, they did not offer even simple help, such as how to place a funeral notice in the newspaper. They also did not give us any information about SIDS, even though we expressed confusion about it. (When we came later to view our son's body, we found an informational brochure in the hallway.)

Just a few of the numerous tips suggested in "Have You Considered?" are

- bathing and dressing your child and wrapping him in a blanket
- remembering that even if you said you didn't want to see your child you can change your mind even up to the grave site
- having a collage of pictures or using balloons and stuffed animals instead of flowers around the casket
- having someone your other children feel comfortable with available during the service in case they choose to or need to leave
- requesting a lock of hair
- considering cremation as an option

Several parents interviewed for this book who have had their babies cremated said they are now comforted by having the ashes with them in their homes. "I didn't want to put him in the cold, hard ground with strangers all around him," says Bernadette Sanders-Dzidzienyo of her son Cameron, who died on Christmas 1993. "It comforts me to have his urn here in our home and to be able to sit next to it and touch it." Another thing you may want to do is to take photographs of your baby in the hospital or in her casket. There is nothing strange or morbid about desiring to do this. Some SIDS parents say they took pictures of their babies after they died because they had so few photos of their babies alive.

Eulogy for Margaret Hood Schuth: A Gift from Her Mother

by Kee Schuth Marshall

I do not know whether I can finish this, but I want this service to be as personal as possible for Margaret.

Maybe because we are so close to the Christmas season, I have thought so much about Margaret and Baby Jesus. One of my favorite Christmas stories is *Amahl and the Night Visitors* [2], an operetta by Gian-Carlo Menotti. It is a wonderful story with beautiful words and music.

My favorite song is one where the three kings—who are on their journey to visit Baby Jesus in Bethlehem—stop at a poor widow's home to rest. Her crippled son has left the house, and the mother is alone with the three kings. She stares at their gifts and gold and asks about them.

The kings say the gifts are for the Child.

Mother: The child? Which child?
          But perhaps I know him.
          What does he look like?

The kings: We don't know, but the star
          will guide us to Him.

          Have you seen a Child the color of wheat,
              the color of dawn?
          His eyes are mild
          His hands are those of a king as King He was born.

          The Child we seek holds the seas
              and the winds on His palm.

          The Child we seek has the moon
              and the stars at His feet.

          Before Him the eagle is gentle,
              the lion is meek.

          Choirs of angels hover over His roof
              and sing Him to sleep.
          He's warmed by breath
          He's fed by Mother who is both Virgin and Queen.

Throughout the song the Mother says she knows such a child:

Mother: The child I know on his palm holds my heart.
          The child I know at his feet has my life.
          He's my child, my son, my darling, my own.

One of my most precious thoughts is of the night before Margaret died. I was giving her a bottle during which I felt her eyes looking at me, and I looked down. She was staring at me, and when she saw me look at her she stopped drinking and just beamed at me. She made me smile, and my smile made her smile even bigger. We egged each other on, and I felt like we were just giggling. And that is one of my last, most precious memories of her.

Finally, I'd just like to say that Sam absolutely adores Margaret and was always giving her a kiss and a hug. He does not understand the finality of death—he talks about her usually as if she is still here with us. He is right, you know. We will always have her love and memories, which we would not trade for anything. Her brief little life was not in vain—it has touched us all, and we hope that we will be better persons for it. She has gone to God as her perfect little self.

And as Sam put it, "Margaret's not afraid. God will take care of her." And He will.

Obituary of Christian Horchler

by Josette Shiner

Christian Gabriel Horchler, two months old, died May 9 of Sudden Infant Death Syndrome at his home in Cheverly. His short life was marked by the great joy he brought to those around him.

Christian was born March 8 to Gabriel Francis Horchler, a manager at the Library of Congress, and Joani Nelson Horchler, a freelance writer and contributing editor of *Industry Week* magazine. "He was like a gift from heaven and will always be with us in spirit," his mother said yesterday. "His sisters and I will write a note to him in a journal every day."

In addition to his parents, Christian is survived by three sisters, Ilona, Gabrielle, and Julianna; his paternal grandmother, Dora Nagy Horchler of Philadelphia; and his maternal grandmother, Doris Guhin Nelson of Aberdeen, South Dakota.

Services will be held at 9 am today at St. Ambrose Church in Cheverly. Burial will follow in Philadelphia.

The family suggests that expressions of sympathy be in the form of contributions to the SIDS Information and Counseling Program in

Baltimore or the Rogers Heights Elementary School French Immersion Program in Bladensburg.

Josette Shiner is managing editor of The Washington Times *and a friend and neighbor of the Horchler family. Her obituary of Christian provides good guidelines to anyone wishing to write an obituary.*

The Funeral Director and Home
An Interview with Melonie Wilhelm Wagner
by Robin Rice Morris

At just the time when you will make one of the biggest "purchases" in your life—a SIDS funeral and all that accompanies it—you are often the least able to think straight, pay attention, or even care. More than a few people have been "taken" in any number of ways because of this and have found that there is little they could do about it. Melonie Wagner explains the process and how to avoid some potential pitfalls.

Melonie is more than aware of the public's opinion of funeral directors. As a funeral director and owner of a small but dignified funeral home, Melonie makes it her business to break out of that stereotype. In fact, her business card reads: "Now, a funeral service that takes exception to the belief that spending more means you care more."

Melonie has handled the funerals of many babies and children, yet it is still a small percentage of her experience. "You expect someone in their 80s or 90s to die," she explains. "But babies? That's backwards. It's really tough to do those services." For that reason, she doesn't even charge for her services if the death is that of a child. "Whatever it costs me out of pocket is what it costs the family, and that's all," she says.

Once Melonie is contacted, she is available 24 hours a day. She arranges for the baby to be brought to the funeral home when the medical examiner is finished with an autopsy. She makes an appointment to meet with the family in their home or church or in her office. During this appointment, a family chooses either a burial or cremation and picks a casket or urn. They select someone to conduct the funeral or, in the case that they have no such contacts, Melonie will provide names she knows to be reputable. Someone must then provide her with detailed historical information on the baby and his family for the official death certificate. She will provide clerical assistance in the completion of various forms associated with a funeral and securing the death certificate and disposition permit.

After the arrangements are made, the family decides if they want to see the baby again. Many families have already held their baby after death at home or at the hospital. If they do not wish to see the baby, it is not required. If they do, embalming and any cosmetic work required take about an hour. Then the family is given all the time they wish with their baby. At this time, children and other family members should be welcomed by the funeral director—although Melonie admits that for some directors children are seen as a threat to the furniture more than a help to the grieving process.

There is little that is not "allowed" in any funeral home except that which is against a funeral director's personal or business policy. Melonie encourages parents and other family members to hold the baby and to place items of sentimental value in the casket to stay with the baby. "Letters," Melonie says, "seem to especially comfort survivors." For the most part, funerals and burial can wait until family members who will be traveling great distances have arrived. The only constraint might be the time slots available from the cemetery. The funeral director will make all of those arrangements on a family's behalf.

Although she did not want to point a finger at anyone in particular, Melonie offers several suggestions so that families are not taken advantage of in this most foggy and dazed time of their lives. Along with these suggestions, she recommends the use of a more distant relative or another less recent SIDS survivor to act as a protector when decisions are made. "But beware," she says, "that some funeral directors do not like such third parties. Whether it be that they slow down the process by asking so many questions or simply make it more difficult for him or her to take advantage of his grieving client is hard to say."

Melonie believes that it is helpful to be aware ahead of time of average costs for funeral services in general and services in your area in particular. These days, the smaller Mom-and-Pop organizations tend to be about 20–25% less expensive than the franchises that are on the New York Stock Exchange. They also provide better service, Melonie believes. Items and services you may elect or will be required to purchase include a casket or urn, outer burial containers, embalming and cosmetic work if desired, the viewing and funeral ceremony, transportation (such as a hearse or limousine for family members), service folders or prayer cards, acknowledgment cards, a shipping container, graveside services, forwarding of remains, receiving of remains, direct cremation, or immediate burial.

Whereas a recent survivor is in no shape to be "shopping" for services, a friend might be, and funeral directors are required to give their prices over the phone. (Few funeral homes offer free services for children as Melonie does, but many do cut their adult prices in half, so be sure to ask for their services in regard to a baby.)

Charges that may be incurred by the funeral home on your behalf may include the cemetery or crematory, obituary notices, certified copies, clergy, church, musicians or singers, cemetery property, flowers, and hairdressers. But beware! Although considered absolutely unethical by Melonie but allowed by the Federal Trade Commission, funeral directors can charge a "commission" on these second-hand services in whatever amount they like (usually 10–20%). They must state that they are doing this in writing, but they do not have to state the percentage they charge unless asked.

Unfortunately, though it indicates human life at its shabbiest, it is not uncommon for a lesser quality product—such as a casket or urn—to be substituted for the one you chose and paid for. In your grief, how will you be aware, let alone certain, of such an event, should you ever even stop to think about it? If you are concerned, plan to take a few pictures of those items purchased so that later on, when you have the strength and if you have the desire, you can pursue justice. Again, an advocate who is less emotional at this time is a help.

Financing your costs is possible through some funeral homes, but the paperwork involved in its application is quite lengthy and burdensome. Some funeral homes on the "better side of the tracks" almost always wait for their payment until after the fact, whereas those on the "other side" usually feel that they must demand payment in advance if they are ever to see a penny of it. Sometimes, a discount of 10% is offered for those who pay up front.

Finally, feel free to ask for your records from the funeral home at a later date. Melonie's home keeps a record of flower cards for the survivors for a full year. Also on record indefinitely is your statement of services and the information that was provided for the death certificate.

Chapter 11

Learning To Live Again

In the early days of mourning, the thought of once again living a life of vitality and fulfillment is impossible. The pain, crashing again and again like steady ocean waves, seems too powerful ever to ease, let alone stop entirely. Joani remembers a time soon after Christian's death when she read that the process of grieving for a child lasted 18 months to 3 years. She was relieved, thinking that if she could only survive three years, she would not be sad any more.

Since then, Joani has learned—as all long-time survivors do—that there is no guaranteed time line on grieving and that its emotional impact lasts far longer than our society recognizes. Moreover, when grief does finally loosen its grip on a survivor, it is not some jarring halt at a magic moment. Instead, it is an ever-lessening strain on your energies, your attention span, and your capacity to cope. You will always grieve to some extent for your lost child. You will always remember your baby and wish beyond wishes that you could smell her smell or hold his weight in your arms. But as time goes on, this wishing will no longer deplete you of the will to live your own life.

When are you ready to live again? There is no list of events or anniversaries to check off. In fact, you are likely to begin living again before you realize you are doing it. You may catch yourself laughing. You may pick up a book for recreational reading again. You may start playing lighter, happier music. When you do make these steps toward living again, you are likely to feel guilty at first. "What right have I," you may ask yourself, "to be happy when my child is dead?" And yet something inside feels as though you are being nudged in this positive direction. You may even have the sense that this nudge is from your child, or at least a feeling that your child approves of it.

Even so, those times are likely to be mixed with bouts of horrible grief for quite a while. When Joani began to emerge from the darkness and numbness of those first few months, she was surprised and dismayed that she still felt the sharp physical pains that had begun when Christian died. "I felt like a nail had been driven through my heart and that it had never been removed and was causing me to bleed inside. As I started to feel a little better over the first year, the bleeding stopped, but the wound felt raw and crusted over. Even three years later, I still feel that rawness. But the pain isn't so sharp, and I can enjoy many aspects of life."

There are many signposts that indicate that you are beginning to move forward. At this point in your grieving, you may not recognize any of them yet. Or, you may recognize a few. Be assured that eventually these and many more will occur on the road to recovery.

■ Once you thought you'd never be able to smile or laugh again when you thought of your baby. But, as you work through your grief, you very slowly begin to be grateful for even the very short amount of time that you had together. You begin to remember little things, such as the funny expressions on his face, and you find yourself smiling.

■ Your loss begins to feel more like one part of your life, and no longer the end of your world.

■ You find yourself facing some of your fears head-on. You can allow yourself to immerse yourself in your grief for a few minutes or an hour, without fearing that you'll lose your mind.

■ You may once again be able to bear to look at your baby's pictures, videos, gifts, and clothes. You can play music that reminds you of the baby. You realize that the only way *over* the depression of grief is *through* it, and you feel some small measure of courage to go through it.

■ You feel in touch with your baby's spirit, and the feeling serves to soothe you. Often one can feel the baby's spiritual presence in one's home, the home in which the baby died, or simply in one's soul.

■ Although there are no more answers than before, a sense of resolution in the battle of answering "Why?" comes.

■ Some people come to believe that their baby now belongs to God. Others believe that the baby's spirit is a kind of guardian angel to the baby's siblings or to the family as a whole. Still others believe that the baby's time on earth was meant to be, for reasons that will be given at some time in the future. Through all these beliefs, the baby has become part of something bigger than both his family and himself.

■ You find yourself selecting a handful of memories you do not want to forget, and you deliberately burn them into your heart and mind. Not wanting to forget is a sure sign that some part of you knows life will move on.

■ You can walk through the baby department of a store, see an outfit or toy like one your baby wore or played with, and not burst into tears. Rather, you feel a little tingle of happiness in remembering.

■ You can drive past the hospital trauma unit sign without that sharp stab of regret and litany of self-recriminations about not getting your baby there sooner.

■ You feel thankful, to God or the universe, for anything.

■ You find that you can give back to others again. This may be as a peer contact for newly bereaved SIDS parents, or simply returning a favor done for you in your early days of grieving.

These signposts may come few and far between, or lumped together like the first day it is noticeably spring. Some can take years, others only a few weeks. And the amount of time it took for certain signposts to come to another grieving survivor is no indication of when they will come to you. All we know is that those who do not abandon the grieving process have these and many other lovely signposts to look forward to.

"How Many Children Do You Have?"

by Joani Nelson Horchler

In learning to live again, you will venture out into work and social worlds. You are likely to find that these worlds feel divided into two groups: those who know about your loss and those who do not know. Both can be tiring. You may find yourself longing for people who do not know, who can let you forget your loss (but never your baby) for a moment or two. And yet, those who do not know can create the dread of that almost unbearable question, "How many children do you have?"

There is no right or wrong answer to this question. You will answer according to what makes you feel the most comfortable. Ruth Skopek's response is, "I'm a mother of five, raising four of my children." My usual response is "I have four daughters and also a son who died of SIDS."

Whether a parent includes the dead child in the count depends not on the parent's wish to forget the child, but more on the emotional investment he or she wants to make in the person with whom he or she is talking. If it is a casual question from a grocery store clerk, the parent of two living children and one dead child might say he or she has two children. However, if the question comes from a new co-worker who is likely to learn eventually about the lost baby anyway, the parent might answer three, with an explanation, in order to establish a firmer and more personal relationship with that person.

If your only child died, you grieve not only for your lost baby but for your lost role as parent. Are you still a mother or father? Of course you are. You always will be. But only you can decide how you want to answer the question, "Do you have children?" When interviewed, many SIDS parents say that they do answer yes in most cases (though they frequently answer no when the question is from someone they will likely never see again). You may find yourself tailoring your reply to the situation and your own inner needs at the time. Whatever your reply, know that for the time being the honest answer is the answer that makes you most comfortable. Eventually you will find an answer that makes you feel loyal to your baby, to your emotional needs, and to the person asking the question.

The Glass Half Full

by William C. Ermatinger

Are you familiar with the saying, "The optimist sees the glass half full, the pessimist sees the glass half empty"? I would like to use a variation of that imagery to illustrate one of the differences that exist between the time before we are healed from a SIDS loss and the time after healing takes place.

Let us represent our child's potential life as an eight-ounce glass, and place in the glass four ounces of water to represent the actual life the child lived. In our grief, we will appropriately focus on the top, empty part of the glass. This represents all that we have lost and all the potential our child had but now will never fulfill. We see only this emptiness in our lives.

Upon healing, we will focus on the bottom part of the glass, where the water that represents the life and purpose of our child is located. We will now be able to see the meaning of our child's life clearly.

While grieving, we are handed this half-empty glass. We want so much to cast it away. But our task is to hold the glass and, starting at the top, work our way down through the emptiness until we come to the healing water that is there. Then slowly, as we drink the water, we are comforted by all that our child was to us, to our family, and to the world as a whole.

And it is a magical glass, for in addition to being comforting, this water can never be fully consumed. It will always be there to refresh us as we continue on life's mysterious journey.

Going Out into the World Again
by Carla Hosford, LCSW-C

One of the many unfair things about a SIDS death is that dealing with it never becomes simple. Yet after the first weeks of constant, unremitting pain, there comes a point when parents can face the fact that there is life after SIDS. You could compare it to families who must rebuild their homes after a hurricane or flood. So parents must begin to rebuild their lives after their baby dies. It is this time of trying to create something solid from the destruction that constitutes the real work of grief.

Three common areas that parents have trouble with are re-entering the world, how long the grieving and healing process is taking, and the fear of forgetting their baby as they move back into the mainstream of life. There are no easy answers to the problems that arise in these areas, but I do have some suggestions to move toward your own personal answers.

Going out into the world again is a real challenge. Aside from the emotional pressure of having to enter a world that is not at all the one you wanted, parents must also face questions like, "What do I say to people who don't know the baby died?", "How can I go back to work with people who knew I was pregnant when I left?", or "What do I say if people get really upset when they find out?"

To begin with, I suggest that you say only what you are comfortable saying, and don't feel that you have to respond in the same way to everyone who asks. It sometimes helps to practice, or role play, a response before an anticipated and potentially awkward situation arises. As silly as this may sound, it can make people feel more comfortable, and more in control, if they have tested out different answers.

Many grieving parents feel guilty for "raining on someone else's parade." Others are surprised at how quickly some people change the subject when the topic turns to a death. At the same time, some people want to ask questions, and to offer help and support. And a few want to know each and every detail of the experience. What is most important for you to understand is that you are not responsible for other people's reactions. Also know that telling your story is sending an important nonverbal message: You have been through a tragedy, but you are surviving.

As far as moving forward goes, parents often report that, some weeks after the baby's death, people begin expecting them to "get over it." The fact is that we live in a society that values speed. We expect things to happen quickly, and we don't always have patience when they don't. SIDS destroys your life in a split second, yet recovering from it takes a very long time. It strikes with the immediacy and intensity of a bomb, yet it is survived inch by painful, crawling inch. Unfortunately, there is no way of making the pain go away quickly. We can switch channels on a remote in seconds and create a meal within minutes in a microwave oven, but human emotions cannot be rushed.

People who have not been through major loss or trauma may not know this. They may apply some timetable of their own to your feelings of recovery. They want you "back to your old self" and for you to "put it behind you." (In fact, you will never be your old self, but a new—and maybe better—self.) You will not ever forget. Nor will you be able to put it behind you without ever looking back, but you will be able to move on while remembering. Grief is individual, and healing takes time. It may feel as if others are giving you a below-average grade in grieving, but be assured that people move at their own pace.

To the extent that you can, try to be kind to yourself. You cannot take away other people's discomfort over the fact that you are still sad six months after the death. That is truly their problem. You need only be sure you have the help and support you need to cope with the sadness.

Those who are fearful of forgetting their baby should read these words from Larry Woiwode's short story, "Firstborn," which appeared in the *New Yorker* of Nov. 28, 1985 [1].

> *And it wasn't until after they had not only a second child but also a third and a fourth (that) he knew that this child had always been with him, at the edges of his mind and in his everyday thoughts, as much as any of their living children.*

This story tracks a father's emotional adjustment, over a period of years, to the stillbirth of his first child. I often think of it when a SIDS parent expresses a fear of "forgetting" the baby when the pain of grief becomes less intense. It is as if pain becomes so closely associated with the infant that we think we won't remember if we no longer hurt.

Events that are traumatic, that shape our lives and give direction to them, seem etched in our minds. Years after the event we can recall how people looked, what they said, and what they did. We remember what the baby looked and felt like. We remember our feelings—the depth of pain, the intensity of anger, and the sense of drowning in grief. As Woiwode indicates, your child will always occupy a little corner of your mind. That attachment never ends. Your child will always be with you, even without the raging hurt that seems so all-encompassing at the beginning.

How I Survived My Baby's Death

by Joani Nelson Horchler

Smiling in the womb! I couldn't believe my five-and-a-half-month-old unborn baby was grinning inside me. But the ultrasound technician snapped a clear photo of it.

That happy image sustained me through the next three-and-a-half months of my pregnancy, during which I learned to my dismay that I would be laid off from my business magazine editing job. Though the firm was downsizing, I felt hurt after 12 years in the same office.

But I still had giving birth to look forward to. And it would be fun to be home full-time for the first time with my three daughters, ages eight, six, and two, and the new baby. Now I would have a career baby!

Christian Gabriel Horchler, a robust nine-pounder, came roaring into the world on March 8, 1991. His father was thrilled to have a son "to help around the house." His sisters couldn't put him down and invited the world over to admire him. We made a special journey to my husband's office at the Library of Congress. In the cafeteria, where Christian nursed as we and our friends visited, my husband and I looked at each other and, without words, wondered how we'd deserved to be so blessed. Our complete joy was marred only occasionally over the next few weeks by a nagging suspicion that things were too perfect.

May 9 was an ordinary day, except for my husband leaving from his job for a weekend conference in a city two hours away. The morning was mellow, warmed by sunshine and smiles from Christian. But after school was hectic, keeping tabs on the baby while watching my three children and a neighbor boy. At about 6:30 or 7 pm, I took Christian upstairs to his bedroom, nursed him to sleep, lay him on the firm mattress of his baby basket, and left the room—anxious to check on the other four kids. I glanced in a few times at Christian, who seemed sound asleep in his darkened bedroom.

I let the time run away, and by the time the kids finished bathing, it was already after 10 pm. We went into Christian's room to get a book, but I told the kids not to disturb him by turning on the light. Ilona, my oldest daughter, touched Christian and said, "He seems cold, Mom." I looked at him; he appeared to be asleep. I quickly touched the long hair that stuck straight up on his head and replied, "He's fine. I'll get him a blanket later." Strangely, I didn't touch his skin; maybe, subconsciously, I sensed that something was wrong, but I didn't want to admit that something could be wrong.

After I put the kids to bed, I went back into Christian's bedroom and touched him. He was stone cold! He was dead! In panic, I grabbed him and thrust him into the hallway light. He had a purple ring around his forehead. Besides that, he looked like he was still peacefully asleep.

I suppressed a scream; the kids were sleeping. I thought I should call 911, but I was confused; any spark of life was long gone. Then I realized in horror that strange people would come and take my baby away from me forever. I had only a moment in eternity to be alone with him. So I carried him downstairs and held him to my breast and rocked him for God knows how long, perhaps a few seconds, perhaps a few minutes. Then I called my mom and a friend, then 911. I followed the dispatcher's resuscitation instructions, though it was so obviously futile. As paramedics rushed Christian away, neighbors came to stay with my kids and to drive me to the hospital.

There I was met by a kindly counselor, who took me to a white room where some examiner told me that my baby had died of Sudden Infant Death Syndrome. I'd heard the term before, but I didn't know what it meant. I had never known anyone who had lost a baby to SIDS. My husband called from his conference, and I had to tell him by phone that our son was dead. By then surrounded by family and friends, I held Christian for two hours until Gabe arrived, and then he and I held him and bid him farewell together. By then, my hardened breasts were dripping with milk he couldn't drink.

I profoundly felt my husband's frustration at not being able to do a single thing to save our son's life. Some parents get to leap into burning buildings or snatch children from train tracks, but we didn't get any second chances—not even a first. There could be no pleading on TV for prayers or money to rescue our child. It boggled my mind that babies have endured being thrown from cars and beaten by parents, but our baby couldn't survive a peaceful evening nap.

Returning from the hospital, we got another huge shock. Detectives were upstairs taking pictures of the baby's room! Did they think we were murderers? Had our baby somehow choked to death in his bed after I nursed him? Our fears eased a little when one detective said that our son had been sleeping in "the safest possible place"—a baby basket inside a larger crib. There were no pillows, blankets, or toys inside on which he might have suffocated, and he had died on his right cheek in the middle of a firm mattress. I'd thought of "crib death" as choking or suffocation, but those causes are ruled out before a death is labeled SIDS. There are more than 400 theories about what causes SIDS. Most researchers now believe that it is caused by brainstem or cardiac immaturities or abnormalities.

My shock moved me physically through the next week, when many people mistook my disbelief at what had happened for some superhuman emotional strength. Over and over I said, "How can WE be the 1 in 650 this happens to?" Luckily, the SIDS Information and Counseling Program, in Baltimore, called me three days after Christian's death to offer help.

At the funeral home, Gabe, our daughters, and I gazed into a little coffin at the still-handsome face of our son and brother. His sisters stroked the lock of hair that curled out from under his hooded white sweater, and we all rubbed his icy folded hands to warm them. With him we put farewell notes, a rosary, his teddy bear, and copies of some of our children's favorite books, such as *Pat-A-Cake* and *The Velveteen Rabbit*.

In the hall, after we left Christian, I found a brochure on SIDS, which said that it is the leading cause of death between the ages of one month and one year, killing more than 5,000 babies annually in the United States alone. It infuriated me that these were the first brochures I'd ever seen on SIDS and that no doctors or hospitals had ever made available to us any information about SIDS.

The usual excuse for not offering SIDS information to the public is that SIDS is considered unpredictable and unpreventable. Well, I say information is always better than ignorance. Like many other parents, I didn't know CPR when my son died. I didn't even know that the breathing or heartbeat of an apparently healthy baby could suddenly stop. Even if I couldn't have saved my son, I'd feel better now if I'd at least had the knowledge to try and save him if I'd been there. I do believe that the vast majority of SIDS cases are unpreventable, but I also feel that knowing CPR never hurts.

Our neighbors in Cheverly, Maryland—a Washington, D.C., suburb—were wonderful, sending complete dinners for three weeks after the death. But no one could know how awful we felt. After the funeral, some people told me I'd gotten through the worst part. How wrong they were. When the shock wore off after a few months, I descended into a living hell. I'd lost the innocence of my youth, my trust that if I "did things right" things would go right for me and my family. One of our family's lowest points came eight months after the death when I miscarried a baby. All our arms ached to again hold a baby, *our* baby. And, after that, it took more than a long, lonely year to conceive again, even though I'd never had fertility problems before.

Every morning, my first thought about Christian's death was, "I can't believe it really happened." Thankfully, I had three other kids to drag me off to the pool or playground. While there, I sometimes burst into tears, and my two-year-old would explain, "My mommy's crying because our baby died." She'd also say, "Big people don't die—only babies die." My six-year-old once said, "God kidnapped our baby."

I was even angrier at God than she was, and I spent many miserable days and nights cursing God for being rotten to His friends. It took me many, many months to come to believe that God didn't do this to us; if He'd wanted to teach people lessons, He could have picked on ax murderers and other people who have done a lot worse things than we have. Nature and bad luck, not God, did our baby in. I want to believe, however, that God was there to welcome Christian's spirit home and to try to comfort us.

I suffered tremendous guilt the first year. I cursed myself for hurrying to leave him that fateful day. I felt a complete failure as a mother because I hadn't sensed he was dead and felt his skin sooner. I found it so hard to believe that a baby could die for no known medical reason that I invented reasons on my own—like maybe he'd died from some mild medication I'd taken while I was pregnant. All the experts said I hadn't done anything wrong, but that didn't stop me from "grasping at straws" to blame myself, as one counselor put it. As awful as it was to shoulder the guilt, it was even worse to feel completely out of control.

I told Gabe that I wanted to die, and I felt my guilt compounded when my two-year-old overheard me and pleaded, "Mommy, don't die." I realized then that my ranting, raving, barking, and self-blaming were robbing me and the children I was still lucky enough to have of the short, precious time we have together on this earth. And that's when I realized that I had to start pulling myself together.

It was a long, excruciatingly slow process because I still couldn't help feeling cheated. I'd put my body, soul, and heart into making that baby. At birth, he weighed nine pounds and got a score of nine on his Apgar test, a general fitness examination. He was completely breast-fed, rosy-cheeked, and chubby-legged. After this ideal little boy died, I'd look at moms with the "perfect" girl–boy families I'd always dreamt of having and be furious at their good fortune. Why Christian? Why me? Yet very slowly I came to ask why NOT me? More than 70% of

SIDS moms, like me, have no risk factors, such as smoking, poor nutrition, or drug or alcohol abuse. Many people suffer pain and tragedies. Why should I be immune?

In my darkest moments, I've wished Christian's life did not happen so that we in his family wouldn't have to suffer. Now I try to be thankful for the time we had him because he changed the way we view life, arguably for the better. Our family is closer. We've made lots of friends we'd never have known. I stand in awe of the majority of the contributors to this book. They've chosen not to wallow in self-pity but to make the rest of their lives testimonials to purpose and faith. They've come to realize that SIDS is as profound an experience for what it gives as for what it takes away.

I used to think I'd awaken one morning miraculously healed. Now I realize that I must learn to live with some amount of grief.

At the same time, I must continue to readjust my vision of what life is and how I can be happy in this world. I am empty, yet full; thirsty, yet satisfied with many aspects of my life. The knife still turns as I see toddlers the age Christian would be and go to family events where a very important person is always missing. Yet I can again enjoy my many blessings—my loving husband and four strong daughters (including our beautiful new baby Genevieve, born two and a half years after Christian died). Too, I've finally accepted that we're not in control of all aspects of our lives and that I did the best I could at the time.

This experience won't make me a saint; God knows I'm far too ornery for that. I do hope and pray that one day we will know how life's puzzle pieces fit together and that this tragedy's higher purpose will be revealed. However, even if this life is all there is, and even if I never get to be with my son again, I still feel blessed, honored, and happy that I was the lucky person who got to be Christian's mother during his short time on this earth.

A Letter to Michael
by Liz Waller

My Dearest Michael,

As my firstborn, you will always have a very special place in my heart. I remember your birthday, August 20, as if it were yesterday. I was nervous, anxious, and very excited. Would you be a boy or a girl? What would you look like? Would I be a good mother? I remember November 18 just as clearly. The phone call at 3:30 pm with the message for me to get to the hospital. I did not know what was wrong, but how I prayed that everything was all right. Had you fallen from your infant seat? Had one of the other kids in day care hurt you?

Never did I think that you would be gone forever. How could this happen? Why?!? Questions to which I still do not have and may never get the answers. However, I now realize that if I had to ask why you were taken from me, then I'd also have to ask why you were given to me, and I wouldn't trade the three months we had together for anything.

It's now been more than two years since your death, and I can honestly say that I have accepted it. I never thought I would reach this point, let alone be able to laugh again. The anger and the pain were immense. It took time—lots of time—for me to forgive myself, forgive God, forgive the world, and in a way forgive even you, for leaving me. I believe that the only way I reached this point was through my involvement in the SIDS parents' support group. Actively participating in these meetings forced me to deal with my grief and the feelings that went with it. I was involved with people who knew exactly how I felt because they too had been in the same position. It's a tough way to have to learn about the grieving process, but I now hope that I can be of help to other grieving parents. As my tribute to you and your life, I will continue to be involved in SIDS events and groups until one day we can say we know why SIDS happens.

Those short three months with you were the best of my life. You will always be our son and Matthew's big brother. You will always be a big brother, a grandson, a nephew, and a godson...and always my firstborn!

All of my love,
Mama

A Prayer for Spring
by Janis Heil

Like springtime, let me unfold and
grow, fresh and new, from this cocoon
of grief that has been spun around me.

Help me face the harsh reality of
sunshine and renewed life, as my
bones still creak from the winter of my grief.

Life has dared to go on around me.
And I recover from the insult of life's continuance.
I readjust my focus to include recovery and growth
in my future.

Give me strength to break out of the cocoon
of my grief. But may I never forget it as the place
where I grew my wings, becoming a new person
because of my loss.

This poem first appeared in Unite Notes, *the copyrighted
newsletter of UNITE, Inc., Philadelphia, in 1984.*

Moving Beyond the Sudden Death of a Child
by Regina A. Rochford

Can time heal the painful wounds of a child's death, or does it just provide the survivors with the insight needed to resume living?

About 10 years ago, I took my eight-week-old baby out for a walk. It was a raw, chilly, overcast day, so I stopped by my parents' house to warm up. While my mother and I were sitting at the dining room table, my father picked up my infant daughter and faced her to me. I immediately noticed that her eyes were squinted closed and her skin had a blue-gray tint. At that moment, I knew that I would never see her open those eyes again. What I didn't realize was how the sudden death of this newborn would completely alter my perspective on life and marriage.

Rosemary was rushed to the emergency room of a local New York City hospital, where the doctors informed me that she had died from Sudden Infant Death Syndrome (SIDS), a diagnosis given when there is no apparent cause of death. One minute my beautiful, healthy baby was resting quietly, and the next she was dead. I was completely shocked. After receiving the tragic news, I shook the doctors' hands, thanked them for their assistance, and left the emergency room in a state of calm, quiet disbelief.

As my father drove me back to my house, all I could think about was how I was going to tell my husband that our beautiful infant had died. Moreover, I was petrified of how he would react. A few minutes after we returned home, I heard my husband pull into the driveway. I asked my parents to stay in the kitchen so that I could speak to him alone. As he opened the door, I noticed that he was carrying Christmas presents for the baby and me. I abruptly blurted out the bad news. He was stunned and began to run up and down the block screaming, until two of our neighbors (who had also lost a child) came running out to help me escort Frank back to the house before he was hurt, too.

Sitting in front of the cradle in the living room, my husband asked me a string of questions about the death that I couldn't answer. I was extremely calm but not at all in control. When my sister-in-law whom I'd just seen that morning walked in the door, I didn't even recognize her at first. Yet my husband, who appeared to be hysterical, mentioned something I hadn't considered: the funeral plans.

As we sat in the undertaker's office, I couldn't help but think about the irony of this whole situation. Instead of baptizing our daughter on Sunday, we would go to a local funeral home to view our dead child dressed in her christening gown in a little white coffin. The following day, she would be buried quietly with only a few close relatives present. There would be no celebration or jubilation over the birth of a baby, but rather only tears from two parents who would kiss their child good-bye and never see her again.

After the burial, my husband and I returned home in our first attempt to weather this storm, but our house was filled with memories, from bottles filled with formula to Rosemary's laundry waiting to be washed. To friends and family, her belongings became a painful reminder of her death. Many people begged us to dismantle her room, but we adamantly refused. In our hearts, it was the only way we could keep her alive a little longer. I relished the smell of her crib sheet, which still contained her faint odor. I even placed a doll in her crib and covered it with a blanket to see if I could feel her presence when I patted it softly, but nothing worked. Rosemary was gone, and even her aroma gradually faded from her room.

One night shortly after Rosemary's burial, my husband and I took a walk after dinner. I was flabbergasted at the gaiety of all the Christmas lights and decorations throughout the neighborhood. I couldn't imagine how people could celebrate a holiday when our baby had just died. The clock had stopped in our lives, but it kept ticking for everyone else. Unfortunately, this was only one of many stabs that grief would give us during our long journey through bereavement.

Three weeks after Rosemary's death, I returned to work in a feeble attempt to get my life in order. Those first weeks were filled with frequent visits and calls, when various business associates awkwardly expressed their condolences. At that time, I was working for a large corporation where people were expected to maintain a stiff upper lip; therefore, I was forced to carefully control my feelings and not let a tear show. Gradually, I began to withdraw from most social functions, for it was becoming extremely difficult to put on a happy face when my world was crumbling to pieces. The most comforting part of my day was entering a stall in the ladies' room to bury my head for a good long cry.

One cold morning in the end of March while I was walking up the long narrow steps from the subway station to my office, the crass reality of Rosemary's death hit me like a ton of bricks. I wasn't supposed to be at work; I should have been at home with my baby whom I hadn't seen or touched in more than three months. On one hand, I was intellectually cognizant of my daughter's death, but the poignant reality had just exploded within me and was about to consume my very existence. Little by little, this revelation turned into rage, and the emotional repertoire my husband and I had maintained for years was no longer effective during this mournful period. We were at a point of no return and either had to modify the way we related to each other and the world around us or end our relationship.

One of the first issues I confronted was the role my husband had been designated within his family. From childhood, he had been encouraged to take care of family members who were dysfunctional or in distress. While my husband had become adept at meeting the demands of various relatives, we had both neglected to address what we needed to sustain our marriage. Ironically, when we craved love and attention, everyone vanished into thin air. As terrible as this appeared to be, it was a blessing in disguise because we finally had to confront each other one on one for the first time in our lives.

In response to my anger and rage, I launched an all-out attack on my in-laws, letting them know how deserted and disappointed I felt by their behavior. I seized this opportunity to shake myself free of relationships that served only to suffocate and stifle our individual and conjugal growth. It was a time for change, but I didn't know that an emotional upheaval had to first transpire between my husband and me before it could ever transfer to the other relationships that made me feel so furious and resentful.

Our incessant battles eventually led us to the couch of a local family therapist, who was able to help us recognize the tremendous love and commitment we had for each other. Yet as helpful as the counseling was, this too was a grueling process because we were simultaneously trying to deal with the loss of a child and straighten out problems that had been festering for years. Gradually, we suffered through this painful period and renegotiated a more mutually beneficial marital rapport, which has brought us extraordinary happiness, intimacy, and another daughter.

I believe that in every cloud there is a silver lining. My husband and I endured one of the most tragic events that could befall a family. As a result, we came out of this experience richer and with more insight into life and each other. Time has moved along. I am no longer angry about my daughter's death or at my husband's family. We all did what we thought was best despite our lack of skills and preparation in coping with such an unexpected loss. I've accepted that Rosemary had a very important mission, which she accomplished in eight short weeks. Her brief life and the terrible pain we experienced after her death have helped us lead more joyful and productive existences than we ever would have known had it not been for that precious little baby who never even uttered a word.

Chapter 12

Happy Birthday? Merry Christmas?

Couldn't we skip
Christmas this year
My baby's dead
and I don't
feel like celebrating

This poem, entitled "Merry Christmas" and published by SIDS mom Sharon A. Dunn in her poetry book, *We Bring Her Flowers* (Fithian Press, Santa Barbara, CA, 1990) succinctly expresses what all parents who have lost babies feel on holidays and anniversaries. How can we celebrate when our babies are not here with us?

Joani has now been through six of Christian's birthdays without him. She has suffered through six death anniversaries. She has spent six Thanksgivings, six Christmases, six Easters, six Mother's Days... the list goes on and on...missing (and remembering) Christian.

Other than New Year's Day, when most people look to the year ahead, holidays are all about remembering. And usually about remembering through celebration. Celebrating great presidents, brave veterans, holy births, and important deaths. Holidays are milestones, times to stop and think—and feel. To consider what was, what should have been, and what still is.

For SIDS survivors, the first year is marked with wrenching milestones and holidays. Often the anticipation is even worse than the day itself. But for each holiday and anniversary that is passed, a degree of strength is added. Each year, the bittersweet day becomes a little less bitter and a little more sweet.

Finding a way to celebrate a SIDS baby's life is an important part of grieving, and holidays provide a good opportunity.

It is spring, and a dozen note-filled balloons ascend to the sky. At first, the Horchler family is quiet, almost whispering, "Happy Birthday" to Christian. How unfair that some balloons get stuck in the trees. Yet how jubilant the atmosphere as they free themselves and dance their way up into the clouds. The Horchlers cheer! "Not everything about our baby had to die," Joani explains. "His spirit can still be celebrated."

After almost 10 years, Jennifer and Ken Wilkinson still remember their daughter Larkin's birthday by purchasing gifts for their other children in her honor. "Oh yeah, it's Larkin's birthday!' they exclaim.

Sam and Nina Sandeen chose instead to honor the anniversary of their son's death. They take a special cake—made of birdseed, peanut butter, and popcorn—to the cemetery. They write "Dwight" in popcorn and present the special cake for the birds to enjoy.

Some people choose to do something for others to acknowledge the loss of their child. For example, Jean Hulse-Hayman and her husband Dale celebrate their son's short life by tying a ribbon on the "Ben oak" and sending a donation to a SIDS organization. Besides supporting research, they have donated about two dozen copies of this book to libraries, pediatricians, ob/gyns, hospitals, SIDS support groups, and others through the sponsorship program run by its nonprofit publisher, SIDS-ES. (SIDS-ES prints a personalized label for the inside cover of each donated book that honors a baby who has died of SIDS and says who has donated the book. More information about this program is on the last page of this book.)

SIDS grandmother Sandra Graben and her daughter Catherine Hulme recently spent the death anniversary of T.J. Hulme delivering the 32 books they donated in memory of him to libraries all over Arizona. "It made us feel better on that sad day to do something that would help others," says Sandra.

Other families have chosen to donate the money they would have spent on birthday or holiday gifts to a charity or to invite a senior citizen or foreign student to share in their families' festivities.

In Maryland, the SIDS Program holds memorial services for area SIDS victims. Parents light candles in memory of their babies, and ornaments with each baby's name are given to the parents. SIDS survivors can stand up and recite poems or articles they've written. A program gives each baby's name and his or her birth and death dates. SIDS parents often provide the music.

Other ways to remember a baby include hanging a memorial Christmas stocking or yearly ornament, buying flowers for a church service, or burning candles on all personally significant holidays to acknowledge the baby's spiritual presence. Joani always includes her baby's name in her annual Christmas letter to family and friends. She signs each letter this way: "Love, Joani, Gabe, Ilona, Gabrielle, Julianna, Genevieve, Stephanie, and Christian in spirit." The Horchler family often includes a photo of Christian in family portraits; a family member holds the photo.

To remember their babies and promote SIDS awareness, many people now wear (and help make) pretty SIDS awareness pins designed by Lisa Werner of Washington state, who lost her son Blake to SIDS in 1995. Lisa now heads a national grassroots volunteer effort to produce the pins. (To obtain a pin or to contribute time or supplies, call 1-800-232-7437.)

Of course, finding your own special way to celebrate in your baby's honor is not the only holiday challenge you will face. Getting through "required" holiday social functions, such as the annual office party or Grandma Tilly's don't-you-dare-miss-it turkey dinner, can also be rough. You may feel too physically, mentally, emotionally fatigued (or all three) to attend such functions. You may not be ready to talk about your loss with co-workers or casual friends, or you may fear that no one will talk about it—the old "there's no elephant in the room" scenario. In any case, it is perfectly okay to suggest to your boss or host that you'd like to accept the invitation conditionally, based on how you feel that day. Explain, if needed, that your emotions are still on a roller coaster, and that you want to be with them if you feel up to it.

Holidays like Thanksgiving, Christmas, Hanukkah, and Easter usually come with some kind of celebration. But for a SIDS survivor, the anticipation can feel more like dread. Often, preparations are put off until the last minute, causing survivors to panic when they realize that the Christmas presents aren't wrapped, the pies aren't baked, and Aunt Matilda has been left standing at the train station!

There are no easy answers to this common problem, but some survivors have found it helpful to plan far ahead, before anyone—especially you—has even thought about getting into the holiday spirit. You can also make a list of things that you usually do and then cross off whatever is not essential. Don't be afraid to make changes in the locations of the celebrations or in the rituals surrounding them, but be sure to consider and allow time and space for each member of the family's emotional needs. You may want to write down any fears you have about the holiday and then consider how you might react if they come true. Some people find that preparing for the worst can head it off.

By meditating and trusting ourselves to be gentle with ourselves, we can use holidays "to make long-considered changes in our lives, allowing ourselves 'to be' instead of feeling pressured 'to do,'" says Patricia Andrus, a social worker in Lafayette, Louisiana. Be kind to yourself, and focus on the peace of the season, she advises. Some practical suggestions: Shop from catalogs instead of fighting the traffic and store crowds, order goodies from food catalogs instead of standing on your feet baking; decorate less; shop earlier; and clear your minds by eating well-balanced meals and drinking plenty of water and avoiding drugs and alcohol. Allow others to help you accomplish the tasks of holidays; this is not a sign of weakness but an acknowledgment on your part that you are busy accomplishing the necessary but physically and emotionally draining job of grieving.

It is interesting and important to note that some holidays appear to be harder for fathers than mothers, and vice versa. William Ermatinger, facilitator of a SIDS parent support group, has observed that mothers often find the baby's birthday more difficult than the anniversary of the death. Ermatinger theorizes that a birthday is likely more difficult for mothers to bear because they were the ones who physically gave the baby life. In addition, mothers are traditionally more involved in planning birthday celebrations and thus feel particularly empty on that day. Fathers, Ermatinger has noticed, usually seem to experience more pain on the anniversary of the baby's death. The reason, he suggests, is that the father's contribution to the family often (although not always) focuses more on the raising and supporting of the child and investing in the child's future. The death anniversary is a harsh reminder that there is no future in which to invest.

It is common for SIDS parents to find that the anticipation of pain on a holiday is often worse than it actually turns out to be. Be warned, however, that many also report that they "crashed" the day after the holiday. Not realizing how much they had psyched themselves up, and in some cases forced themselves to participate in things they really didn't want to, they temporarily reverted back to the confusion and depression of those first few months after the death. Fortunately, though, one thing noted by all SIDS parents is that the birthdays, death anniversaries, and other holidays do get easier with time.

Missing Danny at the Beach
For Daniel C. Roper IV: 9/9/95–12/4/95

by Janice John Roper

My birthday boy. One year old,
smiley red lips, a whisper, like a breath
would have been. Light fingers across my cheek.
An imprint of you.

My baby boy. Chubby pink flesh,
soft wiggly hugs and quiet sleeping
might have been. In my arms,
slipping into my heart. Disappearing
into an ocean of dreams.

My blue-eyed son. Squealing
like seagulls, trying to catch
or follow them.
Sand on your hands and knees.
Disappearing in a wave,
a small indent, then nothing,
a ripple, an invisible shimmer
wet like my tears
bright, blinding like the sun
like my pain, my son,
when I remember
those squeals are not from you
it is another boy
the age you would have been.

He is starting to walk
fat steps, small sandy footprints.

His mother catches him, they are
giggling.
Another wave comes,
grasping at those dark prints,
destroying that imprint,
dissolving my hopes for you
until I cannot see
past the next minute.

I touch my cheek but feel
only gritty and wet
while time drags me
further from you
into its dark ocean
where I might
forget to breathe too.

Surviving Anniversaries and Holidays
by Shelley A. LeDroux

Birthdays and anniversaries are special, and so are the loved ones with
whom we celebrate them. I have learned to find peace and comfort in
celebrating the memory of our daughter Katelin, who passed away to
SIDS on December 8, 1991. On Katelin's birthday I prepare myself
for a long ride filled with a lot of happy and sad tears.

Because the joy of having had Katelin is greater than the sadness of
losing her, these days of celebration are usually beautiful. She was born
in the season of spring, so it's bright and colorful. I place bright balloons
and a pretty bouquet of flowers beside her memorial plaque. Through all
the tears, I pull out a picture of Katelin and sing "Happy Birthday." Back
at the house, I light a candle in memory of her birth and the time we
shared together. The candle is placed in front of her picture.

I and others who loved her also remember the day she died. This
year, I decided to do something a little different. After placing flowers
beside her memorial plaque, and saying how much I love and miss her,
I wrote her a poem. I then had it printed in calligraphy and matted in a
pretty blue with lace. It now hangs on my dining room wall.

Kathy's Day
by William C. Ermatinger

George Washington was a special person to our nation. So, too, were Christopher Columbus, Abraham Lincoln, and Martin Luther King. In our country, we recognize these and other special people with specific days set aside for us to honor their lives and memories. Official events are held, and most of us usually do something different from our daily routine. Often we do something extra special and traditional.

Within a few years after Kathy's death, I decided that I would set aside a special day to honor her life and memory. I chose the anniversary of her death. It was a day I already would be thinking about her in a special way. Over the years, the day has acquired a certain tradition.

If it is a work day, I take it off. In the morning, I visit her grave, talk to her, and bring her up to date on what has happened and what I am doing. Then, for the rest of the day, I do something special. One year I went to the seashore and walked on the beach. Other years I have gone to a museum or art gallery. When I was single, I usually was alone; now my wife (even though she never knew Kathy) joins me. We celebrate Kathy's life and memory. I don't expect the world to join in this celebration, but neither will I let the year be complete without this special day being included in the calendar of hearts.

Marking the Milestones When You Have Lost Your Only Child
by Michelle Morgan Spady

Looking back, I remember being so happy and excited when I found out that I was pregnant with my first child, and even more so when I found out that my child was to be a boy. The first thing I wanted to do was find a charming, unique, but cute name because I felt that he was going to be very special. Armani.

Who would have ever imagined that he would come to me and leave me all within a year's time? I had stopped work for a while, and after

Armani's death in March of 1991 I felt lonely, helpless, in despair, and sometimes even suicidal.

Armani and I used to do everything together: shopping, laundry, singing, dancing, park visits, playing, and sometimes just laying around. I can remember times when I would put clothes in a basket and he would take them out! I'd put dishes in the dishwasher and he'd want to help!

It was hard at first. I felt as though I'd lost my best friend. I had. To facilitate my grieving and to commemorate Armani,

- I kept a diary, though after one and a half years I didn't write as much.

- Since Easter came right after his death, I went to his grave site with a toy.

- On Mother's Day, I bought a locket to put one of his little pictures in. Now I don't leave home without it!

- I had two pairs of his shoes bronzed: his first, and the pair we bought just two weeks before he passed away.

- I went through his baby book, and I framed a few of my favorite pictures.

- At Christmas, it was very hard for me because he was with us the Christmas before. I took one of the pictures of him with all of his toys and placed it inside one of the SIDS Christmas cards and mailed them to family and friends.

- On his birthday, I bought a card and put it in his baby book. I plan to do this every year. I went to his grave and placed a toy there. I also bought cupcakes and a gift for one of his day-care playmates. I burned a red candle in his memory all day.

- I talked to people about SIDS through church and school organizations and with friends. I find it very important to keep talking about Armani to people and to make them realize how important it is for them to talk about him to me. It's all part of the healing process.

- I keep a picture of him on my desk at work, which sparks conversation about SIDS and creates more awareness.

■ I've been very involved in SIDS-related activities, editing our chapter's newsletter, chairing our Family Services Committee and the Minority Outreach Committee, serving on the national SIDS Alliance Committee for Cultural Diversity and Minority Outreach, and more. All of these activities help me to feel a sense of belonging. My attitude is that I should do as much as I can for SIDS because that's the only thing I can still do for Armani.

Portraits for Easter
In Memory of Nigel Christopher Radich: 2/24/94–7/11/94

by Cheryl Radich

Yesterday I decided to take my three daughters to get their picture taken for Easter. It was going to be their first portrait taken together, and I was looking forward to it. Instead, it turned out to be one of the most difficult experiences for me since Nigel died. I guess it suddenly hit me that he "wasn't in the picture." I looked around the walls of the studio and saw portraits of other little boys in their sporty outfits holding footballs and trucks. Each one was like a stab of pain to my heart. I thought of all the cute outfits I had for Nigel that he never got to wear. Now they are in his trunk at the foot of my bed with the tags still on them. There were props and backgrounds of footballs and trucks, but of course the photographer never thought to use them for me.

As I was standing at the cash register, a young nurse was holding her baby boy and was picking up her portraits that she had had taken of him. She held one up for him to see. He looked to be only a few months old, and I thought to myself how lucky she was to have him. But I also thought that it was good that she had had his portraits done. You never know… She looked down at him to see if he was looking at his picture, and then she looked up at me. Her baby boy was looking at me instead. I smiled at him. He smiled the most beautiful smile back at me. I was touched. His mom was proud.

I went home with my three daughters and cried.

Chapter 13

Peer Contact and Professional Help

I found the SIDS Network on the Internet late one night when I couldn't sleep. I immediately felt a connection to others who could understand my feelings. It has since become a comfortable place where I can gather information, share ideas, and talk about my son at any time of the day.

— Cheryl Radich

There are many resources available to help SIDs survivors move through their grief. Lee Hackel, a program specialist with the Georgia Division of Public Health's SIDS Project, notes, "After the SIDS death of their baby, many families have an intense need for more information about SIDS and hungrily 'devour' whatever they can find that will point them in the direction of elusive answers to the standard questions: "What is SIDS? What could I have done to protect my baby? Did my baby suffer?" Information can be found in books such as this one, Ms. Hackel notes, but other sources of information are state SIDS projects (usually located in the maternal and child health program of your state health department), the National SIDS Resource Center, the national SIDS Alliance and its local affiliates, and other SIDS or bereavement support organizations. (See this book's appendix for a listing of resources.)

A new and important source of information and support for both families and professionals can be found on the World Wide Web. The SIDS Information Home Site (URL: http://sids-network.org) has been rated among the top 5% of all sites on the Internet by numerous "surfing" organizations. The SIDS Information Home Site helps in several ways. It ties together the smattering of existing information on the Internet. It provides information not previously available on the Internet: research progress, support information, contacts throughout the world, educational information about risk factors, news of SIDS awareness activities, and stories from those directly affected by the tragedy of SIDS. SIDS families are getting immediate support, researchers are contributing updates on their research, the general public is learning about this terrible disease. This Web site has been viewed by thousands of people from all over the world. The SIDS Information Home Site on the World Wide Web is produced and maintained by volunteers of the SIDS Network, Inc., an all-volunteer, nonprofit SIDS full-service provider in Ledyard, Conn. The SIDS Network was co-founded by Deb and Chuck Mihalko. They have been involved at local, national, and international levels of SIDS awareness, education, support, and marketing since their 38-day-old daughter, Margaret Joy, became a victim of SIDS in 1989.

Another important Internet resource for SIDS families is the Sudden Infant Death Syndrome (SIDS) Mailing List. This SIDS "discussion group" is a place for parents and professionals alike to discuss issues related to SIDS. When you join a mailing list, the "conversations" that happen are delivered to you via e-mail. When you place a message on the mailing list, that message is delivered to everyone else on the mailing list. Families seek and give information and support, share intense feelings, and explore theories of SIDS. Also contributing to the discussions, while gaining valuable insights about the needs and concerns of SIDS families, are SIDS researchers, health educators, and SIDS program professionals. The Discussion Group is a 24-hour-a-day resource for parents who often turn for support to "computer friends" in the middle of the night, when feelings of longing for their beloved baby intensify. You can reach the SIDS mailing list via the SIDS Information Home Site address (URL: http://sids-network.org) or through an improved WWW-to-List interface at http://www.mills.edu/PEOPLE/gr.pages/balzer.public.html/sids.list.html, or through e-mail (balzer@ella.mills.edu). The list owner is Ned Balzer, a SIDS parent (and a contributor to this book) whose son Willie died at the age of four months in 1993.

A very touching way to remember a baby is to place her picture on the SIDS Network's SIDS Information Home Site. Steve Ruggiero, who lost his son Lucas to SIDS in 1995, has offered to scan photographs so that they can be placed on the site. For more information, contact Steve Ruggiero at his e-mail address: steve@cookie.secapl.com or contact the Web site.

Public health nurses, another valued resource for families, are working in almost every county in this country. More specific information about counseling and information services provided by public health nurses can be found in this chapter in an article by Linda Esposito.

Peer contact, offered through organizations such as the SIDS Alliance, SIDS Educational Services, and other SIDS centers, is an important component of SIDS services. Toll-free numbers for these organizations are given in this book's appendix. Providing peer contact is also a mission of SIDS-ES, the nonprofit publisher of this book; its phone number is in the appendix, and it may be called collect. The peer contact volunteer is a parent, grandparent (or other relative), child-care provider, or foster parent who has experienced the death of a child due to SIDS and who contacts grieving family members to offer support during their bereavement. Fellow SIDS family members who have reconciled their own grief are capable of helping newly bereaved families in ways that may be beyond the experiences of relatives, friends, and professionals. Peer contact volunteers are part of, and receive the support of, an established SIDS service network, which includes other volunteers and professionals (counselors, nurses, doctors, and first responders) working to meet the needs of grieving SIDS families. Peer contacts are not considered counselors, nor are they intended to replace professional counselors. They recognize their role—and their limitations—as sympathetic listeners who can share experiences to validate family members' feelings and assist family members in clarifying their options. Nancy Maruyama's article in this chapter further discusses peer contacts.

SIDS counseling professionals may be social workers, psychologists, psychiatrists, or family or marriage counselors, who are experienced and available to help families through complications of grieving. Carla Hosford's article in this chapter gives more information about the types of professionals, how to decide if you need one, and how to choose one.

Many times peer contacts team with SIDS counseling professionals to facilitate a support group for SIDS families. In the introduction to their *Bereavement Support Group Guide: A Guidebook for Individuals and/or Professionals Who Wish To Start a Bereavement Mutual Self-Help Group*, Margie Pike, RN, and Sara Rich Wheeler, RN, write the following concerning support groups: "For many people, it is a tremendous comfort just to learn that they are not alone in the experience of loss and bereavement, that others have journeyed down the rocky road of grief and are making it, and that it is a safe place for them to share their sorrow." This guide is an excellent "how-to" workbook on how to start such a support group.

A Peer Contact Answers the Question: "Are You Still Doing That?"

by Debbie Gemmill

We just sent in our registration for our high school class reunion. It's the first one we'll attend. I was hugely pregnant with Tyler, our second child, when our 10th reunion was held, more in the mood for fuzzy slippers than dancing shoes. We haven't seen most of our high school friends in years, and of course we are eager to see who they've turned out to be and what they've done with their lives.

The registration form was fun to fill out. We were high school sweethearts; John was in the band, and I was on the drill team. The questionnaire asked if we had any high school memorabilia to bring to share, and we answered, "One another!" It will be interesting to see who shows up, who married, who had children.

I was completely unprepared when I came to the line on the form asking about our children. I filled in Jen's name and age, and Jordan's and moved on to the next line, but I returned in a second. What about Tyler?

Except for a few close friends, none of these people even knew Tyler lived, let alone died suddenly and unexpectedly when he was seven months old. Why bring it up?

This got me to thinking about imaginary conversations at a high school reunion. Mostly we've joked about what we'd say when asked what we've been doing for the past 25 years.

"Oh, gee, we spend a lot of time jetting back and forth between our homes."

"Neurosurgery keeps me pretty busy, when I'm not on the pro tour."

"I had to give up modeling. It was just all so vain."

What we've really been doing is working hard to make a living, trying to keep up with the house and yard work, making quality time for our children and one another, keeping the automobile insurance industry solvent with our ever-increasing premiums, ... oh, and somewhere in the middle of all of that, we've been trying to figure out how a perfectly healthy baby could just die in his sleep and how we can come to terms with that.

A friend we haven't seen in many years did know about Tyler. When he called, years ago, to see if we were going to the 10-year reunion, I explained that I was six weeks away from having another child. We sent him a birth announcement, the only correspondence we had until our Christmas card the following year, which contained a note explaining that Tyler had died the previous spring. There was simply no other way I could think of to explain the absence of Ty's name. We did not hear from this friend until recently, when he called to see if we'd be at the upcoming gathering. When it came to the part in the conversation when it was my turn to say what I've been up to, I naturally began talking about my volunteer work within the SIDS community.

"Oh...You're still doing that?"

I am reminded, once again, of my then-four-year-old daughter, who a few weeks after Ty's death was asked by a well-meaning adult friend, "Are you feeling better now?"

"No," Jen said. "He's still dead."

Yes, I am still doing that. I'm not doing it because I can't find other things to do. I'm not doing it because I'm not "over it," and I'm not doing it because I'm stuck, depressed, or obsessed. I'm doing it because Ty's still dead. And because during the time I've been working on this article, approximately one hour, another baby has died, and another family is beginning that terrible journey of living life as the parent of a dead child.

The time and effort I spend as a parent contact and as a writer about SIDS and the family is a tiny fraction of the time I would have spent with my first son. I have missed 14 birthdays, 13 Christmases, 13 Easter baskets, and who knows how many baseball, basketball, and soccer games. This is not time you can make up.

When I first began writing, I remember an instructor telling me, "Write what you know." It was good advice, and my first articles sold to magazines were about toilet training, making baby food from scratch, growing a children's garden, and planning birthday parties. I knew that stuff because it was my life. And now I write about being part of a family with a missing member, because that is my life now. It is what I know.

I remember the exact hour that I had determined that Ty had been dead for as long as he had been alive. I'm not sure, however, when I realized that my address book was more than half full with the names of people I have met since Ty's death. I can't even put my finger on when it was that I decided I had to do more with our loss than just "get over it."

Someone told me a year after Ty died that she completely understood why I was volunteering with our SIDS support group. "Someday," she said, "you'll feel that you have eventually paid them back for what they did for you." Even though I will always be grateful for the help we received, it's not a debt repayment plan that keeps me involved. I do it because.

I don't know if I'll have anything witty to say at our reunion. I'll probably brag about Jen and Jordan, and commiserate with the others about growing older and the drop in real estate prices. I don't even know if the issue of SIDS will come up, although it's pretty hard to imagine that I'll be able to keep my trap shut all weekend. What else am I supposed to say when someone asks, "So what have you been doing?"

I went back and filled in Tyler's name next to Jen's and Jordan's on our registration form. I never pretended before that he hadn't lived and died, and there's no reason to now. I think I'll even bring his picture, and when they ask, I'll simply say, "Yes, I'm still doing that."

This article is excerpted from Getting Through Grief: From a Parent's Point of View. *See the reading list in the back of this book for order information.*

Untitled

by H. Thurman

I know I cannot enter all you feel nor bear with you the burden of your pain. I can but offer what my love does give: the strength of caring, the warmth of one who seeks to understand the silent, storm-swept barrenness of so great a loss. This I do in quiet ways, that on your lonely path you may not walk alone.

A SIDS Parent Counseling SIDS Survivors

by Carla Hosford, LCSW-C

As a parent counselor at the Maryland SIDS Information and Counseling Program in Baltimore, I am often asked what it is like to work with SIDS parents when I am one myself. As in so many situations, I respond with a wide range of feelings. I could say that I like using my personal experience to help others who are going through what I went through. Or I could say that it's like looking in a mirror because newly bereaved parents look and sound and feel the way I did and still do sometimes, even though it has been 18 years since my daughter Susanna died. Finally, I could confess that some of my friends told me I was crazy to take this job, and they were right.

All of the above responses are true, but I'd like to think that the first is most true. My daughter died just before the federally funded SIDS projects were established. The support that existed at that time came from voluntary groups—the SIDS Foundation, the Guild for Infant Survival, and others. The effectiveness of these groups varied with the people who ran them, but the fact that they could offer new parents an ear and a hand made them invaluable.

I remember all too well the days and weeks before I got a call from the New Jersey SIDS Foundation. I didn't think anyone could really survive the loss I'd suffered, and I wasn't sure I wanted to even if it was possible. The voice of another SIDS mother was a lifeline. It didn't lessen the pain any, but it showed me that people do get through it and that they even reach the point where they can support other parents.

Later, I worked with the New Jersey SIDS Foundation and the Metropolitan Washington Guild for Infant Survival. It made me feel good to reach out to SIDS parents and others who had lost infants to other causes. I knew, however, that I was connecting with only a few of the bereaved families that were out there because there was no mechanism for locating bereaved families at that time. Parents who were contacted were the lucky few.

As a counselor at the SIDS Information and Counseling Program, I have access to a much better system for locating SIDS families. The medical examiner quickly passes information to our office about all SIDS cases in Maryland, and we can usually contact parents within a few days of the death. It's extremely important to dispel quickly the wrong information that newly bereaved parents often receive. For example, an anguished mother will say, "My boyfriend thinks the baby wouldn't have died if I hadn't left him with a sitter." Or, "My mom says it's because I didn't feed her the right formula."

Such concerns can be addressed by simply talking about them to a counselor familiar with SIDS and bereavement issues. Professional help doesn't have to be expensive. Special clinics prorate their charges according to what you can pay. A recommendation from a friend, neighbor, co-worker, or your state's SIDS counseling service is a good way to start. Your doctor may refer you to someone with whom he or she works. HMOs and other insurance providers sometimes have lists of people they believe are qualified to provide services. Agencies that deal with death and dying may have names of people who offer counseling. Many professions have referral services of their own, which you can find through the phone book.

Among the types of professionals trained to provide counseling are psychiatrists, psychologists, social workers, psychiatric nurses, pastoral counselors, and mental health counselors. You may prefer to work with someone of your own gender or religious affiliation. You may prefer someone who specializes in a certain type of treatment such as marital or family therapy. Your relationship with the therapist is of primary importance. A therapist may have credentials rivaling Freud, but if you can't relate to him or her, you won't be helped.

Remember that you are the consumer. You can ask, "Do you have training in grief counseling?" "Have you worked with people who have lost children?" "Have you had a loss like this yourself?" This is not to suggest that to be effective the therapist must have had the experience that brings you to treatment. However, for some people it is easier to work with someone who has been through it.

Going to a counselor doesn't mean you aren't strong enough or lack inner resources or whatever other nonsense critical people may come up with. Coping with SIDS is an enormous challenge, and each person brings to it a different set of emotional baggage, a unique history of relationships, and an individual inventory of strengths and needs. People's support systems and their abilities to cope with stress and trauma vary widely, as does their acceptance of outside intervention.

Factors in a person's past or present life situations can make it unusually hard for some people to handle a loss of such magnitude. For example, a woman came to me for counseling because she found herself crying uncontrollably one and a half years after her baby's death. She thought there was something wrong with her, and this feeling was intensified by the response of others, who couldn't understand why she was reacting in this way at this time. It turned out that at the time the baby died, the woman was facing a move related to her husband's new job in another city. Also, her mother was ill with cancer and not expected to live long. Grieving takes a great deal of time and energy, and this woman was so divided—facing so much change and so much real and anticipated loss—that she was not able to grieve fully when the death happened. Later, when her life was more stable, some event or a memory or something she heard or read triggered the delayed grief reaction.

A man whose baby died several years ago found that he was unable to relate to his baby by a new marriage because "I never said good-bye to my son" and "It's not fair to his memory to love another baby." Talking to me, he uncovered several experiences in his early childhood when he had felt abandoned and unloved. He needed to talk about these early losses and to get in touch with the feelings of sadness and anger they brought on. By doing so, he was able to gain some understanding of why he needed to hold on so tenaciously to this child.

If you feel you are "stuck"—unable to talk about the loss; unable to form new relationships; overwhelmed over time by feelings of anger, guilt, fear, or depression—you might consider seeking professional help. Other cues to the need: sleeping or eating too much or too little; reliance on drugs or alcohol; difficulty maintaining concentration; or acting out behavior.

The fact that you are reading this book is certainly a big step in the right direction. I am pleased to have been involved with it as a consultant because it offers nourishment, validation of feelings, and hope to parents. It is also valuable to those of us who are mental health professionals: What better way to get the feel of this unique tragedy than through the (often painful to read) writings of those who have experienced it? A book like this was not available 18 years ago when I lost Susanna. How I wish it had been.

Finding Friends Among Other SIDS Families
by Nancy Maruyama, RN

The peer parent contact plays a vital role in helping families cope with their grief following their child's death. In the early days after the loss of a child to SIDS, the peer contact can offer support, information, hope, and encouragement. Because they are bereaved parents themselves, peer parent contacts have much to offer newly bereaved parents by sharing their own experiences in coping with the death of their child.

Peer contacts are specially trained to provide a safe, non-judgmental setting for the families of SIDS victims. The role of the peer contact is not to offer advice or to provide solutions to problems; rather it is to listen attentively and offer support. The peer contact is not to be considered a counselor, however. He or she usually works in cooperation with SIDS counseling professionals and can make the appropriate referral if necessary. Confidentiality and the right to privacy are respected at all times.

When a SIDS death occurs, it is important to provide peer support as soon as possible. Depending on the local resources available, newly bereaved SIDS parents may be contacted by a peer contact within 24 hours after the death of a child. There are situations in which the family may not want peer support initially, but may contact the local agency weeks, months, or even sometimes years later. Some cultures provide support systems to families, frequently through the families' religious affiliations. Whatever decisions family members make with regard to support are respected, and they are never forced to accept peer support against their wishes.

Referrals come through many avenues. Sources can include but are not limited to public health nurses, emergency room staff, clergy, and family members. An information packet may be sent, with the enclosed pamphlets and books tailored to parents, siblings, grandparents, and primary caregivers. The packet usually includes information on support meetings and local SIDS agencies. The packet now given to each newly bereaved family by the SIDS Alliance of Illinois contains a copy of *The SIDS Survival Guide*. The SIDS Alliance of Illinois bought at discount

300 copies of the book so that each newly bereaved family will be able to have one as quickly as possible after the death of their baby.

Initial contact is usually by telephone or letter. In some areas, peer contacting takes place in person. Large urban areas, such as Chicago, frequently use the telephone as the primary method of contact.

Peer contact continues for as long as the grieving family would like. This may be as few as one or two telephone calls or may last for periods of more than one year. For the peer contact, it is important to remember that bereavement does not end when the grieving family has accepted the loss of their child.

Nancy and her husband Rodney lost their first child, son Brendan, in 1985. They have two subsequent children, Caitlin and Jennifer. Nancy, who served on the Board of Directors of the SIDS Alliance of Illinois for many years, continues to volunteer on a local and national level.

Home Visits by Public Health Nurses

by Linda Esposito, RN, MPH, CNS, CNA

Bereaved families have received nurse counseling services in their homes for the past 20 years. The nurses who provide such services—often called home health or public health nurses—are trained extensively in the pathophysiology of illness and death. They are experienced in promoting positive mental health without moving inappropriately and quickly into psychiatrically oriented treatments or recommending referrals to psychiatrically oriented professionals without due cause. Nurses are licensed professionals in the states where they practice.

Often public health nurses are employees of county or state departments of health. They often provide home visits, including bereavement services, to people within a certain area. Their visits are paid for by the counties in which they are employed, other funding sources such as grants, or by SIDS organizations that contract for their services.

Family members may feel threatened when they hear that a public health nurse is making a visit to their home. Often this panic is due to a feeling that the county or state thinks that the parents have done something wrong and are investigating them. This fear is unfounded;

the nurse is only making the visits to provide support and comfort. Home health nurses also work in private agencies; usually they are employed by organizations that serve homebound individuals in the community, and the visits are paid for by insurance. Home health nurses can also provide SIDS bereavement services through reimbursement from contracting SIDS organizations or grants.

Public health and home health nurses provide bereavement visits to SIDS families throughout the United States. In other countries, they may be called home visitors and have training in nursing or grief counseling.

The initial stages of grief leave families with varied emotions, such as anger, guilt, shock, sadness, and pain. Families find themselves beginning a long emotional journey in the search for answers that may not exist. They are often surprised and overwhelmed by the intensity of these emotions and the depth of the pain they feel. It is described by parents as an emotional numbness. Through the help of nurses making home visits, families often obtain the information and support needed to survive the initial shock. They also obtain guidance concerning where to get additional help within their communities. Some families find support in groups run by other SIDS parents, by just speaking to SIDS parents over the phone, or by continued counseling given by the nurse or SIDS organization. In other cases, families may need therapists and private therapy.

The nurse can help the family to actualize the loss by encouraging the family members to express their feelings regarding their baby and by reviewing the death scenario. The nurse can help validate the family's feelings and offer support. During counseling, the nurse can give valuable insight as to what is considered normal during this tragic time. Frequently, families fear that they are going crazy when they "hear" the baby cry or when their arms physically ache for the baby. Couples, as well as other family members, may grieve differently. Siblings also grieve, and the nurse can give families valuable information on how children understand death at various ages. Also, the nurse is trained to assist parents in exploring ways of helping surviving children go through their grief.

In a typical case, a SIDS mother said, "I must have done or forgotten to do something that caused the death of my child." Upon hearing a statement like this, a nurse will acknowledge such guilt feelings, while offering facts concerning SIDS. Guilt can destroy emotional healing and affect an individual's self-concept.

Nurses have extensive medical knowledge and can assist the family in traveling through the maze of research findings regarding SIDS. Families may feel more intense guilt when they read about the risk factors of SIDS. It is important to note that risk factors in and of themselves are not causes of SIDS.

Grieving can be hard and lonely work. It is important to allow time to grieve. Grief, whenever it occurs, becomes a part of you. To deny the grief is to deny a part of you, blocking any healing. There is no right or wrong way to grieve the loss of an infant. Often well-intentioned family members and friends give suggestions on how the parents should behave or feel and get impatient with parents, encouraging them to get on with their lives. Parents will never get over the death of their child, but the intensity of grief will lessen to the point where the family members can once again go on with their lives.

The goal of grief counseling is to facilitate the tasks of mourning so that the bereavement process will come to a successful termination. Signs that may indicate complicated grief requiring therapy are the continued inability of parents to talk about the infant without experiencing intense, renewed grief and pain; a minor incident triggering a strong grief reaction; unwillingness to move material possessions belonging to the infant for an extended period of time; radical changes in lifestyle; a history of depression; self-destructive impulses; or phobias about illness or death. The goal of grief therapy is to identify and resolve conflicts of separation, which preclude the completion of mourning tasks. The general rule to determine if the family requires therapy is how their daily life activities are affected by the grief process. The nurse has been trained to assess the family's grief response and can recognize when a family needs psychiatric help.

Hitting It Off with a Counselor
An Interview with Mike Hitch
by Robin Rice Morris

Mike and Janet Hitch were blessed with a Christmas Eve baby boy and struck by a spring SIDS tragedy. Of all the things they learned about surviving a SIDS loss, the prospect that their marriage and two surviving daughters could be in real emotional trouble was perhaps the most unsettling. SIDS, Mike learned, could take surviving relationships hostage. The best way to avoid such further tragedy, he was told by many, was to get professional help early.

Less than two months after their loss, they contacted Cyndi Butler, a parent whose child attended nursery school with one of the Hitch's daughters. As a social worker who specialized in bereavement, she was like a gift dropped in Mike and Janet's lap. They had to do some fancy footwork with their HMO, including getting an approved doctor to "prescribe" Cyndi and to label the Hitches with an official diagnosis of adjustment disorder. But that sufficed for approval and thus partial reimbursement, making their weekly visits more affordable.

From their first meeting, Cyndi showed a solid understanding of the bereavement process. She could even identify with SIDS, having lost her younger brother to an infant death some 30 years before. "We really hit it off with her," said Mike. "It's an intuitive thing. It has to be, I think. I found Cyndi to be insightful, especially about the things we needed to talk about." As a "typical" man who had been raised to believe he should not express his emotions, Mike felt that it was easier to talk to a woman about the personal issues his son's death brought up. Over time, the three talked about a little bit of everything, with the topic of the day depending largely on the stages of grief in which Mike and Janet were at the time.

"In the early days it was denial and guilt. Now it is more about the transition to the resolution phase," Mike says. Throughout the process, Mike and Janet talked with Cyndi about their seven- and five-year-old daughters, who are also making their way through the grieving process.

Other than a few times when Mike was out of town, he and Janet always went to the meetings together. The couple found that it was as if they were on an emotional seesaw; when one was up, the other was down. "It was like we were a dynamic unit constantly shifting weight," Mike said.

According to Mike, who admits he's been conditioned not to express his emotions, the best thing about counseling was that it forced him to address his grieving needs on a weekly basis. "I joke that she's my exorcist, pulling those emotions out," said Mike. Often he would leave counseling sessions feeling worse for a few hours, and invariably the next day he would have a "blowout" of either anger or sadness. "She pulled all that to the surface. And at first glance, that's a negative. But in the long run it's a positive."

Mike and Janet saw Cyndi for about four months and then stopped. They felt that they had learned all they needed to learn. But in retrospect, Mike thinks he just got overinvolved in work. Later, as the dreaded time of Christmas approached, both Mike and Janet began to feel pressure, so they started therapy again. "It was odd," Mike said, "but Michael's birthday didn't really hit us so hard. It was almost anticlimactic. But in January, when everything else slowed down, it was miserable."

Today, as the Hitch family is almost upon the first anniversary of Michael's death, Mike and Janet have no special plans to end therapy. "Maybe in the summer," Mike says, "and maybe not. We'll see her as long as we need to."

My Lifeline
An Interview with Gwen Robinson
by Robin Rice Morris

Not long after her daughter Rachel died of SIDS, Gwen Robinson found herself thumbing through the local phone directory in search of emotional support. What she stumbled onto was a lifeline: a social worker named Gretchen Poole who taught a bereavement class called Healing the Loss. The class would meet 12 times in six weeks and take on anyone grieving anything. Gwen and her husband, Kevin, met all kinds of people, from a woman who suffered from 20 years of bottled up grief over the death of her mother to a woman who was suffering over the loss of a relationship with a father who was still living. Gwen and Kevin were the only ones who had lost a baby. Through sharing experiences, Gwen soon learned that "You can't compare your loss to another's loss."

This thought was reinforced when the couple attended a Compassionate Friends meeting, which addressed those affected by miscarriage, infant loss, and stillborns. "Each person in this world experiences their own losses and pain. I learned that even though my daughter died, that did not mean that someone who had a stillbirth or a miscarriage experienced less pain than I did." At the same time, Gwen did find comfort through being able to identify specifically with other SIDS survivors whom she met through a SIDS support group.

Using the *Grief Recovery Handbook* [1] by John W. James and Frank Cherry, co-founders of the Grief Recovery Institute, Gwen followed a step-by-step program for moving beyond loss. Her instructor, Gretchen, offered an alternative style of spirituality and believed in reincarnation. "I liked that," Gwen said, "because Gretchen believed that your child picks you to be his or her parent and that you have a contract with your child and God. It meant that my baby was able to learn what she needed to learn and was able to go on," said Gwen. "That was the most comforting way I have found to think of it."

Since then, Gwen has read several books about people who have survived clinical death and who now believe there is life after death. (One such book is *Beyond Death's Door*. [2]) "Before," Gwen said, I had never really thought about death and what happens afterwards."

In addition to Gretchen, Gwen got in touch with an individual counselor through an Annandale, Virginia, group called Haven. This non-profit bereavement support group offers lay counselors at no cost. Gwen and her husband Kevin were assigned to Peggy Cauley, a woman who knew grief well. Peggy had four children. Of the three with cystic fibrosis, two have already died. Together, Gwen and Peggy would look at pictures, go to lunch, or just meet and talk.

Between her class with Gretchen, various readings, support group meetings, and meetings with Peggy, Gwen has patchworked her way through the grief process. Yet even with these invaluable aids, Gwen still knows what she has always known: "You have to go through the grief process yourself. I knew that I personally had to go through the pain, and do it now, to be able to live and enjoy my life. Above all, I didn't want to be bitter."

Chapter 14

Emergency Medical Responders and the Authorities

When a SIDS death occurs, a whole host of strangers abruptly become integral parts of the survivors' lives. These strangers include 911 operators, paramedics, police detectives, physicians and nurses, medical examiners, SIDS counselors, and funeral directors. Often these professionals are sensitive about the tragedy of SIDS and are helpful to SIDS survivors. However, there are times when the survivor feels that a professional is insensitive, abrasive, or even downright mean. Survivors then have all the more anger to deal with.

Unfortunately, there is evidence that it is becoming more common to blame parents or other caretakers for a SIDS death. *Redbook Magazine*'s March 1996 issue documented a shocking trend among coroners and other officials to question a diagnosis of SIDS. Parents, already filled with "searing grief and stubborn self doubt," now "fear the reaction of friends and family who do not understand SIDS," the article states. Moreover, SIDS parents "fear that authorities, who are growing increasingly suspicious about every SIDS case, will accuse them of killing their own children, through abuse or neglect."

It's not that SIDS parents don't want a thorough investigation of their children's death. SIDS parents and their advocates at the national SIDS Alliance have led efforts to pass laws that would require rigorous investigation of all infant deaths. "Parents want the kind of resolution that a standardized procedure would provide," says Phipps Cohe, director of communications at the SIDS Alliance. Unfortunately, few communities have adopted standardized procedures for responding to SIDS deaths that would help police and other emergency responders pinpoint SIDS during their death scene investigations. In many communities sudden infant deaths are handled by medical examiners who are not specialists in pathology, forensics, or pediatrics.

The police investigation that must follow a SIDS death can be one of the most abrasive and frightening experiences for any parent. Emergency responders should try to keep in mind how bewildering and upsetting it is for parents to have strangers bursting in on them and immediately taking over their parental role. After finding her son Christian so obviously dead, Joani waited a few minutes before calling 911. "I knew they would grab him from me and that I would never, ever again have him all to myself," Joani said. When she did call 911 and the paramedics came, they rushed him into the ambulance and drove away, leaving Joani behind to tell neighbors how to reach her husband, Gabe. Of course, they were only doing what they were supposed to do, looking out for Christian above all else.

Later, having already been questioned by detectives at the hospital, Joani and Gabe were caught completely off-guard when they went home and found two more detectives taking pictures and examining everything in Christian's bedroom. The Horchlers had never before been investigated by the police for anything, and Joani's first thought was, "My God, do they really think we killed our own baby?" Would the police put her in jail for not checking him often enough, Joani wondered, or for not watching him breathe? Joani stayed downstairs while Gabe went upstairs to talk with the detectives. One of them, in a very kind manner, said, "You know, your son died in the safest possible place." While it seemed impossible that anyone could have died in "the safest possible place," Joani and Gabe were greatly comforted by this detective's simple statement. (Later, the Horchlers discovered that they had undergone a "death" investigation, which differs from a criminal investigation. Detective Steve Kerpelman explains the difference in an article in this chapter.)

To aid police officers in dealing with SIDS deaths, a training manual for investigations in Prince George's County, Maryland, where the Horchlers live, urges police officers to display "genuine tenderness and compassion" for parents, whom it calls "the real victims" in a SIDS case. The training book continues:

> *Officers must be particularly careful not to trigger doubts or guilt feelings in the parents. Lifetime emotional problems, divorce, or even suicide are very real threats to members of a SIDS family, and police officers must always conduct their investigations with these threats in mind.*

This manual[1] is well written and compassionate, an excellent example for all police officers and detectives to follow. It is available by writing to the Prince George's County Police Department's Education and Training Division. (The address is in the bibliography.)

Similar manuals are available to all types of emergency response personnel, including 911 responders, paramedics, nurses, physicians, hospital emergency personnel, and funeral directors. Several of these protocols may be ordered from the Pennsylvania SIDS Center[2], or through information obtained from the National SIDS Resource Center (See appendix for address).

Officers are allowed to tell parents during their investigations that the death appears to have resulted from SIDS. However, a final determination of the cause of death must be made by a doctor. Joani was first told that her son had probably died of SIDS by a hospital official, and it helped to relieve her racing imagination and self-recriminations. In fact, she had been so distraught on the way to the hospital that she kept thinking that if she had contributed to her son's death in any way she seriously intended to jump off the nearest bridge.

Once at Prince George's Hospital, a kind grief counselor named Rose Nalley was waiting for Joani. The counselor took her into a small white room, where a doctor told Joani that Christian had died and that preliminary results showed that the cause was SIDS. Father John Hurley, who had been summoned to the hospital by one of Joani's neighbors, arrived shortly after that and stayed as detectives interviewed Joani about how she had found the baby, whether anything had been abnormal that day, and what kind of pregnancy she had had. What Joani appreciated most, though, was that Rose let her stay with and hold Christian for several hours after he had died and made sure he wasn't taken away before Gabe—who had been away on a business trip—could get there to say good-bye to his only son.

Later, other professionals were there to help Joani. Pablo Renart, her obstetrician/gynecologist, reassured her that she was not to blame for the death. So did Christian's pediatrician, Ruth Steerman, who took the time to meet privately with Joani to review the autopsy report when it became available several weeks after the death. Three days after the death, Joani was contacted by a counselor from the SIDS Information and Counseling Program, which routinely receives medical examiners' reports of SIDS deaths and contacts SIDS parents to offer assistance.

Later, when Joani felt the need to consult the state medical examiner's office for more information and reassurance, she was given prompt attention and comfort.

Joani's experiences show the positive way in which a SIDS death can be handled. To encourage these kinds of responses, we begin this chapter with a list of dos and don'ts from the aforementioned Prince George's County Police Department training manual.

Dos and Don'ts for Emergency Responders
(A section from SIDS Training Module 85-2)

by Kerry Day of the Prince George's County, Maryland, Police Department

The Right Things for Emergency Responders To Do:

■ Encourage the parent to be patient with himself and not expect too much.

■ Say you are sorry about what happened to the deceased child.

■ Allow the parent to express grief as often as desired.

■ Allow the parent to talk about the deceased child as much as desired.

■ Reassure the parent that the child received the best of medical care and was well taken care of, if you know that to be the true case.

The Wrong Things for Emergency Responders To Do:

■ Say you know how the parent feels unless you have been a SIDS parent too.

■ Change the subject when the parent mentions the deceased child.

■ Avoid mentioning the child's name when appropriate.

■ Tell the parent how he or she should feel.

■ Try to find something positive about the child's death (such as a moral lesson or closer family ties).

■ Say the parent can always have another child, or say that at least there are other surviving children. (Other children can never replace the one who died.)

■ Make comments which suggest that the medical care given to the deceased child may have been inadequate. (SIDS parents are already bothered by doubts and feelings of guilt, and they don't need further "ifs" to ponder.)

When Emergency Responders Lose Their Own Baby

by Michelle Grogan

My husband Patrick is both a professional and a volunteer paramedic and firefighter (EMT-P). I work as a private, in-home day-care provider and as a volunteer emergency medical technician (EMT-B) with our local fire company and ambulance squad.

Our son, Aaron Christopher, was born June 29, 1996. He weighed 6 lb 15 oz and was perfectly healthy. Patrick and I were overwhelmed with joy.

For the first months of Aaron's life, Patrick worked 24 hours at a time from home on the paramedic unit of Annapolis City Fire Department. On September 22, Patrick was gone most of the night responding to 911 calls. When he arrived home in the morning, he awakened me as he came up the steps. He said, "Good morning" and went to Aaron's crib. He stood frozen, looking into the crib. I sensed that something was wrong but had no idea that I was about to suffer the shock of my life. As I sat up in bed, I remember thinking, "Put your hand on his back." Maybe I even said it. But just then Patrick started screaming, "Oh, my God, Michelle, he's dead!" As he knelt to the floor to do CPR, I jumped out of bed. I ran into my walk-in closet and fell to the floor, crawling around screaming, "No, God, no!"

Seconds, later, I crawled to the phone. As I started to dial, Patrick said, "Its too late!" I called 911 because, as parents, we needed help. As responders, we knew he was gone. Then Patrick again said, "It's too late; he's gone," while crying so hard that I couldn't understand him at first. I said, "No," over and over again, crying and screaming in fear and anger. When Patrick handed Aaron to me, I knew in my head that he was gone, but in my heart I couldn't believe it. Not us. Not our son. We can fix this! We have all the training!

Waiting for the ambulance felt like forever, but in reality it arrived in minutes. Patrick was in shock—shock like I've never seen in all the time I've been riding the ambulance.

I lay Aaron on the bed while I put on some clothes, and then I carried him downstairs. I sat on the couch rocking him, unable to look at his swollen, bruised face. His body was cold and lifeless.

Four of our closest friends arrived on the ambulance: Dottie, who was at the hospital when Aaron was born; Dallas (Patrick's best friend), who drove me to the hospital to meet Patrick when I went into labor with Aaron; and Wayne and Allen, with whom we've been close for years.

As Dallas rushed through the door, I could see the look of determination on his face. I said, "No, Dallas, no. It's too late! He's gone! No CPR. It's too late!" He believed me only when he held Aaron himself.

It's not easy *not* to do all that you have been trained to do. Saving lives is our business. It was not easy to face the truth—that our son was dead—to the point that CPR would have been senseless and cruel.

When the police and medical examiner arrived, I handed Aaron to Patrick and went outside to sit. Dottie sat with me and made some calls to my family for me. I was numb. I didn't cry. I didn't talk. I couldn't move my body, but I couldn't stop shaking.

It was very hard for the police officers to do their job. We've known them on and off the job for many years, some through the fire department, others more personally. As they asked us questions about Aaron, his crib, and other things, I could hear voices cracking and see tear-filled eyes. It was like a dream. My body was there, but I was looking in on this event. I kept saying to myself, "Wake up, Michelle. Aaron is okay; it's only a dream." But this was a living nightmare.

The medical examiner is a very close friend. She took pictures, checked Aaron's body, and filled out paperwork. Patrick helped with everything; I was frozen in the chair. Patrick called the funeral home and then said that I should hold Aaron before he went away. I held him tightly against my chest, still unable to look at him. I couldn't bear to see him like that. Then Patrick took him away in the ambulance to the funeral home just two blocks away.

We had a hard time during the next three days before the funeral: no sleep or food for me, just coffee and numbness. Patrick cleaned and cleaned and re-cleaned. He never stopped eating until he was sick, and we couldn't even look at each other. Actually, this went on for weeks. I was afraid that our marriage was over. How does anyone survive this kind of loss?

At Aaron's funeral, I was overwhelmed by all the flowers and cards. We met at my sister's afterward and then went home. Still very quiet, we lay in the bed looking at the empty space in the room where Aaron's crib used to be. We were still thinking, "How can this be?"

Then the ambulance siren blew, and I started thinking, "What if it's a baby?" I turned on the pager, and to my relief it was not a baby, but someone did need help. Again, the siren blew. They needed an EMT to get the ambulance out on the call. I hesitated, but then I thought, "I need to go and be on the ambulance for me and Aaron." It was hard getting back on that ambulance, the same one that had carried my son away from us to the funeral home.

Patrick wasn't able to go. All he could think about was that while he had been out saving someone else, his own son had been home dying in his crib. He made that statement a thousand times. He told me over and over, "What if I have to tell someone it's too late? I can't do it now, and maybe not ever."

After a few weeks, we returned to work. Patrick was put on the fire truck, not the paramedic unit. He felt that he was unable to make life-saving decisions and he was very afraid that he would go on a SIDS call and fall apart. I needed to ride the ambulance to ensure that everyone who called 911 got help just as we did when we needed it.

It's been three and a half months since Aaron's death. I ride the ambulance often, but I hesitate when it's a baby or a child. My fears overcome me at times. What will I do, what will I say, if the baby's gone? Will I fall apart on the scene, or will I be able to take over? Patrick is also able to ride more often. We both know when we need to step back and let someone else handle the call.

Patrick still cries every day. He visits Aaron's grave every three days and takes new flowers. We both miss him very much.

We both find that some times are harder than others. Patrick was telling me about a time he was in the fire truck and passing by a small boy held by his mother. As Patrick looked over, the boy said, "Fire truck!" and tears came to Patrick's face as he read his lips. We both love the fire department and what we do. We couldn't wait until Aaron could share it with us.

The hardest thing for us to face still is that we weren't given even a slight chance to use all the lifesaving skills we've learned to try to save our son. The ounce of hope that most people get when they call 911 was never given to us.

We find comfort in our belief that Aaron is safe with my mother and that he will never know this kind of pain. But we would give anything to have him back.

SIDS and the Homicide Detective
An Interview with J. Richard Salen and Steve Kerpelman

by Joani Nelson Horchler

More than 75% of the SIDS parents that Detective J. Richard Salen has worked with after a SIDS tragedy did not know what SIDS was when he tried to explain to them why their baby died.

Moreover, "I'm willing to bet that 95% of parents don't know CPR," says Detective Steve Kerpelman, a colleague of Detective Salen in the Prince George's County criminal investigation division.

These officers believe that if the risk of SIDS was better publicized and discussed by pediatricians, parents would feel less guilty in the aftermath of their babies' deaths. "SIDS is not being publicized enough," asserts Detective Salen. The detectives note that many people mistakenly believe that SIDS is due to suffocation, choking, or some other preventable cause. Therefore, when their own baby is found dead, they think they should have somehow been able to prevent it. More education about SIDS would lessen these guilt feelings, the detectives believe.

Because CPR can save the lives of some babies who stop breathing, CPR training should be a normal part of childbirth preparation training, says Detective Kerpelman. "It's strange that so much time is spent teaching parents how to breathe while giving life, and, at the same time, we don't teach people how to sustain that life after it is born," he states.

Detective Kerpelman stresses that when there is a death without obvious signs of foul play—such as a SIDS death—the investigation is a death investigation. "This is one which investigates the circumstances surrounding the death, and no one is suspected of any wrong-doing, as opposed to a homicide investigation, in which there are suspects, witnesses, and so on," he says. When a SIDS death occurs, there is usually no criminal investigation. The investigation turns into a homicide investigation only if during the course of the death investigation it appears that there may have been a criminal act.

Detectives Salen and Kerpelman also discuss how they determine whether a child has died of SIDS. Detective Salen notes that it is routine for detectives to search the entire house to determine whether the infant was cared for properly and had an adequate supply of food, diapers, and other necessities. The condition of baby equipment must also be documented in the officer's written notes because the discovery of a dangerously defective item could be important if an autopsy later reveals that the child died from injury. Officers also need to obtain the names and assignments of all ambulance crew members and make a list of what lifesaving actions were attempted. This is important because CPR efforts can produce injuries that might suggest possible child abuse if not otherwise explained. "Cracked ribs are one of the most common negative side effects of properly done CPR," notes Detective Kerpelman.

Officers walk a thin line when investigating SIDS deaths, says Detective Salen. "Unfortunately there are people out there who do abuse and kill their children, so we have to go in with an open mind while still being compassionate."

Detective Salen stresses the fact that all police officers in Prince George's County learn that SIDS is a death to which any child—including their own—can fall victim. "I have three beautiful daughters, and SIDS was always in the back of my mind when they were babies," the detective notes. "I guess that's why I always make an effort to treat parents the way I'd want to be treated."

Officers are cautioned to be aware that several "suspicious" conditions might be observed in an infant's body that are quite normal in a SIDS death. These include a bloody froth around the mouth or nose and possible discoloration of the face or extremities. The Prince George's County police training manual states that "lividity stains in an infant are more pronounced than in an adult, and apparent bruises on a baby might in fact be exaggerated lividity."

In fact, if there are no fluids on the sheet where the baby died, it would "raise questions," says Detective Salen. Some parents have felt so guilty that they have actually changed the sheets on the baby's bed before investigators have arrived. "But a savvy detective would discover that," Detective Salen says.

Preservation of the scene is, in fact, perhaps the most difficult of the officers' jobs. If the child is clearly dead and is not undergoing lifesaving efforts, the officers are required to keep parents and other family members from handling the child's body and tampering with personal-care items. Officers obviously have to be extremely tactful in separating the parent from the child and are urged to stress to the parent that the separation is only temporary until the proper investigatory procedures are completed.

The task of the detective is not always pleasant, but both Detective Salen and Detective Kerpelman agree that the more the public knows about SIDS the easier their jobs will be.

How NOT To Treat a SIDS Survivor
by Darlene Buth

SIDS is something you read about but think can never happen to you. Then it hits you like a ton of bricks.

I seem to be a normal, happily married woman with two beautiful daughters. But what most people do not know is that I am the mother of three children, not just two. My oldest daughter, Amanda Lynn, is nine. My second daughter, Kayla Ann, is three. My third child was a little boy who arrived on Sunday, July 23, 1995. Although he came three weeks ahead of schedule, he was given a clean bill of health, weighing eight pounds, three ounces. He was the apple of his parents' eyes.

Yes, we thought we were a complete family, with two healthy girls and now a little boy. Our dreams were all finally coming true. We named that little boy after his daddy, James Alan, and his grandpa, Pete. Peter James-Alan. We called him PJ.

Before we knew it, the baby was six weeks old and it was time for Mom to return to work. I loved the time off, but I knew there was no way we could pay our bills unless I returned to work. Fortunately, my husband and I worked different shifts, so we shared child-care duties and didn't have to worry about child-care expenses. I worked during the day and came home to my family at night.

Then one day our world caved in. I got up for work as usual on October 3. I went downstairs, showered, got dressed, and fixed a bottle for the baby. I went back upstairs and fed little PJ. He drank his bottle and dozed back off to sleep. Part of me wanted to stop time and just stay there cuddling him, but I had to go to work. So I gave him a little kiss on his head like I did every morning and tucked him back into his crib with his 101 Dalmatian friends. I didn't know these events were going to be turned into sweet memories...just sweet memories...and never again would I be able to share sweet moments with my son.

At work, talk was about the O.J. Simpson trial. Today the verdict would be in. Would he be convicted of murdering two people or would he be acquitted? Then everyone heard that O.J. was a free man. All the talk about whether it was a fair trial and whether O.J. was guilty or framed was going to have a lot of significance for me in a short time.

Someone from the Personnel Department came in and told me I had to go home due to a family emergency.

"Don't bother with cleaning up. You have to get home and I'm taking you," she said. I had no clue as to why. Thankfully, I lived only three blocks from work. When we pulled up to the side of my house, I saw a police officer standing outside talking with our insurance agent. Yes, I did recall that he was due to stop by with some paperwork, but what did this have to do with the police?

"What's going on?" I asked.

"Just go in the house and you'll find out," I was told. I walked into the house, and you could have heard a pin drop in it. There was another police officer in the dining room. My husband was in the living room dressing our two-year-old. I looked around the room and did not see my son.

"Oh, my...where is my baby?" Complete silence. My husband finally said that the baby was on the way to the hospital. Earlier, my husband had gotten up to answer the door, and he came back to find the baby not breathing, with bluish skin. He called 911 right away and called work for me to come home.

I received no words of encouragement from the police officers. Not even, "I'm sorry for what you are going through." Nothing. All they said was, "We'll be back later to question you about what happened."

Question us about WHAT? I didn't know what had happened or why it happened.

The ride to the hospital was dreadful. Though we lived only 15 minutes from the hospital, it seemed like hours. All the way there my image was of holding PJ that morning and seeing him smile at me when I laid him back in his crib. I thought he had to be all right because I loved him and he was an important part of my life. I hoped he would be crying for his mother when I got there.

At the emergency room we were met by a couple of nurses. I could barely get the words out, "Take me to my baby; I want to see him now." They led us to a small room and said the pediatrician would be in to talk to us in a moment.

All I could think of was, "NO! This cannot be happening to me! Not my little boy! He's a healthy boy."

Well, the doctor came in and told us that they had done everything they could, but they could not bring my little boy back. I just wanted to scream out, "This isn't fair! You can't take my little boy away from me!" They said we lost our boy to Sudden Infant Death Syndrome. No clue as to why—just that he died peacefully. I still have to ask why God took my little boy's life away and gave O.J. his freedom. This just does not feel right or fair to me.

They led us into the examination room where PJ was lying peacefully in a little crib. My husband was by my side carrying our little girl.

They notified my parents. My husband's parents were already on the way to the hospital. They called our minister. They told us to say our good-byes and all I could think of was "How do you say good-bye to your baby?"

I sat down in the rocking chair, and they placed the baby in my arms just as they had done when he was first born. He looked so peaceful, as if he was just sleeping. I just wanted to shake him to wake him up. I needed to tell him that I loved him and that I needed him to be alive, to just please start breathing again for Mommy. I just wanted to take that baby and run as far as I could, but I could not even find the strength to get up. Somehow we found the strength to leave the hospital, only to go home and face more tragedies and pain that would never go away.

Back at home, still filled with shock and disbelief, we were greeted at the door by the police and two people from the Human Services Department. They separated us. A police officer and a worker from

Human Services questioned my husband in the front room, and I was questioned in the kitchen. There was no sympathy or understanding from these people.

"What kind of life insurance policy does the baby have? How much is it worth? Who is it payable to? How is it payable? How does your husband treat the children? Why does your oldest child have a different last name? Where is her father? Does your husband feel angry or bitter that he has to support her? Are you collecting child support from her father? What kind of temper does your husband have? Has he ever lost his temper? Is he violent? Do you feel safe with him? Do you feel that the children are safe?"

During this questioning my in-laws came in with my two-year-old. They were told to leave the house and take the child with them and that they could come back when the questioning was done. But after a while my mother-in-law came back in because she was concerned about what they were doing. She was not allowed to say anything, but at least she was in the room with me.

After they stopped grilling me, they toured the house. My husband led them to the couch where PJ had been. They took pictures and said they needed to check out the rest of the house.

We took them upstairs to the girls' bedroom. There was only one bed set up. They wanted to know why. We tried to explain to them about the recent recall of bunk beds. Our two-year-old had gotten her body stuck in the headboard. We didn't want to take any chances, so we had sent the girls' bunk beds back. We told them that we had to buy another mattress so we could set up the other bed. I couldn't understand what the big fuss was all about because my two-year-old loved the chance to sleep in Daddy and Mommy's bed and to take Daddy's spot when he was at work.

But these people wouldn't listen. They just said it was wrong and that a two-year-old should be sleeping in her bed. They wanted to know what was in all the boxes and bags in the closet. We told them it was clothes that the children needed to grow into. They told us to get them out of there because it was a fire hazard. "And, by the way, we could give you a fine for that."

I just couldn't understand what they were trying to do. Where was the compassion? The caring? Where were the kind words? Why were they treating us this way? What did we do? We had just lost our son. What did all this have to do with it?

We found out the answer to that a long, horrible week later. We were being accused of foul play...insurance fraud. They wanted to remove my daughters from our home because they thought it would be in their best interest. All this threw me completely off balance. How could they think anyone was capable of harming their own baby, let alone killing him? I never could or would harm any one of my children or anyone else's children. I kept telling them over and over that I would not harm my baby for money. Money means nothing to me. If you bring my little boy back I will give you all the money I have. All I want is my son back, alive and healthy. They left the girls with us, but they did not stop harassing us. They continued to investigate for insurance fraud.

We somehow made it through all the funeral arrangements. We picked out an infant coffin and had his bumper pad from his crib cut to fit the coffin. We also had his crib sheet and comforter put in his coffin. This way he looked like he was peacefully sleeping in his own little bassinet with his 101 Dalmatians looking after him. We bought a little miniature yellow Tonka dump truck representing the big one that he was going to get for Christmas. We created a little memory board with all his pictures on it.

The next few weeks were terribly difficult, still being questioned by the police for foul play even after the autopsy showed no signs of foul play and that our baby had died of SIDS. It was just before Christmas that we finally got the police off our backs about insurance fraud. The chief of police called and wanted to come to our house to discuss results of the blood tests. We knew nothing about any tests, so we called the hospital to try to find out what was going on. The hospital could not release any information to us and told us to call our doctor.

Our pediatrician was very confused and shocked when we told him that we were under investigation for foul play in the death of our son. He told us that after the autopsy no further blood tests had been ordered. There were no results because there were no tests. This doctor was not only our children's pediatrician but also the doctor the county used in cases of child abuse. If he had ever seen a problem he would have been obligated to report it to the proper authorities. But he had never seen any signs of child abuse in our family. Therefore, he called the police and told them in no uncertain terms that there had been no foul play and that they were not helping to ease our grief with their handling of the case.

To be accused of killing our own child is something that I will never forget or understand. We loved our baby and would do anything to bring him back. It is obvious that a lot of professionals who should know about SIDS do not know anything about it. Why can't professionals be trained to deal with SIDS properly and compassionately? Why do these people treat parents with so much contempt? If all their questioning is part of their job, why can't they figure out a better way of doing it? SIDS is a very tragic, painful experience, so why do they add to the agony?

The "Suspicious" Loss of Twins

by Joani Nelson Horchler

"I thought I was going to jail for murder, even though I knew I hadn't done anything," Kimberly Panuska said after her twins died of SIDS. "My main concern should have been for my babies," Ms. Panuska said, "but instead I was forced to worry that they were going to break up my whole family."

On February 21, 1993, Ms. Panuska and George Blair of Baltimore tried to wake up their six-month-old twins for their noon feedings and were horrified to discover that they were not breathing. However, instead of receiving sympathy and understanding, the couple fell under suspicion of child abuse. Their four-year-old daughter was taken from them for 10 days by social workers acting on mistaken advice.

Upon discovering their stricken twins, the parents called 911, and Mr. Blair resuscitated them. But the twins, who had not breathed for 15–20 minutes, had suffered brain damage. At Johns Hopkins Children's Center, Todd appeared to be recovering until Brandon died on February 23. Todd quickly began deteriorating, too, and died the next day. "It was like there was some kind of bond between them," Ms. Panuska said.

Returning home from the hospital at about midnight on the first day of their ordeal, the couple were shocked to learn from Ms. Panuska's mother that a male policeman had, in their absence, made their four-year-old daughter pull down her pants and pull up her shirt so he could check for signs of abuse.

The suspicion of child abuse resulted from erroneous reports by a hospital technician who thought an X-ray showed that one of the babies had fractured ribs and misinterpreted the discoloration from resuscitation efforts as bruises. The technician was later shown to be wrong, but his report was enough to prompt the visit by the police officer and subject the couple to hostility from the hospital staff and social workers.

Within just two days of the twins' deaths, Dr. John E. Smialek, Maryland's chief medical examiner, gave the provisional cause of death as SIDS and said that there was no evidence of foul play. Two months later, he made that judgment official. In addition, police found no evidence of abuse, but they told Ms. Panuska that if she didn't cooperate they would put her daughter in a foster home. The child was taken away for 10 days, although Ms. Panuska succeeded in having her placed with her aunt.

The separation was extremely hard on the mother and child. "I'd call her three or four times a day, and she'd beg me to bring her home. When I cried and told her I couldn't, she wouldn't talk with me anymore. She was mad and felt abandoned," Ms. Panuska said. "She was all I had to hold onto, and they wouldn't let me be with her."

Inaccurate hospital reports also led to inaccurate media accounts, which made Ms. Panuska and Mr. Blair afraid to stay in their own home. "I thought a rock was going to come through my bedroom window," Ms. Panuska said. "There were so many reporters posing as me and as doctors that I couldn't get through to the hospital to check on my own babies. I had to start using my birth date as a code to call the hospital and get information."

Many national and local media reports persisted in using incomplete information. For example, based on Ms. Panuska's frantic call to 911 dispatchers saying that she found the twins "wrapped in a blanket," some reports implied that the twins were wrapped in the same blanket and could have suffocated. "Who in the world would wrap two babies in the same blanket?" Ms. Panuska said. Although they were wrapped separately in blankets, the twins were sleeping in the same crib, kept apart by a rolled-up comforter in the middle of the crib. Their pediatrician had said that was okay because they had been born two months premature and weighed less than 11 pounds each at six months of age. They both stopped breathing with their heads to the side and their faces uncovered.

Dr. Smialek's verdict exonerated the couple. Their twins were the victims of SIDS, the most common cause of death for children between one month and one year old. It kills one in 650 infants and is more common among twins than among babies born alone. But simultaneous deaths among twins are rare. Only 11 other cases have been documented in the world.

SIDS, thought to be caused by an immature or abnormal brain stem, is considered unpreventable. But Ms. Panuska said that only one social worker treated her with decency and respect. Two who didn't came to the family's house four days after the twins' funeral when Ms. Panuska was exhausted from her ordeal and running a 101-degree fever. "They nitpicked about a plant in my bedroom and whether it was there when the babies stopped breathing, and then they interrogated me about where I was going to get the puppy I had promised my daughter after her brothers died," Ms. Panuska said.

Officials in the family preservation office of Maryland's Social Services Administration declined to comment, saying only that the procedures followed in the twins' deaths were "according to our policies." Dan Timmel, (now former) director of the SIDS Information and Counseling Program in Baltimore, a support service for bereaved families, said that the state had a mandate to protect the surviving child.

"But the issue is how the removal was done and the degree to which it was done," he said. "Should a male policeman force a young girl to remove her clothes, and couldn't the state's mission have been accomplished by placing the child with a relative overnight instead of for 10 days?" Mr. Timmel also questioned the accusatory, unapologetic attitude that persisted among hospital and government workers even after Dr. Smialek announced that his verdict would probably be SIDS.

Ms. Panuska and Mr. Blair are very angry about how they were treated at the hospital. "You'd figure they would have been supportive, but the nurses and doctors were just mean...and they never bothered to apologize for us about the misread X-ray that was a major reason our daughter was taken away from us," Ms. Panuska said.

"I didn't want publicity at first, but now I want the world to know that all we ever did was love our babies, and we were treated awfully," she said. "We realize how difficult it is to believe that two babies could die of natural causes at the same time in the same place, because we ourselves still find it almost impossible to believe, but that doesn't excuse anyone for presuming we were guilty without any evidence.

"We were just dealt an incredibly bad hand in life, and we've already suffered enough without people inflicting more pain on us," Ms. Panuska said.

After the Blair case was officially labeled SIDS, Mr. Timmel visited Ms. Panuska and Mr. Blair at home to talk with them and their daughter about SIDS and offer support and contact with other bereaved parents. Ms. Panuska said that his visit was "very helpful. I wish everyone would have been as supportive in our time of need."

A small blessing for which Ms. Panuska and Mr. Blair are grateful is that Chief Medical Examiner Smialek happens to be one of the most knowledgeable physicians in the world on the unusual subject of simultaneous deaths among twins. In 1986, Dr. Smialek researched nine cases of twins dying simultaneously of SIDS and wrote an article about how bereaved families are often subjects of suspicion despite medical evidence gathered in both the United States and Europe demonstrating that twins do die simultaneously of SIDS.

"Although SIDS is now widely accepted as a condition that parents have no power to predict or prevent, the occurrence of simultaneous deaths of infant twins is a phenomenon that still evokes bewilderment and suspicion," Dr. Smialek wrote.

In the past, SIDS deaths have often been wrongfully attributed to parental negligence, such as suffocation, overlaying by parents sleeping in the same bed with the infant, or pneumonia. "Such opinions were the result of inadequate investigation, lack of careful autopsy studies, and uninformed human nature, both in the lay and professional community," Dr. Smialek noted.

Although Dr. Smialek did not speculate on what causes twins to die simultaneously, he quoted another researcher as saying that "it is the very quality of being a twin which somehow or other is combined with a predisposition to sudden, unexplained death."

An edited version of this story appeared in The Washington Times *on June 6, 1993.*

The Role of the Medical Examiner

by John E. Smialek, M.D., Chief Medical Examiner of Maryland

The shock and disbelief experienced by parents who find their seemingly healthy baby dead are soon accompanied by an urgent need for answers and explanations as to how this could have happened. Families are not alone in their search for answers to this overwhelming loss. Society also has a very serious interest in the cause of any child's sudden and unexplained death. For this reason, medical examiner and coroner laws exist in all parts of the United States for the specific purpose of authorizing a legal investigation into the circumstances and cause of death of any individual, including infants and children. A proper scene investigation, together with a careful autopsy examination, will in most cases provide an answer to the cause of the child's death. At the very least it will exclude evidence of injury or neglect as factors in the death of the child. However, the autopsy cannot be relied upon as the sole source of answers. Suffocation or strangulation may leave little, if any, evidence on a child's body to indicate that the child has died as a result of an accident or even a homicide. If a proper scene investigation is not carried out, questions will remain unanswered and suspicions unallayed long after the death.

Understanding the purpose of such an investigation can help relieve the baby's parents from feelings of persecution or unfair treatment by law enforcement officials. A professional, objective approach on the part of police officers carrying out an investigation, without an accusatory overtone, would certainly do much to help the parents at such a traumatic point in their lives. Indeed, the author has witnessed increasing recognition by police agencies that infant death investigations often result in determinations that the manner of death due to SIDS was a natural one. As a result, these agencies have modified their approaches to the investigation and interrogation of the family members. (Perhaps this change has resulted from the awareness that children of police officers and other law enforcement agents can be lost to SIDS as well.)

In the investigation of an infant death, the pathologist plays an important role. He or she is responsible for the physical examination of the child, which may include toxicological and biological tests to determine the cause of death. Depending on the experience and training of the pathologist, he or she might be able to reach a conclusion as to the cause and manner of death within 24 hours of the completed autopsy and assessment of the information from the investigation of the scene and other medical records. This prompt completion would allow the pathologist to contact the family and inform them of the results of the autopsy examination and investigation. It also provides the pathologist an opportunity to explain to family members what SIDS is and means and assure them that they could not have predicted or prevented it.

The family should expect to receive information from the pathologist at the earliest possible time. If they have not received communication as to the cause and manner of death, they should realize that they have every right to contact the medical examiner or coroner to obtain the autopsy results. In a minority of cases, questions may still exist at the completion of the autopsy. Additional procedures such as toxicological tests or microscopic examination of tissues may be required to resolve these issues. Several days, or possibly as much as two to three weeks, may be necessary to complete such studies. If further investigation of the circumstances of the death is warranted, however, an even longer period of time may be involved.

Pathologists should realize the key role that they have in the treatment and support of parents who have been victimized by SIDS. They should recognize that the prompt sharing of information about this killer of approximately 4,000 infants in the United States each year means a great deal to a couple struggling to deal with the guilt of having been unable to prevent the death of their beloved child. At the same time, parents should realize that a proper and thorough investigation and autopsy examination are in their own best interest. This is the only way that information can be gathered to answer future questions about the death of their child. Such questions may become even more important if and when other children are added to the family. Parents should also realize that they are entitled to information gathered in the course of this investigation and autopsy. They should not be reluctant to seek answers to questions that trouble them.

Chapter 15

A Subsequent Baby and the Question of Home Monitoring

Whether six days or six years after a SIDS loss, most parents hold their breath when they think of having another baby. Rightly so: Having a subsequent baby after a SIDS death is usually a terrifying proposition. Many, many questions surface. Can a survivor possibly love another baby even half as much as the one who died? Will the new baby be thought of as a replacement for the one a survivor will always miss? When is it too soon to have another baby? Most frightening of all, will this baby die, too?

Once the plans for another baby are actually made, and possibly before, another important question must be answered: Will a home monitor—a source of comfort for some and stress for others—be used to check on the baby's breathing and heart rate? Most of the time, these questions are answered slowly and after much thought and advice-seeking. Fortunately, what feels most right for parents is often best.

When Should You Have Another Baby?

The standard advice of grief counselors is to wait for at least one year so your decision won't be based solely or primarily on your intense grief. Counselors also typically believe that having another baby can interfere with the grief process by preventing parents from allowing themselves to experience the extreme ups and downs of the grieving process that are necessary for healing. Indeed, some SIDS parents who got pregnant shortly after their babies died feel that they "crashed" emotionally several weeks or months after their new babies were born.

One mother explains that she didn't want to allow herself to be miserable about her dead baby when she was pregnant for fear that her emotional state would harm the new baby within her. She also "felt guilty for not being happy" when she was pregnant, and thus put her grief for her dead baby "on hold." After the new baby was born, she felt guilty that she hadn't "grieved completely" for her dead baby. At the same time, she felt emotionally torn between completing the grieving process for her dead baby while trying to "be happy" for her new and very alive one.

Whereas the above potential pitfalls should be considered, many SIDS survivors believe that having a subsequent baby early on is an individual decision. Many couples who get pregnant right away say that the anticipation and arrival of their "healing babies" helped them enormously, not by replacing their lost child, but by giving them hope and filling their empty, aching arms. Several parents explain that they had desperately wanted a baby and had had everything ready for a baby. Thus, they questioned why they should avoid pregnancy and put off the fulfillment of their dreams of parenting an infant. This rationale is augmented by those who have had infertility problems or are moving past the childbearing years.

(A study by Dr. Frederick Mandell found increased rates of miscarriage and infertility after a SIDS death, probably due to the physical and emotional stress related to grieving.)

Should You Have Another Baby at All?

Maybe for you it's not a question of how soon to have a new baby, but whether you can garner the courage to have one at all. For a parent who has lost his or her first child and has not had the experience of raising a child past infancy, the fear can be almost overwhelming. After a SIDS death, you may find yourself amazed when other parents take their eyes from their sleeping babies. You're also likely not to believe it when you hear the news that someone "just had a baby and he's perfectly healthy." You think, "Sure, my baby was perfectly healthy, too, and he died!" However, the great majority of subsequent siblings to SIDS deaths are healthy and do survive infancy.

Is Your Next Baby at Greater Risk for SIDS?

It's a statistic that none of us like to think about, but several studies have indicated that the SIDS risk among subsequent siblings of SIDS victims is about three to five times higher than the rate of SIDS among the general infant population. However, "most, if not all of this increased risk is explained by the fact that, as a group, families that lose a baby to SIDS have an increased number of adverse risk factors at the time of their first SIDS loss, and in many cases those adverse risk factors (e.g., maternal smoking) are still present at the time of the next pregnancy," says John G. Brooks, M.D., professor and chairman of the Dartmouth Medical School in Lebanon, New Hampshire. "Families that have none of the established risk factors were probably at very low risk for losing their first infant to SIDS and are probably at equally low risk for losing a second infant to SIDS," he notes.

If it is of any comfort, one controlled study done in Washington state showed that SIDS families had no more risk of losing another child during infancy than comparable families who had not lost an infant. Some other studies have shown that the risk is less than 1%.

Should a Subsequent Baby Be Monitored?

Home monitors keep tabs on a baby's breathing and heart rate. When either drops below a certain level, an alarm goes off, signaling to caretakers that there is a problem. If the baby isn't breathing or doesn't have a pulse, mouth-to-mouth resuscitation or CPR must be given. However, the great majority of alarms are false, caused by shallow breathing, a baby old enough to play with the wires, and numerous other factors. Moreover, if some researchers are right, an actual SIDS baby cannot be revived in any event.

Indeed, several SIDS parents interviewed for this book cite how their babies appeared to die almost instantaneously despite immediate resuscitation efforts. For example, Martina Murphy tells of how her son Jimmy was alive and alert in his stroller when she bought an airline ticket and was noticed dead just a few minutes later when she went through an airport metal detector. A nurse and a policeman happened to be walking by and immediately gave him CPR correctly, to no avail.

There is much controversy in the medical community over whether home monitoring can actually help save lives. Many experts contend that home monitoring cannot make much of a difference because only 7% of SIDS deaths involve infants who have had either apnea (cessation of air flow at the nose and mouth) or apparent life-threatening events. However, monitors can provide tremendous emotional support for parents who have lost babies to SIDS.

Many parents feel that a monitor, which is prescribed (literally) for valuable research and medical reasons, is really a tool for a parent's peace of mind. And why not, if it helps a survivor sleep through the night? SIDS mother Liz Waller says that she was able to fall asleep feeling reassured that "those flashing lights on the monitor were there to tell me everything was okay."

The University of Maryland SIDS Institute and many other medical groups recommend home monitoring of SIDS siblings, usually for a six-month period. Many commercial insurance companies have agreed to this recommendation. (If your insurance company at first refuses to grant your request for full or partial payment for a rented monitor, obtain letters of support from physicians and keep appealing, because it is likely that you will prevail.)

Dr. Robert Meny, director of the clinical division of the University of Maryland SIDS Institute, has used memory monitors to study changes in the baby before the alarm sounds. His research has shown that the heart rates of babies who died while being monitored were abnormally low when their monitors began to alarm for the last time. Thus, even though the alarm alerted the parents to trouble, they were unable to resuscitate their infants. This means that it is crucial to look for some earlier sign—one that precedes a fall in heart rate—so that parents can successfully resuscitate their babies. Dr. Meny proposes, with further funding, to test the use of oxygen monitors (which also, like currently used monitors, track heart rate and apnea) in the home setting.

Dr. Meny theorizes that because there is evidence that low blood oxygen levels precede a drop in heart rate, oxygen monitors may be able to prevent some SIDS cases by providing earlier warning to parents of babies considered at higher risk for SIDS, such as subsequent siblings to a SIDS death.

What If You Can't Have or Don't Want Another Baby?

Healing from a SIDS loss does not depend upon having another baby. Even if you cannot or choose not to give birth to another baby, you may be able to find other ways to nurture a child. Michelle and Arnett Spady found comfort and joy in adopting an infant boy. Other parents become the favorite aunt or uncle of the family and help out other parents by offering babysitting services. If a couple chooses not to have another baby, they may receive negative comments from others, feel "weak" for not having the courage to face another death, or even question whether they loved their lost baby as much as other parents who do choose to have a subsequent child. Like all of the choices after a SIDS death, subsequent children must remain a choice made by the parents and should be supported by their families and friends.

Thoughts on a Subsequent Pregnancy

by Sheri Laigle

What is it like to be pregnant again after a SIDS loss? There is joy, of course, along with excitement, love, nervousness, and morning sickness—everything there is for any new mother-to-be. There are plans to make, things to buy, changes to discuss. There are people to tell and congratulations to receive. But there is also something different, different from my past two pregnancies and different from the pregnancies of my friends, sisters, and neighbors. Certainly different from the pregnancies written about in books and followed in the magazines. This time there is something else, something that haunts me. It is something that wakes me at night, fades our smiles as my husband and I spread the news, and robs the "pregnant glow" from my cheeks. This time there is fear. There is uncertainty. There is sadness and pain. This time there is the constant ache and longing for another baby, as well as this one. A baby who might have shared this special time with us. A baby who began life in the same womb, in the same way, just months ago. A baby who died.

As I sit and stroke my belly, still round from a previous pregnancy, I am overwhelmed by emotion. My blood, filled with hormones, brings tears to my eyes that spill over and fall into my lap while my vision blurs and my fingers shake. Will my baby live? I can't help but wonder. Will he even be born? If so, will he make it through the night? Will she thrive and grow? Will he learn to smile, lift his head, grasp a toy in his fingers? Will she wear dresses, feel the sun on her face, pick flowers in the springtime? Will he take his first steps on our hardwood floors, speak his first words, feel the thrill of independence? Will she ever feel anger or throw a tantrum? Will he know sadness and rain? Will my baby grow up?

The heat creeps through the window, and sweat breaks out on my forehead. I am not sure I know how to mother you, my child; I fear I will rob you of your birthright, to be loved and raised as any child—normal, healthy, and imperfect. You have the right to a night of undisturbed sleep, a late afternoon nap by the pool in your carriage, and a visit to your grandparents', snoozing dreamily in your car seat while I drive. You have the right to a mother who calmly soothes and reassures you when you sneeze, cough, or catch a cold. You have the right not to spend your infancy in doctors' offices and apnea clinics. A right not to be subjected to tests, tubes, and monitors, or to be shaken and waked when you try to do what comes naturally to you—to sleep.

What will become of the rest of us? Can we ever enjoy you as you were meant to be enjoyed, as we did your brother and sister before you? Can I still smile at you as you twist and sigh in your restless, newborn dreams? Can I lean my head back in the armchair and nap with you after you nurse yourself to sleep in my arms? Can I tuck you into bed with your warm papa at night, then linger in a hot bath while you sleep? Will I ever feel rested, cheerful, grateful? Will that special ease of instinctive, confident mothering ever be mine again? Will I love you for who you are, rather than who you are not? Will I rush you through your first year of life, ignoring the milestones and excitement until you emerge from the "danger zone"? And all those only to look back wistfully as you blow out your first birthday candle, feeling that we've missed you, never known the baby you were, never gloried with you in the special warmth and beauty of infancy?

I stare at you, tiny lump beneath my skin, and as the spinning fan dries the tears from my cheeks, I can only smile. Who knows what the future will bring? I love you now and always will. Just like the bond between every baby and parent, ours is a unique and precious one, filled with its own, individual history of hopes, fears, and expectations and blessed with its own special rewards, for both parent and child. Ours is a wonderful and miraculous bond, one that only you and I will share, healthy, human, and full of promise. May it last forever.

Another Baby with Dark Brown Eyes

by Kandace DeCaro

Eight months after my daughter Kelly Marie died, I became pregnant again. I was still so very depressed that I had no hopes for this new pregnancy. I was sure that I would have a miscarriage even though I had never had one before. Then I did, and it was awful. I kept crying in the hospital that day, waiting for a D&C. I just kept crying for Kelly over and over again. I was so sure that my attitude toward my pregnancy had somehow caused the miscarriage that I discussed it with my doctor. He assured me that that was not the cause.

Two years after Kelly died, I became pregnant again. Again, I was in a state of panic. We wanted this baby so badly, but I was afraid of another miscarriage, and of course, of SIDS. Indeed, it was a difficult pregnancy. Unfortunately, after losing a baby to SIDS, it seems quite impossible to take joy in another pregnancy. You are so torn. You want another baby, but you miss the one you lost. Fear seems to overtake you constantly. I'm afraid that I don't have much good advice for this situation. You can only take it one day at a time. I prayed a lot. We discussed the use of an apnea monitor with the doctor at the SIDS Institute in Baltimore and decided to use one.

The most difficult part came when we had to open Kelly's bedroom for the new baby. The door had been closed for more than two years. This, in truth, had caused some problems for our younger daughter, Julia. She had become afraid of closed doors. She did not want to be in any room with the door closed. I think that she came to associate a closed door with death. Thank goodness, I had the help of a dear friend, whom I had met in the MIS support group. She, too, had lost a baby, a son named Frank. I was so afraid to open that door, but my friend was with me. The experience was not as bad as I thought it would be. Yes, everything was the way I had left it a few days after Kelly died. But, somehow, my friend and I set to work with a vengeance. I took everything out of the room and quickly put it in bags to sort out later. We cleaned the whole room, taking the curtains down and opening the windows. Later, my husband painted the room, and we put up new curtains.

It was strange, yet good, to see the sun shining through that room again. As my pregnancy progressed, I felt that I was more ready now to have another baby. When the time came, I thought about Kelly through my entire labor. I couldn't help it. I wondered if this baby would remind me of her. After having three girls, weren't we surprised to have a little boy! He was beautiful! Yes, he does remind me of Kelly. My daughter Katie has blue eyes. My daughter Julia has hazel eyes. Kelly had dark brown eyes, and I remember thinking when she died, "I may never have another child with beautiful brown eyes." But then I did.

Thomas's eyes are a source of joy and heartbreak at the same time, for they will always remind me of Kelly. It is still difficult at night when I sit in the rocking chair in his and Kelly's bedroom. In the dark, with his dark eyes, he often reminds me of her because I used to sit there and rock her to sleep.

Monitoring Thomas was very difficult, and yet I couldn't have managed without it. It gave me a great sense of security, especially because I was home alone with him most of the time. Of course, you are in constant fear of the specter of SIDS, and even your dreams are affected. Once Thomas had passed the point at which Kelly had died, six and a half months, I started to feel a little better. At seven months, we took him off the monitor. Recently, we celebrated his first birthday, and I'm finally breathing easy again.

It is a very long road, learning to cope with your grief. You die within yourself, and you have to learn to come back to life. It's a slow process, and there's still an empty space in my heart that will never be filled. It has Kelly's name on it, and there's another one for the child I lost after Kelly. I am grateful, though, for the children I have left. They have given me a reason to live.

Celine

by Marie-Pascale Hill

This is the first time I am writing about Celine since her death. It hurts so much to write, maybe because it only happened a few months ago. Celine was my second daughter. My husband and I felt that we had the perfect family (I have always loved girls), and that we should stop with number two. Three months later, we were transferred to the United States from Brussels, Belgium, where we had lived for three years. To make the move easier for the children, we left them for a few weeks with my parents in France until we were settled. Unfortunately, Celine never made it to the United States. Five days after our arrival, my mother called and told me that Celine never woke up for her 9 am bottle.

We were in shock; it was unreal…We were so far away, it was just like a nightmare. The first night, I was physically sick, spending my time on long-distance telephone calls trying to ease my mother's guilt and also figure out what we were going to do. We decided to fly to France the next evening to attend the funeral. Although I was on valium, which did help to relax my body, it was the hardest thing I ever had to do in my life. But it was something I felt I had to do—for Celine, for me, and for my relatives.

I never saw Celine after she had died. In one way, I wish I had held my lifeless baby once again, but in another way I'm glad that I didn't because I fear that I would have been haunted forever by the image of her dead. My remembrance of Celine is one of a healthy baby and moments of happiness. However, looking back, I still can't say whether or not I did the right thing.

At the funeral I touched the coffin, and while in the car going to the graveyard my husband and I kept talking to Celine. God, I felt so close to her. She is buried in a nice little cemetery in our family village of France. The cemetery is surrounded by yellow wheat fields. It is peaceful and pretty. During the week I was in France, I came back a few times a day to talk to her. They were very intimate moments, which I miss now that I live so far away. Perhaps because she was not cremated, it feels like Celine remained at my parents' village. I still talk to her, but she is there, 1,000 miles away.

For my two-and-a-half-year-old daughter, Anne-Charlotte, it was always very clear that Celine would never come back. She believes that Celine is like a little star, and whenever Anne-Charlotte sees a star it is Celine. Six months later, she still claims to anyone that she has a little sister whose name is Celine. We often talk about Celine with joy and remembering, but when Anne-Charlotte sees me crying she knows how sad I am sometimes. "You cry because of Celine," she says, and I always make sure to tell her that I am usually happy because of her. At Christmas, she said, "I want to have a baby, but forever." I am now three months pregnant and tell her that this is forever, although inside of me I am not sure.

In some ways, this new baby has been the biggest relief since last July. But in other ways, my feelings are mixed about this new baby because I carried Celine only a few months ago. It brings back so many recent memories, yet it also brings so much hope. When I think of babies now, it is not just with the pain of the past but also with the hope of the future. I can hold a baby again and touch baby clothes without having tears in my eyes. I thank God for being pregnant again. Although I know Celine will never be replaced, I feel as if a part of her will come back in my next child. After all, my subsequent children would never exist if it were not for the sacrifice of Celine. God knows what those children and future adults will bring to this world. Inside of me—as a proud mother—I will always know that they would not have been if it had not been for their sister's death.

Celine made me aware of all the precious moments I am sharing with my oldest child. You just don't know how long you will have happiness, so you must take advantage of it while you can! Anne-Charlotte has helped me tremendously in coping with my grief, and I enjoy every single moment that I spend with her. I think about how great the pain must be for those parents who lose their first child, and how awful it must be not to have other children to love and hold. Hearing about situations worse than mine, which I always do, makes me feel that I have no right to complain.

Celine's death has definitely changed me. Some for the better, some for the worse. I must say that I have lost a lot of my enthusiasm and joy of living, which used to be so much a part of my character. I miss the innocence and good sense of humor that I once had, and I wonder if I will ever get them back.

Five months later: I am now eight months pregnant and expecting a little boy. Celine's death anniversary is coming this week, and somehow I feel relieved that it will soon be behind me. There is no comparison between how I feel today and how I felt the last time I wrote about Celine. A year later, I am myself again. I am, and have been, extremely happy for the past four months, even though Celine is constantly in my thoughts. I have regained my enthusiasm and sense of humor, and I have so much energy. I feel ready for happiness again and to go on with my life in a very positive way, in memory of my beloved daughter, Celine.

Room for More Angels

by Deneena Herrera

When Kendal was born on March 31, 1989, I considered my life complete and perfect. I had a beautiful, healthy baby boy. I was ready to go off with my husband, Bill, and my son to lead a happy, content life. Our lives were filled with much joy and happiness. Kendal grew so big so fast, and he brought more love to our home than I ever thought possible. I recall many wonderful times together—Mom, Dad, and baby Kendal. We were truly experiencing what unconditional love was all about. Then, on November 15, 1989, Kendal left us for heaven to be with Jesus. This was when I discovered what hurt really was.

For me, it was that aching, empty, lost feeling that wouldn't leave me. My life was shattered, and I didn't know how I'd ever put the pieces back together. I had to redefine who I was. Was I still a mom even though my only child was gone? Were my husband and I merely a "couple" again? After four months of not having Kendal with us, we decided to have another baby. Kendal had been conceived without any trouble, so I fully expected to have another baby in my arms in only nine months. Those nine months came and went before Bill and I would conceive.

In November 1990, we found that we were expecting again. It was a very emotional time for us. We were happy and excited, yet at the same time frightened and apprehensive. I had come to realize over those months of trying to get pregnant that this new baby was not going to be Kendal, that he was in heaven and would not be coming back to us. I also worried whether I could love another baby as much as I loved Kendal. In my heart, Kendal was perfect, and I could not imagine having enough room in my heart for another child. It was such a confusing time for me, wanting with all that was within me for another baby, and at the same time worrying that I wouldn't be able to love it enough.

I now know that God had been listening to my worries. On August 1, 1991, He gave us a daughter whom we named Devon and kissed away all those reservations I had. As soon as I saw her emerge from within me, I fell in such love I could hardly contain my emotions. It felt so right, so wonderful, so perfect. I had worried for nothing because I found there is plenty of room in my heart for two angels: the one in heaven and one on earth. I believe there's even more room for more angels in the future.

The Haunting Memory of SIDS

by Jennifer Wilkinson

The morning after Christmas 1984, I discovered my three-and-a-half-month-old daughter, Larkin, dead in her bassinet.

"We'll have another baby," my husband, Ken, and I had agreed, as we stood clutching one another and sobbing, minutes after our terrible realization. It was an immediate reaction for me, straight from the gut level.

Yet as my family and I set shakily forth into those bleak months of recovery, I felt equally torn between the urge to play life safe and appreciate the family as it now was and the desire to tempt fate by trying to have another baby. I had a very definite wish to defy the force that had taken Larkin from me, but along with that desire went the total conviction that the force in question was bigger than me.

What if it happened again? Would any of us be able to survive it? It was all too real for me to assume, as so many friends did, that this time would be different. In the end, I decided that another baby was the only solution to closing our family's wound. While Ken was initially very frightened by this prospect, he finally came to this conclusion too.

Because a large percentage of SIDS babies die in the winter months, Ken and I decided to aim for a spring birth, which would put the baby's highest risk for SIDS, three to six months, in the summer. I was lucky enough to conceive as planned, with the baby due in early March. My initial reaction was disbelief, followed by overwhelming emotion of every kind—joy, fear, dread, anticipation, excitement, longing. In the course of the pregnancy, these feelings would take turns surfacing, producing in me an exhausting overall emotional state.

When we announced our news, the children were overjoyed. Emily, six, and Claire, five, immediately decided not only that we should have another girl and name her Larkin, but that we would have a girl who would look just like Larkin. There was in me, too, a secret desire to fantasize that we were bringing Larkin back somehow.

I still felt very uncomfortable around children of two different ages—the age Larkin would have been, and even more so around those the age Larkin was when she died. I worried about these fears and wondered if I'd be over them by the time the baby was born.

The first anniversary of Larkin's death was the hardest day for me to get through. We had decided it would be easiest for all of us not to be at home, where she had died, so we rented a house in Vermont with my sisters and their families for Christmas. It was a beautiful place on a hill with lots of snow, and being there was better than staying home. But what a sad day it was.

I woke up around 7:30 as I had the year before and relived every minute of that terrible morning in my mind: my initial surprise at the baby's oversleeping, running to her room, my immediate alarm at her motionless body, the hideous realization. It still makes me almost physically ill to remember it.

By January, I knew I should start getting things ready for the new baby. I was still having trouble focusing on it, though, and felt a certain element of panic. When, on the eve of a baby shower a friend had organized in my honor I found myself sobbing uncontrollably at the thought of having to look at baby things, I realized the depth of my fears. As I opened the gifts of outfits and toys, I thought to myself: "Won't it be nice if the baby lives long enough to use these?"

The shower gave me the impetus to sort through the baby things I already had. It was a task I'd been dreading. One of my sisters had hastily stuffed Larkin's things in bags and put them in the attic after she died. I had to decide what to do with them. With a pounding heart, I climbed the steps to the attic. There was the bassinet, the pink and blue blanket she had been under when I found her, her little blue Christmas dress and the unopened presents to her. I took the blanket in my arms. It still smelled of my baby, my beautiful little Larkin.

Most of the things Larkin wore I discarded, while others I put aside for the new baby. There seemed to be no rule of thumb in the process, but I felt comfortable allowing my instincts to guide me. Strangely enough, I now get great comfort from having the pink and blue blanket folded in my study, though I have never been tempted to put it over the new baby.

As the due date approached, each family member showed signs of strain. I started having nightmares similar to those I had just after

Larkin died, but now there were often two babies in them. There was one particularly horrifying one in which, when I went in to the new baby's room, I found Larkin's dead body next to her.

Our doctors recommended monitoring the new baby as a matter of course for a SIDS sibling. They sent us to Children's Hospital several weeks before the birth to meet with the pulmonary specialist, Dr. Robert Fink. He taught us how to use the monitor and how to perform infant CPR. I fought tears as I went through the motions of resuscitating a life-sized baby doll. Could I have saved Larkin?

We were introduced to the monitor that day. It was physically much less threatening than I'd expected. It measured 9 x 8 x 3 inches and weighed only a few pounds. The nurse familiarized us with the alarm sounds: the constant shrill beep of the machine alarms for technical difficulties and the intermittent loud beeps of the human alarms: heart rate fast, heart rate slow, apnea. When a baby is attached to the monitor, lights flash in time to his or her breathing and heartbeat.

My doctor decided to induce the baby a week before my due date. Larkin's birth had been extremely quick and had some minor complications that required the suctioning of her lungs and stomach. Induction would give the doctors more control over the birth and would allow them to monitor the baby closely in the process.

I was deeply thrilled to have another girl and relieved that she seemed healthy—and did not look at all like Larkin. But I was worried that I did not feel the immediate bond I had felt with the other girls. I was all the more worried when I got my first glimpse of the baby on the monitor.

Her hospital monitor had a TV screen attached to it showing her heartbeat and respiration. I found myself mesmerized by those lines, convinced that if my eyes were to leave them, the baby would die. Time and again, the nurse would come ask if she could take the baby back to the nursery so that I could sleep. But I felt safe only if I could feel her breathing, and I would keep her on my chest all night. Ken and I decided against using either of Larkin's names for the new baby. But using Larkin's initials, we thought, would be a way of honoring her without jeopardizing the new baby's identity. We settled on Lucia Anne—Anne for my mother who had recently died, and Lucia in part for its meaning: "bearer of light." I desperately hoped this baby would see us out of our dark time.

I was still haunted, though. During those long nights in the hospital, three words kept pounding over and over in my head: "Lucia is dead. Lucia is dead." Why was I torturing myself so? I wondered. Then I remembered an article I had read about the Soviet dissident Andrei Sakharov who had recently been released after 10 years in a Siberian prison camp. He said one of his survival techniques had been to repeat over and over to himself: "killed by firing squad, killed by firing squad" so that when his captors did threaten to kill him, he would be immune to fear, so accustomed was he to the sound of the words. Lucia's death was a very real possibility to me. I guess I was attempting to soften the potential blow.

Our homecoming was far less ecstatic than with Larkin. I was exhausted from my sleepless nights in the hospital, and the initial phase of monitoring was brutal. The monitor reinforced everyone's total fixation on this child's breathing. There were the constant flashing lights and signs posted all over the house: "CPR: An Outline Reminder" with bold subtitles, "IF BABY DOESN'T START CRYING OR MOVING" and "IF NO HEARTBEAT FELT."

There was a moment of true panic at the sound of our first real alarm. Doors flew open as each family member came running to save the baby. We never had to resuscitate her, but we did have several apnea alarms in the first month. We learned that short periods of infant apnea are quite common in the first month of any life and don't necessarily lead to apneic episodes later on. But they kept us on our toes.

We also responded regularly to machine malfunction alarms when the electrodes attached to the baby became loose or one of her wires was getting old. Then we discovered that a number of other common alarms sounded enough like the monitor to make at least one of us jump up to check the baby: Ken's work beeper, the washing machine's signal that its cycle is finished, trash trucks backing up. I must have been exceptionally tired the day I responded to a cricket. But in time, in spite of the monitor's constant intrusions both day and night, we all became quite dependent on those little green lights signaling that all was well.

With Lucia's arrival, friends started opening up to me more about what they had been through when Larkin died. I was appalled at the misinformation some heard from their pediatricians. The notion that no baby ever died of SIDS while sitting up was one. Until I reeducated my friend, her baby had spent his nights sleeping upright in his stroller. Another friend was told incorrectly that breast-fed babies never died of SIDS. The most outrageous statement, though, was that most SIDS cases were really attributable to child abuse.

When we passed the three-and-a-half-month mark (the age when Larkin died), I started to relax more and felt myself naturally growing closer to Lucia. Because I had never seen Larkin at that age, the temptation to compare the two babies was gone. I noticed, too, that people slipped up less often on her name, and thus we began to allow her to have her own identity. Interestingly enough, the immediate family had no trouble calling her Lucia from the beginning, whereas friends had routinely referred to her as Larkin and then apologized profusely, assuming I was offended by the blunder. In fact, it pleased me to know that Larkin was not forgotten.

By this time, the monitor was very much incorporated into our lives. I was used to trekking it upstairs and down depending on where the baby was, and I had even mastered the art of getting the baby hooked up without waking her if she fell asleep unexpectedly.

One night when Lucia was about four months old, the machine alarm went off in the middle of the night. I threw open the door to her room to find her absolutely beaming with one of the wires in her hand. She had finally found a use for these silly things that had been dangling from her chest since birth: room service.

Lucia became increasingly wise to the speed with which a grown-up appeared when she tampered with the wires. This meant many, many more false alarms in the middle of the night. Fortunately, she never learned, as some children do, to set off the apnea alarm by holding her breath.

Lucia regularly went through sleep studies that record every breath of an eight-hour period so that the pulmonary specialists can fully examine the breathing patterns of an entire night. The apnea clinic at Children's Hospital advised parents of subsequent SIDS siblings to monitor for six months, at which time the baby can come off the monitor if all the sleep studies have been normal. All of Lucia's tests had been normal.

At about five and a half months, Lucia was setting off so many false alarms that we took her off the monitor on our own authority. We didn't get much sleep in those first monitor-free nights, but we're progressing nicely. She's six and a half months old now, and with each day there is an added sense of confidence. Whereas the presence of the monitor had initially given me peace of mind to get some sleep at night, its absence now gives me faith in the baby's ability to survive on her own.

There are still moments of panic, of course. I have yet to wake up in the morning, for instance, without a sense of dread and a pounding heart. But so far, that dimpled little smile has always been there to reassure me when I open the door.

The above article is excerpted from The Washington Post *of October 7, 1986.*

Forever in Our Hearts

by Nick Missos

Your room was quiet for a while,
      your things all packed away.
Our hearts were heavy all the time.
      We thought that's how they'd stay.

Our days were filled with darkened skies;
      our grief was at its height.
Then God smiled down upon us
      and sent a beam of light.

A new babe sleeps in your crib now,
      who's brought us joyful tears.
He's brought us peace and happiness
      but also many fears.

A baby sleeping quietly
      is not the joy it used to be.
Anxious moments every night,
      afraid to check and see.

Your loss has taught us many things;
      now we cherish every day.
You'll never be forgotten.
      In our hearts you'll always stay.

A Clinical View of Monitoring

by Robert Meny, M.D.
Director, Clinical Division, University of Maryland SIDS Institute

SIDS claims almost 4,000 victims per year in this country. It has intrigued me for 20 years, and I have been speaking to groups about it for 15. Whenever I lecture, especially to bereaved parents, a conflict arises between providing information and my fear of causing pain and inflicting guilt on those in the audience.

The greatest conflict comes when discussing whether SIDS can be prevented. It is compounded by the often expressed belief that because SIDS has no cause, it can't be prevented and because it can't be prevented, parents need not feel guilt. This credo was created by well-meaning people, but it makes little sense because all diseases ultimately have causes and, we hope, ultimately can be treated or prevented. It also had a negative effect on research aimed at the prevention of SIDS.

As both a SIDS clinician and a neonatologist, I have always felt that at least some SIDS deaths can be prevented. This belief originated during my fellowship years in the neonatal intensive care unit, where I saw nurses routinely stimulate, and sometimes resuscitate, preterm babies who had apnea, bradycardia, or color change. Most, but not all, of those resuscitations were successful. Had there been no intervention, some of these babies probably would have died. At autopsy, some of them might have had no sufficient cause for death: hence, SIDS.

Intellectually, the idea that a monitor, which follows both breathing efforts and heart rate, could prevent SIDS seems plausible; on a very simplistic level, death occurs either because breathing stops or because the heart stops beating. Indeed, I have met dozens of parents who are convinced that monitors saved their babies' lives. Moreover, I have reviewed memory monitor printouts that initially appear to be recorded deaths because they exhibit several minutes of a low heart rate, dropping further despite stimulation. This is a feature I have seen in many death recordings. But with administration of oxygen, there is a gratifying increase in the heart rate and an apparent saved life. I use the word "apparent" because one cannot prove a negative.

For these devices to "save a life," a train of events must take place. First, the monitor must be used, and its alarm must occur early enough and be loud enough so that the caretaker can hear it and act on it soon enough. Next, the caretaker must be able to resuscitate even though panic-stricken and even though resuscitation training may have occurred months before. An ambulance with well-trained attendants who can provide oxygen must arrive within minutes if the resuscitation by the caretaker is not effective in reviving the infant. Finally, for the most severe events, hospitalization in a pediatric intensive care unit must be available for those infants who require mechanical ventilation. There are a number of infants who meet all these criteria.

To play devil's advocate, I must admit that there is no widely accepted, prospective study that proves that home monitors do prevent SIDS (or, for that matter, that they do not prevent SIDS). However, one study in Baltimore showed a declining SIDS rate for babies born at University Hospital.[1] A program at that hospital selected many babies for home monitoring based on abnormal sleep and feeding behavior. During the same time period, the SIDS rate for babies born at Johns Hopkins University Hospital was stable, whereas that hospital was not monitoring nearly as many infants born there.

In addition, Drs. Spitzer and Gibson[2] in Philadelphia evaluated more than 11,000 patients over a 13-year period and monitored 7,700 of them. Assuming that the average death rate for SIDS was two per 1,000, of these more than 11,000 patients, at least 22 would have died. Because many of these infants were at increased risk, the authors suggest that their risk was considerably higher than two per 1,000, that it was 5.5 per 1,000, and that more than 60 SIDS deaths would have occurred. Instead, only 9 SIDS deaths were reported in this retrospective review, a statistically significant decrease from both 22 and >60. Of the 9 SIDS deaths, 7 occurred in association with noncompliance. I should add that there is also no controlled study proving the efficacy of hospital monitors.

Unfortunately, some infants have died while being monitored whose parents began resuscitation quickly and performed it to the best of their abilities. These relatively rare and tragic cases may be telling us that cardiorespiratory (apnea) monitoring is not good enough for all infants. Perhaps some infants require an oxygenation monitor instead of, or in addition to, the more traditional cardiorespiratory monitor because a decrease in oxygenation may occur long before the cardiorespiratory monitor sounds an alarm. By the time the monitor alarm rings, resuscitation may be impossible because the alarm occurs so late in the dying process.

Three separate studies, however, show that most infants who die with a cardiorespiratory monitor prescribed die when they are not on it or when it is inappropriately used.[3-5] For example, we reported[5] on the deaths of 10 infants who had monitors prescribed at the time of their deaths. Six to eight of those infants were either not on their monitors or their parents did not respond to the alarm at the time of their death. This correlation between noncompliance and death is consistent and striking; it implies to me that had the monitors been used appropriately most of those infants would not have died.

In addition, there was a drop in the nationwide occurrence of SIDS during the decade of the 1980s, especially in New York City.[6] No one is certain why this decrease occurred, but monitors may have played a role. Finally, approximately 75% of all SIDS deaths occur in "low-risk" babies: full-term, healthy babies whose parents and doctors have no clue that their baby is destined to die. Even among premature babies weighing less than 3.5 pounds, a "high-risk" group, most clinicians do not advocate universal monitoring. Rather, we attempt to identify individual babies who require intervention. The bottom line is that the great majority of SIDS victims cannot be identified before death.

Another conflict-ridden topic is whether parental behavior influences SIDS risk. For example, all epidemiologic studies that look at cigarette smoking during pregnancy show that SIDS risk is increased for babies whose mothers smoke during pregnancy. Even more striking is the existence of a dose-dependent relationship: In other words, the more cigarettes smoked, the greater the risk of SIDS. Such a relationship implies that smoking does contribute to SIDS. A recent publication states that there would likely be a 30% decrease in SIDS if smoking could be prevented during pregnancy in this country.

I am concerned when presenting this information to an audience of SIDS parents because I know that some mothers in the audience smoked during their pregnancies. Although it is important to be truthful, I do not want any parent to feel that a specific action such as smoking caused the death of his or her infant. Indeed, most parents who smoke do not lose their babies to SIDS, and smoking by itself does not put a baby in the "high-risk" group, although it does increase risk to about three times normal.

Frustrating for both parents and physicians are the many uncertainties about SIDS. The recommendation in 1992 by the American Academy of Pediatrics that babies be put to sleep on their sides or backs is a prime example. That recommendation fueled debate among pediatricians about its validity. Many of us thought that it was premature for a variety of reasons. When parents hear this debate, they don't know how to position their babies, and they feel real frustration. Fortunately for parents and for us physicians, too, it has become clear since 1992 that the proper sleep position is on the back. In the United Kingdom, the "Back to Sleep" campaign led to a 50% drop in SIDS in the span of a few years. We are making progress in combating SIDS, but uncertainties will remain, and medicine is not an exact science.

Tips for Home Monitoring

An Interview with Barb Follett of Kirson Medical Equipment Company

by Joani Nelson Horchler

When you need a home monitor, you may be confused about where to go and what to ask. You may also be overwhelmed at just the thought of having a machine in your house that is likely to occasionally send you bolting upright at 2 or 3 am, running to answer what you hope is a false alarm.

However, once families get used to home monitors, "You can hardly drag them away from the parents when the baby no longer needs one," says Barb Follett, a professional services representative for Kirson Medical Equipment Company in Baltimore, who brings rented monitors into homes and teaches parents and other family members how to operate them. "Parents often say they can sleep better knowing that the monitor will alert them to any problems the baby might have with breathing or heart rate," notes Barb. In fact, she says, some parents get so attached to their babies' monitors that "they actually become hostile when doctors and insurance companies say it's time for the baby to be taken off!"

Business is booming for rental companies like Kirson because, as Barb notes, "We're seeing a lot more premature babies being sent home on monitors rather than kept in the hospital."

Barb tells the story of one "preemie" whom she believes was saved because the monitor alerted her and other emergency response personnel to his cardiac distress. The baby's very young mother, who was living with her parents in a rural area of Maryland, had the baby over her shoulder when Barb walked in to download the monitor routinely. (Monitors must be downloaded at least once a month so that doctors or nurses can analyze the data they collect on the baby's heart rate and respiration.) The "low heart rate" alarm kept going off as the mother patted her baby and walked him around the room, but the mother thought it was just another false alarm and asked Barb for help in stopping it. "The baby's color was gray," Barb recalls. "I threw the monitor on the computer and saw immediately that the alarms were true. The baby was literally being kept alive by his mother tapping him and stimulating him. We got him to a local hospital where they stabilized him, and then he was flown to the University of Maryland Medical Center, where he recovered."

In telling this story, Barb hastens to add that this baby was considered at high risk for cardiac problems. By contrast, as Dr. Meny notes in this chapter, about 75% of all SIDS deaths occur in "low-risk" babies—full-term, healthy babies whose parents and doctors have no clue that they are destined to die. Thus, parents have no cause to feel guilty that they were not monitoring their babies who died. There is also no guarantee that a monitor could have alerted SIDS parents quickly enough for them to have been able to resuscitate their babies; babies have died while being monitored even after being given expert CPR within minutes of an alarm signifying trouble.

Many parents say that their insurance companies have told them they won't help pay for a monitor, especially in cases where a monitor is requested for a subsequent sibling to a SIDS death. However, Barb advises parents to "keep appealing" because, with persistence, parents will usually prevail. Some parents have switched pediatricians to get one who will go to bat for them with their insurer. Many parents have the University of Maryland SIDS Institute or similar organizations write letters and make phone calls to insurers for them.

Once a monitor is recommended, it should be used religiously, says Barb. In fact, there are compliance logs built into monitors so that doctors can tell whether and how often it is being used. If parents or guardians repeatedly neglect to use a prescribed monitor, they can be reported to state protective services. However, both she and the prescribing doctor normally "go to great lengths to work with people" before such drastic measures are taken, stresses Barb.

Sometimes a parent has a problem with the patches that connect the baby to the wires from the monitor. Occasionally, they cause skin irritation, and in such cases Barb usually recommends that the patches be replaced with a soft belt that goes around the baby's chest area. She says that even six-pound babies can be hooked up to the monitor with a belt.

Barb sees her role as being wider than just as a downloader of the monitor. For example, she notes that "lots of nurses are still not telling new moms that it's thought to be better to place babies on their backs" and thus sees it as part of her job to educate patients about such pediatric recommendations.

Barb advises parents who are inquiring about a heart and respiratory monitor to ask the following questions:

- Which monitors do you make available to patients? (There are several manufacturers. You may want to see their product brochures and instruction manuals.)

- Does the monitor you recommend have a memory? If so, what does it record? (Heart rate? Respiration? Oxygenation?)

- Do you accept all insurance and medical assistance?

- Does my insurance company have a contract with you?

- Who follows the baby's progress? A nurse or respiratory therapist?

- How often are visits?

- Is there a charge for additional visits?

- What will be my total out-of-pocket expense after insurance companies and medical assistance pays?

- Can the equipment company read and analyze the printouts for the doctor if necessary? (Normally, a doctor at a hospital will analyze data from your monitor.)
- Does the equipment company teach CPR?

When You've Lost Your Only Boy or Only Girl

by Joani Nelson Horchler

I was browsing at a yard sale recently when the friend hosting the event came up to me and said, "You don't need any of this stuff. You don't have any boys."

If you're a bereaved parent who has lost your only boy or only girl, you know how much this comment hurt me. It's horrible enough to have lost my only son Christian to SIDS five years ago (as of this writing). But it's salt in the wound to have people (many of whom know we lost our only son) always making comments like the following:

—"You're lucky you have only girls. Boys are just a lot of trouble." (What I would give to know how much trouble boys are!)

—"You have *five* girls? I bet your husband is really disappointed he doesn't have a son." (Go jump in a lake!)

—"Some people just can't make boys." (Hey, buddy, we *did* make a boy. It's not our fault he died.)

—"Maybe your husband has only girl sperm." (As if girl sperm is inferior to boy sperm! Anybody have a good comeback to such an incredibly rude, insensitive, and stupid comment?)

—"You shouldn't care if you have girls or boys. It doesn't matter a bit." (This comment typically comes not only from someone who has never lost a child but from someone who is lucky enough to have both sons and daughters. Of course, such fortunate people don't think it matters. They'll never think it matters unless they ever become unlucky enough to lose their only son or daughter. Then they'll find out how much it matters the hard way.)

I know I sound bitter, and I really try hard not to be. But I miss so much my masculine little boy. He looked and felt so different from my little girls. Even as a baby, he seemed like a little man to me. His hands were so big—like bear paws. He was my miniature version of my husband. He was the promise of the continuation of my husband's name. I could see in him characteristics of my brother who had died and my father who had died. I imagined my son with swimming trophies and out on the soccer field, the best player ever.

Now I am proud to see my smart 14-year-old daughter winning swim meets with incredibly fast times and my intelligent 12-year-old and 8-year-old daughters excelling in sports and acting. The two youngest daughters, born after Christian, have brought much laughter and fun back into our lives.

Both my husband and I adore our five girls, and we try to give them our best. We are grateful for the joy and the pride that they continue to bring us. Our children are our greatest gifts, and we are lucky to have them.

But one of our greatest gifts is gone, and we cannot pretend not to miss him and all the emotional and spiritual wealth he represented to us. Although he could never be replaced by any other child, male or female, I still think it would be easier if we could have another son someday. Then I would feel that God—or fate—was at least making an effort to replace some of the precious things that died along with our son—such as the continuation of my husband's name within our family and my only chance to be the mother of the groom. Unfortunately, we will never have another son. We cannot afford to have more children. SIDS stole our only precious chance to have a son.

Almost six years after my son's death, I still feel that it's okay to feel some remorse at finding out you're expecting a child who is not of the same gender as the one you lost. It's only natural to want to come as close as you can to replacing what you had. Not being able to replace the dreams for either a boy or a girl represents a huge additional burden not faced by those parents lucky enough to have other children of the same gender as the ones they lost.

We love our five daughters more than I could ever put into words, and they have made us happy beyond measure. But I refuse to pretend that I don't miss the only son I'll ever have, the son who was wrenched from our lives for no good reason.

I correct people when they say, "Gabe and Joani have only girls" because it's not true. We have a beautiful son whose spirit will always live within our hearts. That's why I always include, when signing our family letters, "and Christian in spirit"—so people will remember (and I hope, say) that we have "five daughters and a son who died of SIDS."

Chapter 16

Guilt and Risk Reduction

That hated "P" word is burning SIDS parents' ears more and more often these days. Much is being written and discussed about how SIDS can be "prevented." At least one book even uses the words "preventing SIDS" in its title. This usage has caused additional anguish for many newly bereaved families, who are being led to believe that they could or should have done something to prevent their babies' deaths.

The controversy over the "P" word can be heard loudly and clearly over the Internet. Dr. John L. Carroll, a contributor to this chapter, decided to stop using the word after he was lambasted by e-mail from SIDS parents that accused him of both inaccuracy and insensitivity. "You seem to be quite out of touch with what happens when the headlines proclaim, 'SIDS CAN BE PREVENTED,'" said one SIDS mom. "It casts suspicion on those of us who have suffered the loss of our babies to SIDS."

It's "not an issue of trivial semantics," raged another SIDS parent. "I can't tell you the number of parents who are so filled with guilt because they didn't turn the baby, or they let their friends smoke around him. They have internalized this message 'prevent' as that they didn't do it right."

As the first article in this chapter clearly shows, SIDS can and often does happen against all odds, when the parents have done everything right. This is the message that is being lost in the media flurry over SIDS "prevention." We SIDS parents have a message for everyone concerned with this issue: Don't say that SIDS can be prevented until there really are specific measures that SIDS parents can take to *guarantee* that their babies won't die of SIDS. To do otherwise is to do a deep disservice to those of us who have done everything by the book and yet have been cheated out of raising our children. Risk reduction is the accurate and compassionate term.

As Dr. Carroll told *The Baltimore Sun*, "I don't use the term preven- tion in connection with SIDS anymore. I think the message [to reduce risks] can be gotten out just as powerfully without using that word."

Dr. Gary Hoffman, an obstetrician whose own daughter died of SIDS at age 16 months, also strongly favors the term risk reduction. As presi- dent of SIDS Resources of Oregon, Dr. Hoffman has observed that some recent diagnoses of SIDS have "implied that the cause of death was sleeping on the stomach." He warns that such diagnoses—which are based on the erroneous belief that SIDS can be prevented—can lead to false accusations that parents or caretakers actually caused a baby's death by putting him to sleep on his belly. "Putting a baby on its back to sleep is not preventing SIDS, but is just reducing the risk of SIDS," he stresses. "You can do everything perfectly and still have a baby die of SIDS, and you can do everything wrong and yet have a baby live."

To publicize compassionately the risk-reduction message, Dr. Carroll and others have contributed to an excellent video. *SIDS: Reducing the Risk* brings together SIDS researchers, physicians, and policy makers to give parents the most current and important steps that can be taken to reduce a baby's risk of SIDS. This video can be ordered for $19.95 plus $3.50 shipping and handling by calling 800-450-6530.

Against All Odds

by Chris Brink

For all SIDS survivors, retrospect is inevitable. All parents relive the details over and over, investigating every avenue, trying to see where we went wrong or what we could have done differently. We wish that our little Emily's story might help remove some of the horrendous guilt that we as SIDS survivors carry unnecessarily.

It was December 28, 1996, three days after our first and only Christmas with Emily and three days before my birthday. Todd and I were four and a half months into our new role as parents when our world suddenly caved in. I had quit my job to be a full-time mom, and living on just one paycheck was an adjustment. We were getting by, however, and marveling at how life really didn't get any better than this. I had recently taken a part-time job on Saturdays, so Saturday had become Daddy's day to spend alone with Emily and play Mr. Mom.

On this particular Saturday, Todd surprised me by walking to my work with Emily in our new baby backpack. I took a break, and the three of us went outside to talk and spend some time together while I nursed Emily. I recall how warm and beautiful the day was and how hard it was to let go of my daughter when it was time to go back to work.

After walking home, Todd and Emily drove to a friend's apartment to stay until I left work. Emily became fussy shortly after they arrived, so Todd thought that she might be getting hungry. He was holding her and trying to calm her, when suddenly she arched back in his arms and instantly started turning gray. At first he thought she might be choking, but her limpness indicated that something more serious was wrong. He started CPR, and our friend called 911 immediately. The paramedics arrived quickly and tried to stabilize her condition before transporting her, but they could not find a pulse, and she was brought to the hospital with the paramedics still trying to start her heart.

Meanwhile, our friend paged me at work and told me to go to the hospital, saying, "Something is wrong with Emily." I could not drive fast enough as my mind raced over the possibilities. All the way there, I was assuring myself that it would be okay.

It was not okay. The doctors and nurses worked on Emily for about two hours. I worked on God for the same two hours, praying for a miracle. My request was denied. Paddles, injections, and other methods were used to try to restart Emily's heart, but nothing worked. We were informed that "it does not look good for Emily," and we were finally allowed to see her in a last attempt to have her respond to our voices and touch. However, it turned into a time to say our good-byes.

When we walked into the room, Emily's eyes were slightly open, and from a distance I thought she was looking at me. But as I moved closer, I realized that her eyes were lifeless. I held her hand, which felt nothing like I knew or remembered. I begged my little one to hang on and assured her that I loved her. I knew at that moment that she was gone. I left the room in a state of shock, leaving Todd and my mother alone with her. Todd held her hand and kissed her on her forehead, telling her how much Mommy and Daddy loved her and quietly saying a loving good-bye. After a nurse asked Todd about organ donation, the hospital allowed us to leave with little guidance and no answers.

The rest of that day and the next two weeks passed in slow motion. Nothing mattered, and nothing made sense. It will never make sense! The autopsy, as well as further requested research, ruled her cause of death as SIDS. But, "How can that be?" one might ask, "She was awake." Although it is rare, SIDS does not always strike when babies are asleep. Emily was not only awake, but she also defied all the odds based on the epidemiological statistics of SIDS victims. Although this did not matter in our case, she never slept prone. She was full-term. And she was breast-fed by a nonsmoking mother. Supposedly, SIDS is more common on the West Coast, and we live in Florida. It is also more predominant in males. The list of contradictions goes on. SIDS knows no boundaries.

Please do not think that I am saying not to heed the words of prevention. By all means, until a cause of SIDS is found, anything that is thought to reduce the risks should be followed. Todd and I merely want to share Emily's story in the hope that it will help other SIDS survivors end the guilt and stop them from endlessly asking the "if only" and "what if" questions. SIDS has proven, in our case and almost all others, that it occurs without prediction or possibility of prevention. Feelings of guilt for not noticing any signs or not being present when the SIDS death occurred will become destructive if not laid to rest. Without sounding trite, the hardest thing to accept is that sometimes bad things just happen, and we don't know why.

For a Subsequent Child: Reducing the Risks as Much as Possible
by John L. Carroll, M.D., and Ellen S. Siska

The discussion of risk-reduction measures is an emotionally charged experience for parents who have lost a baby to SIDS. Many babies who have died of SIDS had no risk factors, yet they still died. For a couple planning for a subsequent baby, the relatively low risk of SIDS occurring again is no comfort, because they have already "been" the statistic. Despite their risk-reduction efforts, they know that there are no guarantees. Having gone through the devastation of losing a beloved child once, it is not easy to simply follow the risk-reduction guidelines and hope for the best. Often, parents are torn between their desperate desire to have another baby and the gripping fear that SIDS could strike again.

Complicating the matter further are other considerations. Perhaps families were unaware of recommended risk-reduction measures and therefore did not practice them in caring for their deceased baby. They may be angry with the obstetrician, pediatrician, childbirth instructor, or hospital staff, believing that if only they had been informed, maybe their child would be alive. Perhaps they followed risk-reduction practices in their own home but failed to emphasize them to their child-care provider, and their baby subsequently died while sleeping prone at the sitter's, for example. Or perhaps they just didn't believe that SIDS could happen to their baby, and they didn't pay attention to risk-reduction measures.

A natural and normal part of the grieving process is guilt. No matter the circumstances surrounding the death of their baby, parents are likely to feel extreme and prolonged guilt. After all, parents are responsible for the care of their children. When a child dies of SIDS, it is common for parents to search for answers, despite the fact that with SIDS there are, by definition, no answers. It is a diagnosis of exclusion.

It is typical for parents to seek out as much information about SIDS as possible, analyzing every theory and how it might relate to their own child's death. Added to the guilt and confusion is the common misperception from the general public that risk factors are causes. Therefore, if the baby was sleeping on its stomach, or if the baby was bottle-fed, or if there was smoking in the household, then they are likely to believe that these things must have caused the baby's death. Whereas these practices may increase the risk of SIDS, they are not in and of themselves causes. As many people have pointed out, a substantial proportion of babies who died of SIDS had no risk factors. And of course, most babies who do have risk factors do not die. We are encouraged by the reduction in the numbers of SIDS deaths in recent years, and we encourage following the risk-reduction strategies outlined below, but the fact remains that the cause or causes of SIDS are still unknown.

Why the Focus on Risk Factors?

Tremendous changes have occurred in SIDS research during the 1990s. Until the past few years, researchers focused mostly on finding the cause or causes of SIDS, usually assuming that the best hope for reducing the rate of SIDS was to find some sign of physiologic abnormality or predictor that would allow doctors to identify infants with an increased risk of SIDS. This hope has never been realized. After more than three decades of intensive research and the publication of more than 3,000 research papers on SIDS, scientists still cannot predict the occurrence of SIDS in individual infants.

Recently, however, SIDS researchers realized that we do not need to know the root cause or causes of SIDS to do something about it. Studies had shown for many years that certain factors, such as sleeping on the stomach or exposure to cigarette smoke, were associated with a greater chance of SIDS occurring. Researchers decided, therefore, to see if the rate of occurrence of SIDS could be reduced by changing some of these practices. Large-scale public health campaigns were undertaken in several countries. The early results from countries such as New Zealand were striking; the SIDS rate fell quite soon after the inception of public education efforts. As the data emerged, it became clear that measures could be taken that would result in a decline in the SIDS rate. This result led to a major shift in the focus of research and public health intervention to risk reduction, where it remains today. So what is risk reduction, and what does it mean for a subsequent child?

The Concept of Risk Factors Applied to SIDS

Although individual infants likely to die of SIDS cannot be identified, numerous studies looking at SIDS in large groups of infants have shown that certain factors about a baby's environment are associated statistically with an increased chance (risk) of SIDS happening. It is important to point out that these studies examined large groups of infants and identified factors that were statistically correlated with an increased likelihood of SIDS occurring in the population. The presence of a risk factor does *not* mean that there is a high likelihood of SIDS; rather, it means that the chance of SIDS occurring is increased above the usual chance, which is very low to start with.

But how do we apply these concepts to individual infants? We've all heard a common refrain that goes something like, "My babies all slept on their stomachs, and they turned out fine." Those who understand the nature of SIDS risk factors would expect this to be true for the great majority of infants. The current SIDS rate of about 1.1 SIDS deaths per 1,000 infants means that approximately 0.11% of infants die of SIDS and 99.89% don't. A risk factor that fully doubled the current U.S. SIDS rate would still leave 99.78% of infants surviving. The vast majority of infants, sleeping in whatever position, don't die of SIDS. However, this fact does not mean that the prone sleeping position is not associated with an increased risk of SIDS—it is. It simply means that when a risk factor only affects a tiny fraction of a population, one cannot assess the impact of risk factors by looking at surviving individuals. The old "my babies all slept prone and survived" refrain turns out to be meaningless from a scientific stance; one must look for the impact of risk factors in large groups of infants and in the fraction that die of SIDS.

When one focuses on the small but significant fraction of infants dying of SIDS, an entirely different perspective emerges. In the United States, 1.1 SIDS deaths per 1,000 infants adds up to about 4,000 SIDS deaths per year. A risk-reduction measure that reduced the SIDS rate by a modest 25% could translate into 1,000 saved lives per year! On the survivor side of the equation, this is a change of a few hundreths of 1%; on the SIDS side, sparing 1,000 families the horror of SIDS is an immeasurable gain.

It is also important to note that not all babies dying of SIDS have identifiable risk factors. SIDS has struck many families who followed all available risk-reduction guidelines. This fact doesn't mean that risk-reduction measures are not important or that they can't have a major impact—they can and do. It does mean, however, that risk reduction is just that—reduction. An intervention that reduced the current SIDS rate in the United States by 50% would save 2,000 lives per year, but 2,000 babies per year would still die. When risk-reduction measures work, the family cannot know whether their infant would have died had they not followed risk reduction guidelines. Like SIDS risk factors generally, the effects of risk-reduction are best measured in large groups. For the individual family, risk-reduction boils down to reducing the risks as much as possible and hoping for the best. There are no guarantees. Not smoking doesn't guarantee that one won't get lung cancer or high blood pressure; eating a low-fat diet and exercising doesn't guarantee that one won't have heart disease; but wise people reduce the risks as much as possible and hope for the best.

Specific Risk-Reduction Measures

The major risk-reduction measures supported by available scientific research at the time of this writing are (1) having healthy babies sleep in the supine (back) position; (2) not exposing the baby to cigarette smoke, either during pregnancy or after birth; (3) making the sleeping environment as safe as possible; and (4) breast-feeding.

Sleeping Position

All available research indicates that the prone (on stomach) sleeping position is associated with the highest risk of SIDS; the supine, or back, position with the lowest risk; and the side-lying position in between. Basically, "back is best" from a SIDS risk-reduction point of view. This is the current recommendation of the American Academy of Pediatrics and the National Institutes of Health for *healthy infants*. Parents of infants with medical conditions should consult their doctors for specific recommendations concerning sleeping position.

The connection between the prone sleeping position and SIDS is unknown. Studies suggest that the prone sleeping position may increase SIDS risk by (1) blocking breathing passages; (2) increasing the chances of the baby rebreathing his or her own exhaled air, leading to carbon dioxide buildup and low oxygen levels; (3) interfering with body heat dissipation, leading to overheating; and (4) a variety of other proposed mechanisms. Whatever the mechanism, there is now mounting evidence from numerous countries around the world, including the United States, that changing from the prone to the supine sleeping position results in a substantial decline in the SIDS rate.

Although vomiting and pneumonia do not appear to be a cause for concern, there are other side effects of the supine sleeping position of which parents should be aware. Infant development may be affected, with minor delays in the maturation of motor skills. However, there is no evidence that these changes in motor development have permanent or adverse effects. Similarly, when a baby sleeps exclusively in the supine position, some transient changes in head shape may occur, such as flattening of the back of the head. Again, although this factor is still being studied, there is presently no evidence that this flattening is harmful for infants or associated with any permanent effects on head shape.

Orthopedic specialists recommend simply varying the baby's head position during sleep to minimize the effects. Finally, some parents have gone a bit overboard with the supine position recommendations and kept the baby supine even when awake and playing. It should be emphasized that the supine position recommendation applies only to sleep. When awake, the baby can and should spend time in the prone position, which is important for infant development.

Cigarette Smoke Exposure

Smoking during pregnancy exposes the developing fetus to toxins and other potentially harmful effects of cigarette smoke. Numerous research studies confirm that smoking by the mother during pregnancy increases the risk of SIDS. In addition, evidence is mounting that exposure of the baby after birth to cigarette smoke also increases the risk of SIDS. Studies have even shown that the increase in the SIDS risk is related to the amount of smoke exposure; that is, the higher the exposure to smoke both before and after birth, the higher the risk of SIDS.

Although there are several reasonable theories potentially explaining how cigarette smoke exposure could increase the risk of SIDS (e.g., by toxic effects of nicotine, carbon monoxide, lowering oxygen levels to the fetus, effects of smoke on babies' lungs after birth), the link or links are still being explored. However, the weight of the epidemiological evidence linking smoke exposure and SIDS is strong.

Mothers should not smoke during pregnancy or after giving birth. Studies suggest that smoking anywhere in the home may increase the risk, so just going into another room to smoke is not sufficient. In the authors' opinion, no one caring for an infant or child should smoke at all; in addition to increasing SIDS risk, smoking endangers the health of all family members by increasing the risk of lung disease and cancer, and it directly endangers the health of the smoker. However, as smoking is addictive behavior, it is not enough simply to tell individuals to stop smoking. Ongoing smoking cessation counseling throughout pregnancy is an important part of prenatal care for both the expectant mother and the father and should be a major component in risk-reduction efforts. This counseling should continue postnatally as needed.

Safe Sleeping Environment

The baby's sleeping environment also appears to be linked to SIDS in some cases. A recent study from the U.S. Consumer Products Safety Commission (CPSC) indicated that as many as 30% of deaths diagnosed as SIDS may have been related to unsafe sleeping environments or unsafe bedding material. Studies going back three decades have indicated that soft bedding material may be hazardous for young infants. A recent resurgence of research in this area has confirmed that soft mattresses, pillows, and other bedding material can be hazardous and may be associated with infant deaths diagnosed as SIDS.

The CPSC has recently been active with public education efforts concerning crib safety. Some of the recommendations are just plain common sense. These measures include making sure that the crib is in good working order with no missing or broken parts; being sure that the mattress is approved, in good condition, and the proper size for the crib; and positioning the crib so that curtain or blind cords do not hang down into the crib and pose a possible strangulation hazard.

Recommendations against using soft bedding, thick blankets or comforters, sheepskin blankets, pillows, bumpers, and soft crib toys are based on mounting evidence that use of these items is also associated with an increased SIDS risk. Finally, because of the potential hazards of overheating, it is generally recommended that for sleep a baby should be lightly dressed, covered with a sheet or thin blanket, and the room temperature should be such that it would be comfortable for an adult in a short-sleeve shirt. Swaddling and tight tucking in of infants is not recommended.

Current recommendations state that infants should never sleep on adult beds. This recommendation raises obvious questions about infant–parent co-sleeping, which is believed by some people to be potentially beneficial to both parents and infants. Research data on this topic, at the present time, do not provide a clear answer. Some studies have found infant–parent co-sleeping to be associated with a higher risk of SIDS, while others have not. In addition, several studies showing a correlation between co-sleeping and increased SIDS risk also find that co-sleeping appears to be linked with other risk factors, such as smoke exposure. However, there is no question that adult bedding material can be dangerous for infants, and infant–parent co-sleeping exposes an infant to this risk. Studies are ongoing in an effort to answer questions concerning the risks vs. benefits of co-sleeping and whether it can be done in a manner that does not increase the SIDS risk. Until this information is available, it would seem prudent *not* to expose infants to the well-documented hazards of sleeping on adult bedding materials.

Does Breast-Feeding Help?

After numerous studies on breast-feeding and SIDS, results are conflicting, and the relationship is still not clear. Several research studies have found a relationship between not breast-feeding and an increased SIDS risk, while others have not found any relationship. Still other studies have found a lower rate of SIDS in breast-fed infants, but statistical analysis suggests that it was not the breast-feeding per se that was responsible for the apparent relationship. Contrary to the common view, there is no evidence that breast-feeding per se is protective against SIDS. Of course, there are many potential physiological and psychological benefits to mother and infant and, in general, breast-feeding is preferable to bottle-feeding and is recommended.

How Much Can the Rate of SIDS Be Reduced?

We don't yet know the answer to this question. In other countries, following energetic public health risk-reduction campaigns targeting sleeping position, smoking, and breast-feeding, the SIDS rate has been reduced more than 60%. Provisional data available at the time of this writing indicates that the SIDS rate in the United States has dropped about 20–30% since 1992, when the American Academy of Pediatrics began recommending the nonprone sleeping position and with the inception of the "Back to Sleep" campaign and other public education measures. Many experts agree that in the United States it is likely that such risk-reduction measures, if widely practiced, could reduce the rate of SIDS by 50%, and possibly more. How much more, only time will tell. It is worth remembering, when talking about reducing the present SIDS rate, that every percentage point equals about 50 infant lives.

John L. Carroll, MD, is Associate Professor of Pediatrics at Johns Hopkins Children's Center and is a frequent contributor to Internet discussions about SIDS. Ellen S. Siska, mother of Edward David Siska (6/25/91–9/15/91), is executive director of the SIDS Network-

Chapter 17

Dreams and Premonitions

A young pregnant woman dreams that she is standing at a bay window holding her baby against her shoulder. Random bullets suddenly spray the baby in the back, killing him instantly. The same young woman delivers a healthy baby boy months after this dream. But her happiness doesn't last long. He dies of SIDS. She recalls the horror of her dream—what she believes was her premonition that her baby would die.

A lay minister dreams that he and his wife are in a fatal car accident. Even though they don't have a baby, he remembers asking over and over, "Does the baby have to die?" and hearing a voice, as if from God, respond, "Yes, the baby has to die." The minister is so upset by the dream that he can't sleep, and the next day, he checks in on his own grandchild. He almost faints when he is then told the news that his nephew, little Michael Carroll Hitch, has died of SIDS.

Two weeks before Christian died, Joani canceled a scheduled tubal ligation only hours before it was to be done. "I just had this feeling that everything was too perfect. I didn't focus on the baby because he seemed so healthy, but I had a feeling that something terrible was going to happen to someone in the family."

Denise Dickerson had recurring dreams throughout her life that she would have a baby who would die. In her dream, she was first in a hospital being told that her baby died (but never *why*) and later at the baby's funeral. Denise had always attributed this dream to the fact that her mother and father had lost a baby (a girl, Michelle) to an illness. But when her own baby (also named Michelle) died of SIDS, Denise had "a sense of *déjà vu*; that this had already happened to me." Since the death, Denise has never again had the dream.

After her baby died, Denise's brother had a vision of the baby surrounded by a white light and being cared for by a young woman and a young man. Her brother's description of the woman was very similar to how Denise had always imagined her older sister would look. To Denise, this was a comforting sign that her baby was being cared for by her sister.

Interestingly, according to a new study, premonitions are more common among parents who eventually lose babies to SIDS than among parents who do not lose babies. Yet so rarely is this talked about, we were able to obtain only one contribution to this chapter. In this contribution, researchers present examples of the premonitions they uncovered in their recent study.

The Effect of Premonitions of SIDS on Grieving and Healing

by Patricia Christenson, Richard Hardoin, M.D., Judith Henslee, Frederick Mandell, M.D., Melvin Morse, M.D., and Carrie Griffin Sheehan in a study conducted through the Southwest SIDS Research Institute.

"If Only…"

"My baby had another monitor alarm... May I schedule a sleep study for next month?... I... I...", Wendi hesitated. She had lost an infant two years earlier to SIDS and had monitored her subsequent sibling from birth. From the sound of her voice, it was clear that she was still worried and concerned about the well-being of this infant. "I... Something happened... It's hard to talk about... Maybe I'm going crazy... Do you have a minute?" The poignant story that unfolded that summer afternoon would have a lasting effect on our approach to the anxious parents and SIDS families with whom we come in daily contact.

Two weeks before my baby died, I had a vision, a premonition of her death. I was wide awake, working in her closet, when I saw an image of my baby in a small white casket at the front of our church. The vision was horrible! I dropped what I was holding, and the image went away but recurred 10 minutes later. Everyone thought I was crazy... When my daughter died and we went to the funeral home, my baby was placed in a small white casket identical to the one I had seen. It was the only infant casket available... I knew!... If only I could have done something...

The agony in Wendi's voice revealed the depth of her pain, as she discussed the anger, confusion, guilt, and massive grief she continued to experience. Grief resolution was hindered by her belief that aggressive action, following the vision, might have prevented her daughter's death. Although anger is a normal part of the grieving process, Wendi's anger was intensified by the almost uniform lack of support she received from others when she discussed her premonition prior to the loss. Society's discomfort with death and inexplicable events made seeking help difficult. Wendi felt isolated and impotent to prevent her baby's death, leaving her with a deep sense of guilt and many "if onlys."

The Study

The Southwest SIDS Research Institute houses a nationwide database consisting of comprehensive prenatal, birth, neonatal, and developmental histories on babies who have died of SIDS and control infants. Information contained in this database was used to answer the following questions: Are premonitions a normal occurrence among SIDS parents? If common, what is their impact on grieving and healing? Can anything be done to help affected families cope with their losses? Do parents of healthy infants also experience death premonitions that do not come true?

To answer these questions better, SIDS and control parents, responding to a 273-field questionnaire, were asked if they ever "sensed" that something was going to happen to their infants. Parents who answered positively were asked to complete written questionnaires describing their experiences and the effects of these experiences on their lives. Telephone interviews were then conducted with these families to validate the questionnaire and expand upon their answers.

Two additional control populations consisted of 197 parents of healthy infants seen consecutively in a Seattle pediatric practice and 207 parents of every other healthy infant born in a hospital on the Texas Gulf coast. Both groups were asked if they felt that something was going to happen to their infants. Seattle parents were questioned at 2, 4, 6, 9, and 12 months of age. Texas parents were questioned when their infants were 2, 4, 6, 8, 12, 16, 20, and 24 weeks of age. As participants in a study of normal infant sleep physiology, the Texas babies were closely followed throughout their first year of life, all medical records were obtained, and outcome was determined within two weeks of their first birthdays.

Results

In the database study group, 38 of 174 SIDS parents and 4 of 164 control parents stated that they did feel that they would lose their babies. Of the SIDS parents, 94.7% were contacted and agreed to be interviewed versus 75% of the control parents. Of the two SIDS parents who were not participants, one was lost to follow-up and one refused to participate.

Interestingly, three of the SIDS parents who had written about premonitions in the original questionnaire, completed shortly after their infant's deaths, could no longer recall their premonitions. Consequently, SIDS study results were based on responses from 33 parents, representing 34 SIDS deaths. Control study results for database participants were based upon responses of three parents. Follow-up with these parents revealed that two of the three children did develop problems considered to be potentially life-threatening. Review of their medical records showed polygraphic documentation of gastroesophageal reflux and apnea. Both children were treated with monitors and medication. One recovered completely, and one, though four years old, continues to have documented prolonged apnea with oxygen desaturations.

Five (2.5%) of the Seattle control parents stated that they did sense that something was going to happen to their infants, yet nothing had happened. Six (2.9%) of the 207 Texas control parents stated on a questionnaire administered during their infants' sleep studies that they felt that something was going to happen to their babies. Four of the six parents were available for verbal interview. One of these six infants developed significant cardiorespiratory control problems, documented by polygraphic evaluation and in-home recording. She required monitoring and use of theophylline, a respiratory stimulant. The mother of this infant reported concerns about her baby's well-being prior to the baby's birth.

Study findings suggest that premonitions of death are a common occurrence among SIDS parents and an uncommon occurrence among control parents. Statistically significant differences were observed between SIDS and control parents, with 21.8% of 174 SIDS parents compared to 2.6% of 568 control parents sensing that something was going to happen to their infants. Of the 15 control infants whose parents reported a premonition, three (20%) did experience an event believed to be "life-threatening" in nature, and all three had significant cardiorespiratory abnormalities that were well documented.

The Impact

Despite requests for help, many of the SIDS parents were unable to obtain support before their infants' deaths. Anger and guilt were common, even years after the SIDS event.

The majority of SIDS parents experiencing a premonition described a "vague, uneasy feeling without any obvious cause." A few had observed a physical event, such as a choking or blue spell, or had personal knowledge of a SIDS loss, occurrences that may have triggered their uneasy feelings. More than half of those interviewed described a vivid dream or an auditory or visual hallucination while awake. Don, a physician in a large metropolitan area, experienced vague, uneasy feelings as well as auditory warnings about his son's impending death.

During the first trimester [of the pregnancy], I sensed that the happiness his birth would bring would not be long lasting. A few months before birth, I would, on occasions, find myself contemplating a nearby cemetery, now where my son is buried. The day he was born and [I] first held him in my arms, I felt, for no apparent reason, he, my son, was not supposed to be with us. Probably two to three weeks before his death, I would be awakened from my sleep and think about SIDS. The day before he died, a voice sounding very similar to my own, would repeatedly say, "Take a good look. This is the last time you will see him."

According to Don, his fears intensified when his wife planned to visit her parents and take the baby with her. Her parents lived in another state, and a flight was required. The night before she left they argued about whether the baby should go. Don stated that he desperately wanted his son to stay but still didn't relay his fears to his wife. When he took them to the airport, he was flooded with negative feelings. As they walked to security, he heard a clear voice warn him that he would never see his son again. Don stated that he knew that his baby would die while he was gone. Even as he walked to the parking lot, the voice kept telling him to go back, to get his infant. As Don kept walking, the voice got softer, then stopped. His wife called early the next morning and was hysterical, relaying the fact that their baby was dead. Later, Don's aunt shared the fact that she had had similar feelings about the infant. When asked what effect, if any, the premonition had on the grieving process, Don replied:

> *The process has not been a shock to me since I knew before-*
> *hand this [death] was going to happen. The only thing I didn't*
> *know was when and where... I have no idea of its meaning. The*
> *only thing I can say is that perhaps if I would have listened to*
> *"my heart" many mishaps could have been prevented... I think*
> *people have the ability to perceive things and give it a purposeful*
> *meaning which can be used for any future event.*

Another SIDS parent, Mary, described physical symptoms in her infant that triggered her fears. Her baby was frequently congested and colicky. Unlike most parents experiencing a sensation that something was going to happen to their infants, Mary repeatedly sought the assistance of physicians. Unfortunately, they all felt that the mother's concern was disproportionate to the infant's symptoms. Mary was consequently reassured and sent home, most likely dismissed as an overreactive, nervous mother.

> *He had trouble breathing and [was] congested since day one.*
> *[He] cried around the clock, and sometimes he seemed like he*
> *was in severe pain. We did let the doctor know all this, but he*
> *said that he was just an unhappy baby.*

The night before their baby died, Mary and her husband took him to their local emergency room. Again they were reassured that he was fine. Prior to leaving the emergency room, Mary's husband told her that he would press for hospital admission if she didn't feel comfortable with the physician's assessment. Mary, with some misgivings, decided to take her baby home.

Mary continued to feel nervous and uneasy, with heightened concern for her infant. As she walked toward the baby's bedroom with the sleeping infant over her shoulder, she saw their reflections in a mirror. According to Mary, she knew, at that moment in time, that her child would die that night.

Frustrated by her attempts to obtain medical care for her son, Mary felt powerless to avert the impending tragedy. Unable to sleep, she cleaned the house until 3 am so that it would be clean for the family members she knew would attend her baby's funeral. Arousing from a fitful sleep early the next morning, Mary found her son dead, a victim of SIDS. The pathologist's report confirmed his healthy appearance.

This three-and-a-half-month-old boy was found dead in his crib... He had no significant prior illness and had been a healthy baby... [He]... had a minor upper respiratory infection for a week. He was a healthy infant from birth except for a few episodes of colic. On the early morning of August 26th, the parents found him dead in his crib. Clinical and pathological diagnosis: SIDS.

Did the special bond that exists between mother and child allow Mary to sense that her baby had a fatal condition? Certainly neither the doctors who examined the infant before his death nor the pathologists who performed the autopsy were able to document any significant abnormality. Yet Mary knew that her baby would die, with a certainty that defies understanding. Mary's experience strengthened her belief in trusting her own instincts.

Mary has subsequently had two children, a boy and a girl. Both, though beautiful, healthy appearing infants, had severe sleep apnea and gastroesophageal reflux documented by in-hospital sleep studies with esophageal pH measurements. Both children were placed on monitors that recorded breathing and heart rate patterns, and both required surgery because of reflux that was resistant to conventional treatment. These children are doing well, and all symptoms of apnea have disappeared. Mary continues to feel that medical intervention might have saved her son's life. "If only they had listened..." remains a daily thought.

The Role of the Medical Professional

How can a physician distinguish between the new parent who is simply nervous and the parent who strongly senses that he or she is going to lose the baby? Study findings suggest that only about 3% of parents of normal, healthy infants have premonitions about their baby's death. A significant percentage (17.6%) of the infants in this group did experience a life-threatening event during the first few months of life.

When questioned further, many of the control parents who "sensed" that something was wrong and reported a "vague, uneasy feeling" could pinpoint the cause of their fear. Previous knowledge of a SIDS event or direct observation of an unusual or frightening episode were commonly cited. Anxiety tended to be less diffuse than that observed in parents of SIDS infants, remaining relatively constant throughout the newborn period, then tending to decrease with time.

As seen in the control population, the majority of SIDS parents reported sensing an impending loss on multiple occasions; more than half experienced the premonition more than five times. In contrast to the control population, however, there was a strong increase in anxiety as the death approached. One-fourth of the parents reported a premonition during the pregnancy; three-fourths sensed the loss immediately preceding the death.

The majority of SIDS parents felt that the premonitions had a negative effect on the grieving process. Although interviews took place an average of four years following the death, SIDS parents continued to feel anger, fear, and guilt.

Feelings of guilt are common in SIDS parents. However, for the subgroup of parents who "sensed" that they were going to lose their infants, guilt feelings were intensified by their inability to save their children. A 30-year-old teacher said

> *I called the doctor's office Thursday afternoon, but he was out, and the nurse said if the baby wasn't crying not to worry... I wanted to [see the doctor], but the doctor was unavailable at the time. I was told to come in the next day if I was still worried— but my baby died the next day.*
>
> *At first, I blamed myself for not taking him to another doctor. Then I was angry at the nurse who told me not to worry and at the doctor...*

Another parent found herself looking for an excuse to contact her baby's physician. She was hesitant to contact him on the basis of her "feelings."

> *Brandi died on Friday. All day Thursday (Wednesday night, too) I just "felt" like something was wrong... She wouldn't eat, just wanted to sleep and seemed behind [delayed]. All evening*

*Thursday, I cried... Friday morning, I took her temperature
a dozen times. I hoped she would have a fever or something
so I would have an excuse to take her to the doctor.*

*It [the premonition of loss] has frightened me so that I cannot
allow myself to lose control and cry. If I go on a crying jag, I
might lose Michael, too...*

Self-blame was common among respondents. A 28-year-old
mother elaborates:

*I told the doctors that B.J. didn't act right. I knew there was
something wrong with my son. But the doctors said he was all
right... I had B.J. in the doctor's office every week because he
just wasn't right...*

*I blamed myself [for his death] for a long time. I should have
made the doctors run more tests on B.J. and just maybe he would
be here today.*

This mother felt that support from the medical profession would have
eased her pain, even if death was inevitable. When asked if others could
learn from her experience, she replied:

*Yes, if they feel like their child isn't right. Make the doctors run
tests and if that doesn't work, cherish every day you have with that
child, because one day he or she might not be there.*

Parents who reported a premonition of impending death to a medical
professional, spouse, or friend were rarely taken seriously. One-third
of the SIDS parents visited their baby's physician following the premonition. Despite requests for medical intervention or evaluation, nonrou-
tine medical follow-up was not recommended for any of the SIDS
infants studied. This lack of follow-up probably resulted from the very
normal appearance of the infant before death (confirmed at autopsy)
and the tendency to downplay parental fears in an effort to reduce
anxiety. Furthermore, the majority of parents did not report observ-
able physical symptoms and, when done, physical examinations were
within normal limits.

When, despite a normal exam, the parent expressed concern about
the future death of the apparently healthy baby, responses ranged from
outrage ("How could you say such a thing?") to denial ("Your baby's

perfectly fine! Relax and enjoy him!"). These reactions tended to inhibit further verbal communication about the premonition, both before and after the death. Although the premonition often resulted in intensified feelings of guilt ("I knew something was going to happen. I had the responsibility to do something to prevent it..."), respondents seemed relieved to discuss their feelings, and, as a group, were left with a strong belief in trusting their instincts.

Study findings suggest that caring, supportive health-care professionals, who are willing to listen to affected parents and who take their concerns seriously, have the potential to make a tremendous effect on the resolution of their grief. Whatever the outcome, this approach should diffuse the intense anger and guilt so often reported and should provide the parent with a peace of mind not found in the study population.

Those parents who also described some contact with their infants after death (dreams, visions, or feelings) were uniformly positive about the experience and were left with a firm belief that their infants are well cared for and in a better place. These findings, although not previously described in the medical or SIDS literature, are not entirely unexpected. Elizabeth Kubler Ross and Melvin Morse have presented clinical case studies documenting that acknowledgment of such premonitions, and using them to interpret the child's death, can be useful in grief therapy.

The health-care professional's reaction to parental feelings of impending death strongly influences the grieving process. Anticipatory grief, when allowed to occur, may positively affect the grieving family member. It must be understood that the subjective nature of such experiences makes it seemingly impossible to judge their objective reality, nor is it necessary to do so. Simply acknowledging that such premonitions are a natural and normal event can be comforting and validating to parents who have lost a baby to SIDS.

Chapter 18

Moving Forward

[The grief healing process] attempts to seal and protect the space of the dead child for the sake of the parent's integrity and to preserve the relationship with the child.

Joan Hagan Arnold and Penelope Bushman Gemma
A Child Dies: A Portrait of Family Grief [1]

SIDS, a seemingly random and senseless external event, will change a survivor's life forever. In losing a baby—a huge part of both the physical and emotional self—a survivor loses part of his connection to the future. It is likely the ultimate tragedy possible. Through her loss, Joani has discovered that just as a parent's love for a child is without limits, so will be a parent's grief. For her, moving forward has meant, and today still means, that she must actively seek peace and joy in life— even in the face of a grief that will never completely end.

SIDS survivors, like any survivors of a cherished loved one, are likely to feel less than whole for the rest of their lives. After all, how can anyone feel whole when a part of their expected future remains nothing but a permanently blank space? With a vital part of a survivor's inner self ripped out, the space that held the hopes and dreams for the dead child remains empty.

Even so, a survivor can heal and move on. As the opening quote to this chapter indicates, the child is never to be forgotten but will remain a cherished part of a survivor's inner self forever. In effect, survivors fill that remaining empty space with all the memories and love they have for the child and carry that space with them as they move forward and enjoy everything that the rest of their lives has to offer.

Any SIDS survivor would prefer that things had turned out differently. After all, who would not choose a secure, happy, and predictable life surrounded by all of their children? Instead, survivors face powerful blows of sorrow, pain, and helplessness. The only choice then—and it actually will feel like a choice eventually—is to be miserable forever or face grief head-on.

Many survivors make this choice by thinking of what their baby would have wanted for them. Wouldn't the lost baby have wanted the survivors to tackle a project, find a cause, or attempt to fulfill some other dream? Wouldn't everyone be better off if survivors could devote their energies and frustrated love to things that will give the lives and deaths of their babies some personal meaning? As Viktor Frankl, a man who suffered greatly in Nazi concentration camps, wrote: "Suffering can be tolerated only when we are able to find meaning in that suffering."

Many years ago, a 14-year-old boy injured his head in a skating accident and died of a brain hemorrhage. Refusing to accept a future without him, his mother took to her bed. Her other son, age seven, began writing stories to read at her bedside. That boy, James Barrie, grew up to immortalize his brother—and delight the world—by writing *Peter Pan: The Boy Who Never Grew Up*.

Of course, given the choice, any survivor would trade just one more day with his or her healthy baby for all of the published writings, charitable successes, or new levels of understanding in which a SIDS death results. Sadly, that choice is not given. The only choice that is given is whether to die, actually or emotionally, or to move forward by seeking peace and joy in whatever the survivor can salvage and create from the ruins of the loss. In forging ahead, a baby's life and love will not be forgotten but instead will transcend the conditions of physical and even emotional apartness. A survivor can grow and pass on to others the love and other gifts the baby brought. Through a survivor's moving forward, a baby's spirit can live and thrive forever.

Life After SIDS: What Is Possible?

by M. John O'Brien, M.D., Retired Director of the SIDS Institute, University of Maryland School of Medicine

As director of the University of Maryland SIDS Institute, it has been my privilege to come in contact with numerous SIDS families. In this piece, I want to share my thinking on how I see the effect of a SIDS death on the future lives of the parents.

Without necessarily being conscious of it, our experience of life now, in the present, is a function of whatever our vision of the future is. In most cases, we are not aware of this fact. My point is that when a baby is born, and even before birth, a very distinct and specific expectation of the future is generated. We even talk about pregnancy as "expecting." What are some typical expectations? The parents expect their child to be healthy, to be born after nine months of pregnancy and not sooner, to grow and develop into a happy, well-adjusted child and a successful adult, to marry a nice partner, and to start the cycle all over.

This vision of their child's life contributes in very large measure to the parents' own experience of meaning and purpose. The vision of nurturing the growth and development of one's child is an extraordinarily powerful force shaping the parents' sense of what their own lives are all about. Small wonder then that when a well baby is found dead, the effect on the parents is unimaginably devastating. When a child dies unexpectedly, the parents' sense of what lies ahead, of knowing where they are going in life, however unarticulated that sense may be, is abruptly lost. The future, so real in the present imagination of the parents, ceases to exist. All that remains is a void, nothingness. The shock is total because so much of the parents' future was literally the future of the child. The child's future had become the parents' future, and because we are always living into some self-designed future or other, the child's death leaves the parents without any future. I think that this is why the sense of desolation, emptiness, hopelessness, despair, of life being meaningless, is so profound. It is as if one were traveling on a clear highway, with the correctness of one's route being confirmed regularly by reassuring road signs repeating the name of one's destination and indicating that, yes, one is getting closer and closer to that destination, and suddenly one is plunged into total darkness and becomes totally disoriented.

In my view, the main challenge for parents who have lost an infant to SIDS is to generate a new vision of what their lives are all about, one that will give them a sense of satisfaction, fulfillment, joy, and vitality. Although this may seem to be a strange way to speak about a tragedy, it is possible to view the death of an infant to SIDS as the greatest opportunity for personal growth and transformation that any parent can possibly experience.

The opportunity derives from the fact that the SIDS experience forces the SIDS parents to confront head-on the most fundamental questions concerning what it is to be a human being. It forces them to confront the issue of death, something that most of us in the developed world avoid doing as much as we possibly can. We avoid it even though all the world's great thinkers and teachings emphasize that until human beings acknowledge fully the reality and inevitability of death, they are not able to freely embrace their own humanity and take full responsibility for their own lives. When one's baby dies, one can no longer escape the issue of death.

What starker experience of death can there be than to find your own baby, whom you last saw a short while ago alive and vigorous, now lying cold and lifeless? Or to get a phone call from a babysitter or day-care center with the dreadful news that your baby is on the way to the hospital, already probably dead? One minute, death is the farthest thing from your mind. The next minute it is there, inescapable, implacable, irreversible, undeniable, and unyielding. Life at that moment is altered, changed utterly. Small wonder that SIDS parents go through an intense and in many cases prolonged period of questioning why, why, why, why, why, why, why?

Peace and tranquillity are possible only when acceptance of the reality of what has happened replaces the agonized protestation about the unfairness of the occurrence and of life in general. Whether the person is religious or not, the capacity to live life powerfully and joyfully returns only when the person can say simply, "Yes, my baby died suddenly. There is no explanation, and I no longer need one. Life is neither fair nor unfair. Life happens the way it happens. Death happens when it happens. Life is a great adventure. I will invent a new purpose for my life, a new future, one that calls me to be great."

I can illustrate this by referring to my own life. After many years of inquiry and experiencing my own share of setbacks, I am sure that what calls to me, what gives me the greatest sense of satisfaction and fulfillment, is to do or say something that enhances the quality of another person's life. I see that the true joy in life comes when I contribute to others, when I am being of service to others. When I am engaged in that kind of activity, in a manner of speaking, "I" disappear. I become so engrossed in that activity that my personal concerns and grievances cease to demand my attention, and I am totally engaged with whatever it is I am doing. My vision is of a world that works for everyone, where all are taken care of, where all children are treated with reverence and absolute and unconditional love. This vision is not yet how things are. But it is sufficient for my enjoyment of life that I have a really clear sense that creation of such a world is possible. Nothing that happens can shake that vision. As long as I live, that possible world where all people live in harmony with each other, and people honor and celebrate each other's uniqueness, and diversity is welcomed as enriching, the vision of that possible world will be what drives my actions.

Of course there are breakdowns along the way. There are many moments when I experience despair, when I want to give up, perhaps when I want to die. I may get sick or have an accident. As time goes by, people I love may die or move away. War may break out. New and strange diseases may wipe out whole populations. In other words, life will continue to happen as it always has, and much of what happens is completely out of my control. But I have a huge say nonetheless in how my life goes, how I relate to others, how I spend my time, how I care for myself, and how I cherish others. I know now that I will always choose to live as intensely as I know how. I will ask for support when I need it, acknowledging the fact that no great enterprise is ever accomplished alone, even dying gracefully and with dignity.

My invitation to you, the reader, whether you be a SIDS parent or not, is to think deeply about what possible future excites you. What is your unique and distinct vision? Make it something big, something that will really stretch you and challenge you, but definitely something about which you can be passionate. Rediscover the spontaneity of your childhood—before you learned that self-expression was a risky business. It is, but the cost associated with not expressing yourself is much greater.

For a recent SIDS parent, the possible but risky new future may involve having another baby. For a non-SIDS parent, it might be a career change to something you always wanted to do but were never sure you could succeed at. Remember, your notions of yourself come from the past. Take on the radical thought that even though you have a very fixed idea of who you are and what you are capable of, perhaps you don't know yourself at all. Let some big purpose take you over, like ending world hunger, transforming life in America's inner cities, or preserving the earth for your great-great-great-grandchildren. If the cause is big enough, your concerns, pains, sadness, and despair will lose their grip on you. You will be gripped by the future again instead of by the disappointments of the past. You will be fulfilled without having to work at it. You will enjoy life again. You will simply get back to being like a child, passionately engaged in exploring and inventing life.

Twenty-Four Years Later: The Arlette Schweitzer Story
by Joani Nelson Horchler

In 1991, a junior high school librarian in Aberdeen, South Dakota, suddenly found reporters from the *New York Times*, *Time* magazine, *Newsweek*, and all the major television networks practically camped on her doorstep, their next articles and broadcasts hinging on her every word.

The next year, this young grandmother, named Arlette Schweitzer, watched her life story played out "95% accurately" and very sensitively on a CBS prime-time television special called "Labor of Love."

What propelled this ordinary person into the limelight? A true labor of love. She became the first American woman to bear her own grandchildren as a surrogate for her daughter, Christa.

Christa had discovered as a teenager that she had been born without a uterus, which made it impossible for her to have children. Christa's primary goal in life had always been to be a mother, and the whole family was shattered by Christa's grief over losing her childhood dream. So almost immediately, Arlette set about finding a way to fix things for her daughter.

New medical technology, Arlette believed, would be the answer, enabling her to have implanted in her own uterus fertilized eggs from Christa and the young man she would someday marry. Arlette felt that this would be Christa's only hope of having a baby that would genetically be her own. After Christa married, she and her mother set about overcoming the many obstacles society set before them. And today Christa and her husband have a son and a daughter who would never have been born without advances in medicine—and a strong-willed 42-year-old grandmother who carried the twins for nine months despite the amazement of conventional society.

What made Arlette go to such extremes to grant her daughter's dream? A SIDS death had a lot to do with it, as the movie poignantly portrayed. Twenty-four years ago, Arlette found her own five-month-old baby—her third child and second son—dead in his crib.

Baby Chad had cold symptoms the day before, and Arlette—a self-acknowledged worry-wart—whisked him off to the doctor. "It's no big deal—probably just allergies," the doctor said. But Chad fussed all night, and Arlette stayed up rocking him. "I had an ominous feeling that scared me to death," recalls Arlette. "I know it sounds crazy, but I felt something like an emotional chill in the house. I was carrying Chad around, and remember shaking Danny [her husband] awake. Then I called the doctor." It was 4 am.

"You're spoiling him, Arlette," Chad's doctor admonished her. "He just has a little cold or allergy."

Somewhat embarrassed that the doctor was now "kind of mad at me," Arlette finally lay Chad back in his crib at 6:30 am, and she herself went to sleep. At 7:45 am, Danny went into Chad's room as he always did before work. Chad smiled at his dad and took his pacifier. Chad's big brother, six-year-old Curtis, was sleeping in the same room.

About two hours later, Curtis and four-year-old Christa romped into their Mom's bedroom to wake her up with their usual bounce on her bed. "I'll go check on Chaddy," Curtis said. "I don't know why, but I suddenly said very adamantly, 'No, I will,'" said Arlette. "And, thank God I did. I got three steps from the crib and I saw he was dead and it was just awful. I wanted to run and scream and throw myself out a window, but it's amazing how the Lord walks you through this stuff. I managed not to scream and to get the kids (who were still bouncing on the bed in my bedroom) and take them by the hand and walk them to a neighbor's house."

But "what about Chaddy? We can't go without him," insisted a confused Curtis, who knew Mom was incredibly upset but didn't know why.

"The angels came and took Chad to heaven," replied Arlette.

Back at the house, the young mother was "like an animal" waiting for the ambulance to arrive. "Everything is so indented in my brain after that," she recalls. "I remember the mud footprints across the carpet as I watched the ambulance people come in and out. I remember the cars coming and going.

"I rode in the ambulance with Chad to the hospital, and once at the hospital, I lost it. I remember looking at the big window in the hospital room and thinking, 'If I just walk out this window I won't be in this pain.' And the cold, searing, piercing breaths—I felt like I was breathing through a hole in my stomach. I couldn't take a breath without the cold air getting through that huge, gaping hole gouged out of my stomach. For years, I felt that searing cold and sick pain in my stomach every time I breathed.

"Twenty-four years later, I still sometimes wake myself up at night catching my breath. It's still a cold breath, but there's not that big hole in my stomach any more."

From that moment, says Arlette, "I just had to will myself forward from each minute to the next, from each hour to the next. It was more than five years until I could get through a day without hurting for Chad."

After the hospital, Arlette went to a friend's house, but she found it extremely difficult to be there because she and the friend had children of similar ages. When the baby who was Chad's age woke up that day from a nap, Arlette's friend "almost apologized." Arlette just wrapped herself in a fetal position waiting for her husband to be notified by the highway patrol and return from a business trip. "When he opened the door and saw me, tears came to his eyes and his voice broke and he said 'Chad is dead, isn't he?'"

Arlette and her husband held each other, but even though they had always been very close they were not able to share their grief. "He would hold me, but it was like we were in two separate voids of pain. The pain was so immense that it seemed it couldn't overlap to anyone else. I felt all alone even though I knew Danny hurt just as much."

There were no parent support groups available in South Dakota in those days, so Arlette and Dan weren't hooked up with anyone who had experienced a similar loss. The local library, where Arlette searched for information on SIDS, was of little help.

Arlette was able to cry, but Dan felt that he had to be the stoic, strong man, and his therapy was planting rose bushes. It wasn't until some 20 years later, when a television writer came out to interview him for the movie, that Dan broke down and cried uncontrollably.

When being interviewed about Chad's death for the movie, Arlette, too, "bawled and bawled" and "almost couldn't recover" from it.

"It was like 20 years had been suppressed," says Arlette. "Before that, whenever I had brought up Chad, Danny would just close up. He just could not share his emotions. The interviews were like a catharsis for both of us."

For those 20 years, Arlette rarely talked with her friends or relatives about Chad's death. Especially around her friends with babies, "I felt I had to stifle myself because I didn't want to pass on that ugliness and those fears." And of those friends who knew, "No one wanted to ever mention Chad's name; they were uncomfortable, embarrassed, and I don't know what all. They just wanted to get on with their lives, and they wanted me to get on with my life. I was so lonely and felt this had happened to no one else but me. It really affected me mentally; I thought I'd lose my mind. I had to continually remind myself that Christa and Curtis needed me and that I had to try to be a normal mother."

But normalcy was practically out of the question. In time, her gatherings with friends for coffee dwindled. "Everything seemed stilted and stressful and, since no one wanted me to mention Chad, I felt I didn't have anything to share."

Moreover, a few people had made cruel and insensitive comments. One young mother had horrified Arlette by saying, "My baby isn't awake yet. I'd better go check and see if he's dead."

Others would say, "At least it wasn't one of your older children." That comment made Arlette bristle. "There would be more memories to miss, but people need to realize that the moment a baby is born you love that child as much as a 10-year-old. Losing that child is just as profound as losing a 10-year-old to something else."

For years, Arlette couldn't believe how people could look at her and not realize the pain she was going through. "I was so wounded that I thought I must look different externally, that total strangers in a store or on the street should be able to look at me and see how much I was suffering. I felt like I was in a different dimension and that I therefore looked different, too."

The guilt was crushing. "Over and over I thought IF ONLY I'd taken him to the doctor in the middle of the night...IF ONLY I'd stayed up all night...IF ONLY I'd gotten up earlier...I felt I'd been forewarned by my premonition that something terrible was about to happen, and yet I hadn't done anything to save him."

Through it all, "I had to just will myself forward—through every minute, every hour, every day. The pain stayed so fresh. I kept thinking, 'How long will I feel like this? Will it be this bad every day for the rest of my life?' The next day would be just as bad as the day before, and I'd get scared for myself, wondering how I could survive this constant pain."

After about five years, "I remember finally feeling there were little lapses when I didn't think about it so much. I'd feel guilty in one way and relieved in another way. But it was five years before I finally had a full day of relief."

Even now, Arlette sometimes wakes up hearing Chad cry.

And sometimes she dreams about him dying or dreams about him in a box. "Even though I can talk about it now, I still have tears, and I can never just get completely over it. Your child should never die before you die. Life isn't meant to be that way."

Chad's life and death have had "an incredible impact on our lives," Arlette says. "I had my tubes tied after he died when I was only 23, and, being a Catholic, that was a big, traumatic decision for me. But I just didn't think I could live through another SIDS death if it had happened again."

Arlette never stopped worrying that SIDS or another tragedy would strike the family again, and she became "very overprotective." In fact, whenever her grandchildren by her son Curtis would spend the night, Arlette literally stayed awake all night watching them breathe. Of course she never told her son and daughter-in-law about it because she didn't want them to stop bringing the kids over to sleep. (Arlette had not been able to find much information about SIDS and still thought that SIDS always could be prevented if caught in time.)

After she gave birth to her grandchildren, Arlette insisted that they be put on monitors, and doctors agreed because they had been born five weeks prematurely. "It was a wonderful relief to me," Arlette says.

Many SIDS parents wonder how their lives will be affected by the death decades down the road. In 1994, 24 years after Chad's death, Arlette feels "like it was meant to be, like we've just come full circle. We really feel there's a connection between us losing Chad and all that has happened to our family in the past four years."

Christa and Kevin named the boy twin Chad, so now Arlette has another very special Chad in her life who will know about the baby for whom he was named.

"The very first time I called him Chad, I was all alone in the room with him, and I remember curling around him and saying, 'Hi Chad,' and my voice cracked. Now it's just wonderful to have another Chad, and I believe Chad in heaven is so honored, proud, and pleased."

Being a strong Catholic, Arlette also believes the Virgin Mary intervened to facilitate the twins' birth. "Danny, Christa, Kevin, and I went to Mass at a church in Sioux City, Iowa, shortly before the implantation was scheduled to be done. When I went up the side aisle to Communion, I saw the statue of the Virgin Mary looking down at me, and her eyes bore into mine. There was a thrilling, unbelievable experience of telepathy between us, and tears started to run out of my eyes. She was telling me, 'I'm with you; you'll be all right.' It was such a profound experience that I didn't tell anyone about it. Then, a few weeks later, on the way to Rapid City, Christa started telling me my story. It turned out that she'd had exactly the same experience when she looked at that statue!"

Chad's brother Curtis believes that his guardian angel Chad helped save him from being electrocuted last year. (Curtis tells his story in Chapter 6.)

Would Arlette have had the twins for her daughter if she hadn't had the SIDS tragedy? "I think I would have because Christa had always wanted more than anything to be a mom, and there isn't anything Danny and I wouldn't do for our kids," says Arlette. However, she adds, "because I had lost a baby, I felt Christa's loss much more acutely than I otherwise would have. Christa was grieving for the babies she would never have the opportunity to have, and I didn't want her to have that terrible hurt I'd had."

Arlette now makes a point of writing notes of understanding to newly bereaved SIDS parents and has also been in contact with several SIDS parents from around the United States who were touched by the movie's sensitive portrayal of the importance of the SIDS death on Arlette's life.

This "little baby who came to earth for such a short time has affected all of us forever," says Arlette. "People think we had him such a short time, but this baby's life will go on and on."

How Therapy Can Help Us Move Forward
by Patricia W. Dietz, LCSW

A few people who experience major losses in life do not heal. They continue virtually permanently in a state of mourning, bitterness, or despair. Most often, such people have experienced a deep psychological wound to their own identity or self-concept that the loss appears to confirm, or even magnify. Such individuals can struggle long, in therapy or in other ways, to find and understand the route to their own reconstruction. Such people may live in the past, experience grave psychiatric illnesses, or lose contact with any other source of meaning—human, inanimate, or spiritual—in their lives.

Fortunately, most people eventually do heal. Tragedy and trauma are strengthening to the human psyche, as well as damaging. We can be drawn deeply into ourselves to recognize what is important in the brief—sometimes unfathomably brief—moments of which life consists. Ultimately, everyone needs to identify for himself or herself a sense of meaning in life: People who experience a major loss can find, change, reject, or revisit religion or a particular faith community. Frameworks of meaning don't necessarily include a concept of God: Secular humanism and Buddhism are two examples of moral and meaning systems that don't include a concept of a higher being. Other individuals find a creative or expressive outlet to help them clarify for themselves, or share with others, what they have come to know as true. Loss does cause us to confront existential realities, though: Our powers as humans are limited, but we must exercise them well; our lives are finite, but with the capacity for infinite experience.

People who are ultimately able to grow through tragedy are those who expand themselves and their understanding of who they are. They use their understanding to help others—as volunteers, as professionals, or just informally among their own friends and loved ones. They see commonalities as well as differences among people, regardless of background and circumstance. They see beyond the objective, immediate, limited material reality of the everyday to experience profound moments of love, unity, and purpose. If we are open, formative experiences such as major losses take us beyond our "ego," which houses our personality and our self-defined goals. Shape, depth, and individuality of character come from loss. Undoubtedly we are permanently changed by an event as enormous as the death of a child. Yet, peace and even joy can follow in time, as long as we see that the contours of life are not as we first imagined, or even insisted upon, them to be. The lifelong process of changing and adjusting our vision of life can be fostered at certain times by professional therapy.

Letter to Justin

by Norine Blanton

Dear Justin,

When we lost you two years ago, I thought my whole world had come to an end. It was only the love of your father and brother and our families that kept me going. I remember one woman asking about you after you died, and I was sobbing uncontrollably trying to tell her what had happened. As she left she said, "I hope I didn't ruin your day," and I remember thinking that every day for the rest of my life was ruined. I never believed that I'd ever smile or laugh again, let alone dissolve into helpless giggles.

But I was wrong; time and tears are great healers. And with the birth of your little sister, my days are once again full of joy and laughter. I will always miss you, my precious little one, but life goes on, and the pain has subsided until I can giggle again, even while I hold your memory close to my heart.

With love,
Mommy

Letter to Michelle Elizabeth Dickerson

by Denise Michelle Dickerson

My Dearest Michelle,

It has been 17 months since your joyous birth. How much we had wanted you, our first child! However, it has also been just 14 and a half months since your tragic death. I will never forget that Tuesday afternoon.

So much has happened since your leaving us. Do you know we live in a new house? Your picture is still by my bed. I miss your old room, but you would have been happy here, too.

Do you know you now have a little brother, Patrick? But of course you do—you are his special guardian angel. Thank you for keeping him safe. I tell Patrick about his special sister often. He is four months old now and doing things you never got a chance to do.

I wonder so much what you would look like now. I'm sure you would be walking and talking. Would your eyes have stayed light like Patrick's or gotten dark like mine and your Dad's? Patrick has your expressive eyes. They bring me such joy when he smiles, just as yours did. Would your hair be light, or dark like mine? Would you be tall like your Dad? I think you would have been; you were growing so fast!

I want you to know that I hurt less now. I realize that you are close by, watching over us and caring for us. When I think of you now it is mostly with the joy and laughter of happy memories rather than the pain and sorrow of that fateful day in June.

How I miss you, my first born—my little girl! You will always have that first place in my heart; that little hole is yours. I wait for the day when I will see and hold you again. Until then, remember that I love you very, very much.

Love,
Mom

Letter from My Child
by Dolly Guess-Colvin, RN

Dear Mommy and Daddy,

Though I am gone from your view, do not mistakenly think I am gone from you. I am here with you, even now as I am thinking. Surprised? Follow my thoughts and allow me to explain.

Even though I became real to you only as I was born into this world, in essence my reality existed long before this. In fact, you were MY essence. I was your happy thoughts, your loving thoughts. I was "you" longing for a greater and higher expression of love and being. Yours was the dream that birthed me from the world to this. What a glorious

transition that was! All those months you nourished my "self" inside
you, lavished me with your attention, your hope, and even your aspira-
tions. Each day was ours to fill and share. You laughed and I smiled,
you ate and I grew, you slept and I rested, too. Even when you talked, I
listened. You created a world of bliss for me that is difficult to describe.
I only do so now because you are saddened, and once again I am affected. I am saddened for you.

I rest now in perfect peace, and I see much that is hidden from your
view. Do not confine my identity to an earthly body. I am freer and larger than that. I always have been. To become more real to you I became
confined within a tiny frame. Now, I find myself again unbound and
completely free. My scope is limitless, yet I find myself drawn to you,
this time to comfort you, to share with you, to lend the best of myself
to you. If you can feel a sense of peace with me—accept it. This is my
gift to you—just like in the beginning…

I am your happy thoughts
I am your loving thoughts
I am myself…
At home within you.
I LOVE YOU.

Thirty Years Later, a Look at Peter's Gifts
An Interview with George Keeler, M.D., and Kay Keeler
by Joani Nelson Horchler

How could one little baby who never talked, never walked, and lived
for only six weeks have such a tremendous effect on the next 30 years
of a family's lives?

"Before Peter's death, I was an innocent," says Dr. George Keeler,
a family physician in Chevy Chase, Maryland. "I thought I had an
angel on my shoulder and that nothing bad would ever happen to me.
All of a sudden, I wasn't safe, and tragedy occurred right in my face.
Peter's irrational death shook me up, made me search, made me reorder
my life."

George was doing his residency at Andrews Air Force Base Hospital
near Washington, D.C., in 1964 when his fifth child and second son,

Peter, died of SIDS. Being a doctor, George's first reaction was, "Why didn't I notice something was wrong with him?" The base chaplain was no help. "So I wandered around trying to find someone to make sense out of this stupidity and ended up at the Andrews Department of Psychiatry staff meeting. All they did was listen and hear my story, but it helped me realize that this had happened to other people—even doctors—and helped relieve my guilt."

Other people who were comforting to George were his older cousins, who were pediatricians. "They were able to tell me many instances in which babies had died suddenly and nothing could be done about it."

But his life was "still shattered," and he and his wife Kay were moved to start a "theological journey" via a confirmation class at St. Mark's Episcopal Church on Washington's Capitol Hill. It provided the first community where they could discuss their loss. "Until then, I didn't think one could talk about unpleasant things," reminisces Kay. The class "honored despair as a positive thing that could enable us to make value changes in our lives," says George. "I came out knowing that I could stand on my own feet."

In fact, resolving his grief over Peter "got me on a path that literally created the rest of my life," says George. "If I could choose to have him back, I still would, but looking back upon our tragedy 30 years later, I can honor Peter's life and appreciate the difference he made in mine."

George says that losing Peter gave him coping skills that he could not have attained in any other manner. For example, five years after their son died, George's brother was killed in Vietnam. He had been "the star of the family." He had also been a popular professor at the Air Force Academy whose career goal was to be Air Force chief of staff. "My brother's death was on the same level of stupidity and loss as Peter's," says George. "But I wasn't overwhelmed by it, and I consider that to be part of Peter's gift to me. Peter had given me the opportunity to move far enough along in dealing with the ambiguities of life that I was able to deal with my grief and be a bulwark and support to my parents in their grief."

Kay was only 27 years old when Peter died, but she never had another child after him. "We were careful not to have a replacement child," she says. Instead, Kay threw herself back into her studies and earned a master of arts degree, which equipped her as an educator. "But, along with those things, we've also always had the experience of having a great family, and Peter woke us up to that fact," she notes.

Ten years after Peter died, Kay took the Landmark Forum, a three-day course that helps people gain insight into ideas and beliefs that shape and govern their lives. Kay felt guilty about Peter's death before doing the Forum training. "I thought I'd unintentionally caused his death by having him up at our vacation lake house exposed to too many people and sleeping on an old bed with a soft mattress. I moved from self-blame to acceptance of reality."

Through these insights, Kay has learned to be more powerful and effective in working with people. For many years now, she has served as a Landmark leader, assisting students in "leaving the past in the past and inventing a future shaped by what is possible, not by what has been." Risk and change, "no matter how traumatic, can be greeted as opportunities rather than as problems," she says.

By participating with Kay in both the confirmation class and the Forum, George went from being totally clammed up and unable to talk to even his wife about Peter's death to now being "open to the full expression of my emotions and my love of people. When I express my emotions about Peter, it's the honorable and appropriate thing to do... The possibility of being able to do that is another of Peter's gifts."

Before Peter died, George thought he had to be in control of everything. Since then he has come to realize that "being in control is restricting and builds barriers. Being available to life as it shows up is ultimately more fulfilling."

Peter's death has also helped George be more helpful to his patients. "I can look at the whole person better, deal with death and tragedy, be open to new possibilities. So, really, in my career and personal life, in honoring life in the family, I honor Peter's contributions to our lives."

Kay, too, has found that Peter's death has equipped her to be with and assist people who experience deaths in their families. When her son and daughter-in-law had a stillborn baby girl (and when the autopsy later turned up no clues as to why the baby had died), they couldn't talk to anyone but us," says Kay. "They knew we could understand."

Like George, Kay stresses that she never would have gone through Peter's death if she'd had the choice. "But I accept, with gratitude, Peter's many gifts."

Moving Forward by Raising Money To Fight SIDS
An Interview with Susan Hollander of the CJ Foundation for SIDS
by Bob Raissman, New York Daily News

There was nothing unusual about the scene. It was a normal weekday afternoon in a New Jersey suburb, and Susan Hollander had her two kids in the car, doing some errands. Sammy, seven, sat in the front seat, and his sister, Jackie, four, was in the back.

The mother was talking to the kids when Jackie interrupted. "Where's my sister? I want to know where she is!"

Last April 10, Jackie's sister, four-and-a-half-month-old Carly Jenna Hollander, died in her crib, a victim of SIDS. This tragedy has forever changed the lives of Susan and her husband Joel Hollander, the general manager of WFAN.

WFAN held a radiothon to raise funds for the new CJ Foundation for SIDS. (CJ stands for Carly Jenna.) Don Imus, Mike Francesa, Chris Russo, and Russ Salzberg made heartfelt appeals to support the cause.

As hard as they tried, it was impossible to convey the pain the Hollanders still feel. A few months ago, Susan could not sit alone in her own house. She would get in her car and drive. "I didn't want to come home because the house was empty," she said. "I would do anything to avoid coming home. I wouldn't come back until I had one of the kids with me. For about four months, I would drive to a destination and not even know how I got there. I couldn't remember even stopping at red lights."

She was numb and couldn't eat. "It was like all life had been taken out of me," she said.

The memory of the day her daughter died can never be erased. She remembers being in bed with her husband that Saturday morning. It was about 8 am, and she heard Sammy and Jackie playing. She didn't hear Carly. The baby had just begun to sleep soundly through the night, so everything seemed all right.

"I told Joel to get the baby because I was going to nurse her," Susan said. "Within two seconds he came back. I looked at the doorway and he was holding her and she was completely blue. I jumped out of bed. It was like a blur. I looked at Joel and said, 'It's crib death. I know it is.' We started shaking her. She was gone."

Susan remembers telling her husband to call 911. She remembers telling her two children to go into Sammy's room while her husband tried to resuscitate Carly. Suddenly the house was filled with police and emergency responders. Upstairs in the bedroom, the paramedics continued to try and breathe life back into the baby. Susan tried to go back into the bedroom, but the police wouldn't let her in.

"In less than 10 minutes, Joel came out and said Carly was gone," she said. "I walked back in the bedroom, and Carly was lying on the floor on a board. They had ripped her clothes off. Everybody was standing around, and no one knew what to do. No one wanted to pick her up off that board. The policeman didn't know what to say. Nobody knew what to say. They just all looked around."

The emergency responders left the house. Two policemen stayed with the family; they didn't want the parents to be alone. "We just sat with her in our bedroom," Susan said. "We were with her for about an hour." The days after Carly's death are still a blur. The funeral. Friends coming to the house to sit shivah. Susan could feel nothing. "I kept thinking to myself, 'Well, it feels just like she's in the hospital; she hasn't been gone that long.' I just kept thinking that someone was going to knock on the door and bring her back.

"A few days after she died, I went up to her room and got into her crib. I went into her crib because her smell was still there. When Joel saw me in there, the crib came down the next day. It wasn't until lots of things got cleared out of that room that the reality set in." The reality that she still had two children to care for. The reality that she would somehow have to deal with the guilt that lands on all SIDS parents. The reality that she had to find a way to start living rather than just existing.

"There's nobody who can take the pain away or tell you it's going to get better because it doesn't get any better," she said. "Maybe it gets better with time. There are just some things you have to go through to make it get better."

The Hollanders participated in therapy sessions and group meetings with other SIDS parents. Sammy Hollander was part of a SIDS sibling group session. "A week after the group was over, he came into our room one morning and said, 'I just want you to know it was nothing I did. I just wanted to make sure you weren't mad at me.' This was five months after Carly died."

Susan shakes her head. The idea of a seven-year-old boy having to carry guilt isn't easy to fathom, let alone talk about. But this is another part of life for a SIDS parent. Her story can never have a happy ending. She accepts that. This isn't some made-for-TV movie about a brave woman. This is her life, and it's a day-by-day thing.

She is president of the CJ Foundation for SIDS. The radiothon is important to her. "But if I could go back a year and change things, I would. I'd rather have my old life back than do this."

She's been organizing fund-raisers for months. "I'm doing this because I feel I have no choice," she said. "Joel has this vehicle to raise money; other SIDS parents don't. Maybe God took Carly because he knew we could do something about this. We can't sit back and not do something. We can't sit back, just trying to go on with our lives. I wish I could, but I can't."

© New York Daily News, *L.P. used with permission.*

Do Not Stand at My Grave and Weep

Author unknown

Do not stand at my grave and weep.
I am not there, I do not sleep.
I am a thousand winds that blow.
I am the diamond glints of snow.
I am the sunlight on ripened grain.
I am the gentle autumn rain.
I am the rainbow in the sky.
I am the eagle soaring high.

When you awaken in the morning,
I am the swift, uplifting rush
of quiet birds in circled flight.
I am the soft stars that shine at night.

Do not stand at my grave and cry.
I am not there. I did not die.

The Sailing Ship

Author unknown

I am standing upon the seashore. A ship at my side spreads her white sails to the morning breeze and starts for the blue ocean. She is an object of beauty and strength, and I stand and watch until at last she hangs like a speck of white cloud just where the sea and sky come down to mingle with each other. Then someone at my side says, "There she goes!"

Gone where? Gone from my sight...that is all. She is just as large in mast and hull and spar as she was when she left my side and just as able to bear her load of living freight to the place of destination. Her diminished size is in me, not in her. And just at the moment when someone at my side says, "There she goes!" there are other eyes watching her coming and other voices ready to take up the glad shout, "There she comes!"

Rise Up Slowly, Angel

by Diane Robertson

Rise up slowly, Angel.
 I cannot let you go.
Just drift softly 'midst the faces
 In sorrow, now bent low.
Ease the searing anger,
 Born in harsh, unyielding truth
That Death could steal my loved one
 From the glowing blush of youth.

Rise up slowly, Angel.
 Do not leave me here, alone,
Where the warmth of mortal essence
 Lies replaced by cold, hard stone.
Speak to me in breezes, whispered
 Through the drying leaves,
And caress my brow with raindrops
 Filtered by the sheltering trees.

Rise up slowly, Angel,
 For I cannot hear the song
Which calls you through the shadows
 Into the light beyond.
Wrap me in a downy cape
 Of sunshine, warm with love
And kiss a tear-stained mother's face
 With moonlight from above.

Then, wait for me at sunset,
 Beside the lily pond,
And guide me safely homeward
 To your world, which lies beyond.
Just spread your arms to take me
 In reunion's sweet embrace,
And we shall soar, together,
 To a different time and place.

The above poem is reprinted with permission of Bereavement Publishing Inc., 8133 Telegraph Drive, Colorado Springs, CO 80920.

From Juliet's Speech

by William Shakespeare

   and when he shall die,
Take him and cut him out in little stars,
And he will make the face of heaven so fine
That all the world will be in love with night
And pay no worship to the garish sun.

—*Romeo and Juliet*
Act 3, Scene II, lines 21–25

Chapter 19

More Stories and Poems

SIDS
In memory of Thomas Lee Schlomer, who died on 9/25/89

by Jeannette Colyn-Cadriel

I've been so lonely since you've been gone
Why did you have to die?

I don't know why yet either, Mommy, but please do not cry!
I'm having such a good time, you should see this place
It's filled with others just like me; I have friends of every race.
We get to swing on angels' wings and run through fields of joy.
Jesus said that you'd be proud 'cause I'm a special boy.
He said Our Father picked me to come into this place
Just to bring Him pleasure, to look upon my face.
Now there's a special work we do, but yet, I cannot say
I whisper to you this much, it's a surprise for you some day!

Oh, how I wish I could see you now and hold you in my arms
But I know that heaven's blessed with my own little charm!

You were the best on earth I ever could have had.
There's no greater love down there than from a Mom and Dad.
But here things are different; you'll really be amazed
At the difference of how earthly and heavenly kids are raised.
We don't talk back or cry at all 'cause we never do feel pain
We only know of love and peace that on earth is not the same.
Now I look forward to the same thing that you and Dad do, too
When we can be together, 'cause I really do miss you!
So keep your eyes upon the Lord until that special day
That He takes you and you take me; forever then, we'll play!

Trevor's Secret

by Lori R. Dickey

Some people believe that angels exist for all of us, but that many are too busy to "tune in" and listen. I don't know, but I do know that for quite a while after my son died, I hoped and prayed for a sign from him that he was okay and that we would be together again some day. I never saw him, but Rachel, the daughter of my dearest friend, said she did. This is Rachel's story.

Rachel had been visiting from Chicago two weeks before T.C. was born, and I had sent her family videotapes of his first bath, first bottle, that sort of thing. When T.C. died, Rachel took it pretty hard. She told her mother that sometimes when she looked up in the sky she could see him racing with the other angel babies, and that he always won. "They're too young to have wings, so they can't fly yet," she patiently explained to her older brother. When Rachel became worried that T.C. would outgrow his shoes and not be able to run any more, her mother assured her that he would get his wings before that happened. Gradually, Rachel's dreams and visions subsided, but I remained touched by her caring and the concept of heaven from the perspective of a five-year-old.

When Rachel discovered that I was expecting Trevor, she announced that he would have a birthmark. She went on to explain that birthmarks are from angel kisses, so Trevor would have a birthmark where T.C. kissed him. Rachel's mother grinned and said that she thought T.C. would kiss him right in the middle of Trevor's forehead, so he would have a constant reminder of his older brother. Rachel, quite exasperated, explained that T.C. was a good angel and would never do that. She announced that the birthmark would be on his head, under his hair— Trevor's secret.

When Trevor was born, I unwrapped him, and while taking inventory of fingers and toes, I must admit I looked for a birthmark. I found none. So, feeling disappointed and a little silly, I never mentioned it to anyone.

Over the next several weeks as Trevor packed on the pounds, I got in the habit of holding him in a sitting position on my lap to burp him. It was much easier on my back. One night, as I was burping him after "dinner," I smiled at the loss of brown newborn hair, being replaced by blond peach-fuzz hair. It was then that I noticed the newly visible strawberry-colored birthmark on the back of his head. Rachel was right.

Lori R. Dickey is president of the Arizona SIDS Alliance.

Kollin Michael Hughes
by Tracy Hughes

Our dear sweet son,
    Oh, how we miss you so
You were taken from us so quickly,
    Why, we will never know

You were our little miracle
    You brought us so much joy.
To have you in our lives,
    Our only little boy.

You brought us so much happiness
    For just a little while
We'd give anything to hold you again,
    And see your great big smile.

We had the perfect family,
    You were the little brother.
Your big sister Jordyn
    Loved you more than any other.

You'll never be forgotten, little angel,
    You are thought of in every way.
We love you and we miss you.
    We wish you were here with us today.

Ode to Jasmine
In Memory of Jasmine Ferne Stamps: 10/29/90 - 3/22/91

by Lisa Murphy

My heart's greatest joy,
You're all of my dreams come true,
My little bundle of life,
My God, how I'll miss you.

Your laugh,
Your cry,
Your curious sigh,
Your wonderful gurgling smile,
My little Jasmine, always remember
You are the apple of my eye.

All of the days of summer we'll miss,
All of the new flowers of spring,
All of the frosty snowballs of winter,
All of the crisp autumn leaves,

I'll never know your first step,
I'll never know your first birthday,
I'll never know your first crush,
I'll never hear you say,
The love we share will always be
something special between you and me.

But I will remember the good times you brought,
I will remember all of the joy,
I will remember all of the laughter,
I will remember MY LITTLE GIRL, Jasmine
from now till eternity.

I LOVE YOU.

Where They Are Now

This book would not be complete without an update on how the individual contributors are coming along in their grief work since having written their poems or articles. SIDS parent Darlene Buth, a contributor, took on the big task of phoning contributors to get updates. Because of the difficulty of locating and contacting everyone before going to press, some of these brief biographical updates have been taken from the first edition of *The SIDS Survival Guide*, which was published in December 1994. Although this epilogue is thus not completely updated, we think that newly bereaved families and friends will find hope in reading about how our book's contributors have bravely and successfully forged ahead with their lives while never forgetting their babies who died.

Jean A. Andre's grandson, Daniel Andre Prater, died of SIDS in 1989. Jean writes, "We haven't put away his pictures, nor have we forgotten the impact of his life and his death on our lives. We have chosen to salvage our memories. On the anniversary of his death we light a candle and give a silent thanks for the time we had with him. He has a "big" brother now (six years old) who understands the ritual: To remember is to keep him still in our lives, but not to mourn, for mourning serves no purpose."

Ned Balzer and Margie Stewart, who lost their son Willie to SIDS in 1993, have another son, Benjamin, who is now two and a half. Ned is finishing graduate work in computer science at Mills College and administers an Internet discussion list focused on SIDS (sids@earth. mills.edu). Margie is a special education teacher in an Oakland (California) Elementary School.

Norine and Jamie Blanton have moved to Orange Park, Florida. Justin Eli, born January 17, 1991, passed away on October 25, 1991. Five years later, they say they are doing well. Norine is involved with the Florida SIDS Alliance and is now a facilitator for a Jacksonville support group, where she also serves as a peer contact.

Darlene and James Buth relocated to Miami, Florida, in February 1996. They left the small town of Lake Mills, Wisconsin, which turned its back against them when they lost their only son, Peter James-Alan, to SIDS on October 3, 1995. Darlene is an active volunteer for the Florida SIDS Alliance, currently serving as a peer contact, and she still keeps in touch with the Wisconsin SIDS Center. Amanda is now nine, and Kayla Ann is three. Darlene and James are expecting another child on July 28, 1997, two years and five days after the birth of little PJ.

Kandace DeCaro is a co-leader of a MIS (miscarriage, infant death, and stillbirth) support group. She and her husband Tom have two older children, Katie and Julie, born in 1982 and 1986. The family lost Kelly in 1989 and had Thomas in 1992.

Denise and M. Lee Dickerson breathed a huge sigh of relief when their subsequent child, Patrick, turned one year old in 1994. Denise's mother, Julie Beaulieu, who, like her daughter, had lost a baby named Michelle to an infant death, was also thrilled when Patrick reached that milestone.

Patricia W. Dietz, LCSW, currently works in a small psychiatric hospital in Chestertown, Maryland, and also has a private practice.

Chuck and Terre Dohrman, who lost Zachary to SIDS in 1991, have since had two children. They are Luke Jackson Dohrman and Jacob Charles Dohrman.

William C. Ermatinger, whose daughter Kathy died because of a mislabeled prescription many years ago, continues to serve as a facilitator of a SIDS support group.

Gail Fasolo has had a subsequent baby boy, become a speaker on grief, published several poems and articles, and helped many women with losses since her daughter Christina was stillborn in 1991.

Deborah Gemmill has a subsequent child who is now 13. Her oldest child is now 18. She is a volunteer peer contact with the California SIDS Program and conducts writing workshops for bereaved families. She has written three books dealing with grief. Her newest book is entitled *Getting Through Grief: From a Parent's Point of View.* Her two other books are entitled *The Chance to Say Good-Bye* and *Beginning Again.* (The last book mentioned is about the issues facing SIDS families in a subsequent pregnancy.)

Janis Heil, Ph.D., continues as executive director of UNITE Inc., a nonprofit group in Philadelphia that offers support services following miscarriage, stillbirth, and infant death.

Deneena Herrera and her husband Bill have two subsequent children, Devon Leslie, born in 1991, and Caroline Alicia, born in 1993. They lost William Kendal to SIDS in 1989.

Jean Hulse-Hayman and her husband Dale Hayman, who lost Benjamin Dale to SIDS in 1987, rejoiced in the birth of another son, Dillon Michael Hayman, born in April 1994. Jean and Dale also have a daughter Evelyn Anne (Evie), who was born in 1989.

Dora Nagy Horchler lives in Philadelphia and writes wonderful (and often humorous) recollections of her eventful life for her grandchildren. About Christian she wrote, "His memory should be the guiding light that shines in the real perspectives of life and the way that leads to eternity."

Gabrielle Horchler, age 12 in 1997, is a budding professional actress, playing the understudy to the lead role of Addie in *Paper Moon* at Ford's Theatre in Washington, D.C., and acting as a stand-in for young Ellie in the Jodie Foster movie *Contact.* She has also played major roles in several community theater productions.

Ilona Horchler, age 14 in 1997, is an honor student at a private Catholic high school in Washington, D.C., and also excels at swimming. She speaks French and Hungarian fluently and has lived with families in France and (like her sister, Gabrielle) in Hungary.

Carla Hosford, LCSW-C, still serves as a parent counselor at the SIDS Information and Counseling Program in Baltimore. She also has a private practice in psychotherapy, specializing in perinatal and infant loss. After losing Susanna to SIDS in 1975, she had a subsequent daughter, Lindsey, in 1983. She also has a college-age son, Matthew.

Father John J. Hurley, Jr., is currently working at St. John the Baptist Church in Silver Spring, Maryland.

Dr. George Keeler continues as a family physician in Chevy Chase, Maryland, and he and his wife Kay continue involvement in the Landmark Forum.

Pascal, Sheri, and Jessica Laigle delighted in the birth of a baby girl, Solena Samantha, 16 months after the loss of their son, Samuel. Their search for reconciliation has led them through many life transitions, and they continue to strive toward a deeper, more meaningful, and more peaceful existence.

Jay and Sandy Lamb welcomed Jenna into their family in 1994. They also have Rebecca, who was born 13 months after their son Benjamin's death, and Sara and Sheila, who are Ben's big sisters.

Gina and Steve Lawrence are expecting another baby in June 1997. They have one child, J.V., who is nine. They have grown closer as a family since Brianna's death and have leaned on family, friends, and each other when they needed to.

Shelly LeDroux and her husband, Clayton, have a subsequent daughter, Kristy Michelle Zingo LeDroux, who was born in 1992, less than a year after their daughter, Katelin Marie Zingo LeDroux, died. They also have an older daughter, Brittany Nicole, born in 1988. "I enjoy my children more than life itself," says Shelly. "I participated in the first edition of *The SIDS Survival Guide*. I am now a manager of a convenience store. I miscarried a baby on December 28, 1996, at 12 weeks. I plan to have another child, but at a later date."

Robert and Christina Lopez have two subsequent daughters: Crystal Bonnie, born in 1994, and Rachel Claire, born in 1995. They have a son Daniel, born in 1989. Angelique died of SIDS in 1992.

Millie Lutz, grandmother of Zachary Lutz Dohrman, is enjoying her subsequent grandchildren, Luke and Jacob.

Kee Schuth Marshall has remarried and moved from Baltimore to North Carolina since losing both her daughter and her husband in 1992. Sam is now eight years old. She and her husband Jim Marshall have a two-year-old son, Frank Moser Marshall. Kee has become involved with the North Carolina SIDS Alliance and is working to implement a toll-free hot line for both North and South Carolina.

After the death of her first child, Brendan, Nancy Maruyama became active on a local level, serving as a board member for the SIDS Alliance of Illinois. She has also participated on a national level as a committee person. Nancy and her husband Rod have two beautiful subsequent daughters, Caitlin, age nine, and Jennifer, age seven.

Jennifer McBride is manager of the Customer Service Labs for Alcatel Telecom, a global telecommunications provider located in Richardson, Texas. Since Max's death in 1992, Jennifer has contributed to the daily operations and programs of the North Texas SIDS Alliance. These contributions have included speaking to day-care professionals, editing the bimonthly newsletter, *The SIDS Source*, serving as vice-president of public affairs, establishing a SIDS support group in the Plano area, providing peer contact support, working health fairs, and hiring staff. Jennifer views these activities as her "Max activities," in lieu of attending soccer, baseball, and other activities that would have occupied her time if Max had lived. Jennifer was blessed with a subsequent child nine months after Max died. J.B. is now a very active, special three-year-old and, according to Jenny, "the best decision I ever made."

Jon Arthur Mihalko is a seventh-grade student at Ledyard Middle School in Ledyard, Connecticut. He has one older brother and two younger brothers. Jon was five years old when his only sister, Meg, died of SIDS in October 1989. Jon is an active volunteer with the SIDS Network. He has donated hundreds of hours in the fight against SIDS.

Nick and Reny Missos have one subsequent child, Hayden, born within a year of Kevin's death in 1991. They also have an older child, Nicholas.

Terri Bolander, whose five-year-old son Tony Paik wrote a poem in Chapter 6 in memory of his sister Stephanie (who died of SIDS in 1993), has a subsequent child, Gregory Aaron Paik, born in 1994. She also has a child by a previous marriage, Dana Bastianelli.

Beverly Powell continues to enjoy her granddaughters, Kelley and Shelby, both born after the 1989 death of her grandson, Christopher. She and her son John and his wife Alice remain active as SIDS Institute volunteers. The girls are now eight and five.

Nancy and Ken Purcell moved from Baltimore to Florida in the summer of 1994. Before the move, Nancy won an education award from the SIDS Information and Counseling Program for her volunteer work as editor of the program's newsletter. Since then, Nancy and Ken have had a subsequent child, a son.

Regina A. Rochford and Frank A. Rush lost their daughter, Rosemary, 10 years ago to SIDS. "The year following the death, my husband and I struggled to reorganize our lives and relationship," says Regina. "We were blessed with another baby, Theresa. We've learned to live without Rosemary, yet more peacefully with each other and ourselves. Had it not been for this little baby, I don't think we would have been as happy as we are today. Rosemary's life brought us around a full circle. We began with the joy of her birth, then suffered through the painful years of grief and bereavement. Finally, we began to return to a happy state with the birth of our next child and a more powerful loving relationship."

Donna and Dicki Schlomer lost Thomas Lee Schlomer on September 25, 1989. "Ours for a moment—the Lord's forever!" They had Jennifer Lynn on October 16, 1990, and Laura Ann on May 4, 1993. Currently Dicki is vice-president of Grigg's Paint in Phoenix, Arizona. Donna is a full-time mother, happily devoted to her family.

Bob and Stephanie Shaw, who lost Benjamin to SIDS in 1991, have a subsequent child, Emily Victoria, born in 1992.

Carrie Griffin Sheehan retired as a consultant to the SIDS Alliance in December 1993. She serves on the board of the Jubilee House, a Seattle shelter for homeless women, and works on other women's issues.

After losing Armani to SIDs in 1991, Michelle Morgan Spady and Arnett Spady adopted a baby in 1994. His name is Bradford Olander Spady, and he was born December 21, 1993. Michelle took Bradford along when she testified before Congress (in place of Lloyd and Dorothy Bridges, who were not able to attend) for increased SIDS research funding.

Désirée and Ronald Stamps, who lost their daughter Jasmine Ferne in 1991, now have a son, Spencer Ewing Clyde Stamps, born in 1992. Désirée and Ronald are both active volunteers with bereaved parents at work and in their communities.

Liz and Bill Waller lost Michael to SIDS in 1991. They have a subsequent son and a subsequent daughter. They head up a golf tournament sponsored by Bell Atlantic Mobile that benefits the Maryland SIDS Information and Counseling Program.

Richard A. and Leonie S. Watson, both doctors, have moved from Virginia to Georgia. They lost Mark Thomas to SIDS in 1981 and have eight children ranging in age from 24 to 8. Richard is a professor of urology at Medical College of Georgia, and Leonie has a family practice in Atlanta. He is active in the Catholic church and the pro-life movement.

Jennifer and Ken Wilkinson, who lost Larkin to SIDS in 1984, have a subsequent baby, Lucia, born in 1986. They also have Emily, born in 1978, and Claire, born in 1980. Jennifer was president of the Virginia SIDS Alliance for several years. She is now an artist and a freelance food writer who has been published in *Mid-Atlantic* and *The Washington Post*.

Appendix

National and International Organizations That Provide Information, Counseling, Research Data, and Grants on SIDS and Related Topics

- AGAST (Alliance of Grandparents)
  2323 N. Central Ave., Ste 1204
  Phoenix, AZ 85004
  800-793-SIDS

- American SIDS Institute
  6065 Roswell Road, Ste 876
  Atlanta, GA 30328
  404-843-1030 (local)
  800-232-SIDS (toll-free)
  800-847-SIDS (in Georgia)

- Association of SIDS and Infant
  Mortality Programs
  630 W. Fayette, Rm. 568
  Baltimore, MD 21201
  410-706-5062, 800-808-SIDS

- Center for Loss in Multiple Birth
  c/o Jean Kollantai
  P.O. 1064
  Palmer, AK 99645
  907-746-6123(4 hrs earlier than
  East Coast since it's in Alaska)

- CJ Foundation for SIDS
  Hackensack Univ. Medical Center
  30 Prospect Avenue
  Hackensack, NJ 07601
  201-996-5111

- [The] Compassionate Friends
  P.O. Box 3696
  Oak Brook, IL 60522-3696
  630-990-0010

- National SIDS Resource Center
  2070 Chain Bridge Road, Ste 450
  Vienna, VA 22182
  703-821-8955

- Pregnancy and Infant Loss Center
  1421 East Wayzata Boulevard, Ste 30
  Wayzata, MN 55391
  612-473-9372

- SHARE Pregnancy and Infant
  Loss Support Inc.
  St. Joseph Health Center
  300 First Capitol Drive
  St. Charles, MO 63301
  314-947-6164

- SIDS Alliance
  1314 Bedford Ave. Ste 210
  Baltimore, MD 21208
  410-653-8226, 800-221-7437

- SIDS Educational Services
  Box 2426, Hyattsville, MD 20784-0426
  301-773-9671 (fax: 301-322-2620)

- SIDS International
  C/-SIDA (NSW), PO Box 2307
  North Parramatta NSW 2151, Australia

- SIDS Network
  9 Gonch Farm Road
  Ledyard, CT 06339
  800-560-1454
  E-mail: sidsnet@sids-network.org
  Internet: http://sids-network.org

- Southwest SIDS Research Institute
  Brazosport Memorial Hospital
  100 Medical Drive
  Lake Jackson, TX 77566
  409-299-2814, 800-245-SIDS

Stop the Mail and the Callers *by the Virginia SIDS Alliance*

Unwelcome reminders of your baby's death often come by phone or mail in the form of advertisements for baby products. If you would like to reduce this assault, write to the following organizations and tell them of your desire to have your name deleted from their lists. Give your name, address, and phone number. Allow 90 days.

- Mail Preference Service
  Direct Marketing Association
  P.O. Box 3861
  New York, NY 10136

- Telephone Preference Service
  P.O. Box 9014
  Farmington, NH 11735

Bibliography

Chapter 1
1. Bergman, A. B. *The "Discovery" of Sudden Infant Death Syndrome.* University of Washington Press: Seattle, WA, 1988.
2. Beckwith, J. B. "Commonly Asked Questions About SIDS: A Doctor's Response." Colorado SIDS Program: Denver, CO, 1983. (Pamphlet available from 6825 East Tennessee Avenue, Building 1, Number 300, Denver, CO 80224-1631. 303-320-7771.)

Chapter 3
1. Lightner, C.; Hathaway, N. *Giving Sorrow Words.* Warner Books: New York, 1990.
2. Buechner, F. *Wishful Thinking: A Theological ABC.* Harper & Row: New York, 1990.
3. Lewis, C. S. *A Grief Observed.* Bantam Books: New York, 1976.
4. Schwartz, L. Z. "The Origin of Maternal Feelings of Guilt in SIDS: Relationship with the Normal Psychological Reactions of Maternity." In *The Sudden Infant Death Syndrome: Cardiac & Respiratory Mechanisms and Interventions.* New York Academy of Sciences: New York, 1988; pp 132-144.
5. Schiff, H. S. *The Bereaved Parent.* G.K. Hall & Company: Boston, MA, 1977.
6. Ranney, M. D. "SIDS and Parents." In *Sudden Infant Death Syndrome: Who Can Help and How.* Springer Publishing: New York, 1990.
7. Spock, B. *Baby and Child Care.* Pocket Books: New York, 1976.
8. Beckwith, J. B. "Commonly Asked Questions About SIDS: A Doctor's Response." Colorado SIDS Program: Denver, CO, 1983. (Pamphlet available from 6825 East Tennessee Avenue, Building 1, Number 300, Denver, CO 80224-1631. 303-320-7771.)
9. Toder, F. *When Your Child Is Gone: Learning To Live Again.* Capital Publishing: Sacramento, CA, 1986.
10. Epston, D. "Strange and Novel Ways of Addressing Guilt." In Walsh, F., McGoldrick, M., Eds. *Living Beyond Loss: Death in the Family.* W.W. Norton & Co., New York, 1991.
11. Angelica, M. *Mother Angelica's Answers, Not Promises.* Pocket Books, a divison of Simon & Schuster: New York, 1987.

Chapter 4
1. Kushner, H. S. *When Bad Things Happen to Good People.* Schocken Books: New York, 1981.
2. Bramblett, J. *When Good-Bye Is Forever: Learning To Live Again After the Loss of a Child.* Ballantine Books: New York, 1991.
3. Weiss, B. L. *Many Lives, Many Masters.* Simon & Schuster: New York, 1988.

Chapter 5
1. Mandell, F.; McAnulty, E.; Reece, R. M. "Observations of Paternal Responses to Sudden and Anticipated Infant Death." *Pediatrics* 1980, *65*, 221-225.
2. Staudacher, C. *Men and Grief: A Guide for Men Surviving the Death of a Loved One.* New Harbinger Publications: Oakland, CA, 1991.
3. Bramblett, J. *When Good-Bye Is Forever: Learning To Live Again After the Loss of a Child.* Ballantine Books: New York, 1991.
4. Biebel, D. *Jonathan, You Left Too Soon.* Thomas Nelson: Nashville, TN, 1981.

Chapter 6
1. Isle, S.; Burns, L. H.; Erling, S. *Sibling Grief.* Pregnancy and Infant Loss Center: Wayzata, MN, 1984. (Booklet available from Pregnancy and Infant Loss Center, 1421 East Wayzata Boulevard, Suite 40, Wayzata, MN 55391. 612-473-9372.)

2. Fitzgerald, H. *The Grieving Child: A Parent's Guide*. Simon & Schuster: New York, 1992.
3. Skeie, E. *Summerland: A Story About Death and Hope*. Brethren Press: Elgin, IL, 1989. (Brethren Press, 1451 Dundee Avenue, Elgin, IL 60120.)

Chapter 10
1. "Have You Considered?...Planning Your Child's Service." The SIDS Foundation of Washington: Seattle, WA, 1990. (Pamphlet available from the foundation at Children's Hospital, P.O. Box 5371, Seattle, WA 98105. 206-526-2110.)
2. Menotti, G.-C. *Amahl and the Night Visitors*. G. Schirmer (ASCAP): New York. Copyright (c) 1951. (Renewed) by G. Schirmer, Inc. (ASCAP) International copyright secured. All rights reserved. Reprinted by permission.

Chapter 11
1. Woiwode, L. "Firstborn." *The New Yorker*. Nov. 28, 1985.

Chapter 13
1. James, J. W.; Cherry, F. *Grief Recovery Handbook: A Step by Step Program for Moving Beyond Loss*. Harper & Row: New York, 1988.
2. Rawlings, M. *Beyond Death's Door*. Bantam Books: New York, 1978.

Chapter 14
1. Day, K. "SIDS Training Module 85-2." 1985. (Pamphlet available from the Prince George's County Police Department, 7600 Barlowe Road, Landover, MD 20785.)
2. Pennsylvania SIDS Center. Publishes several SIDS study outlines and protocols for police officers and other emergency responders. (Available by writing Pennsylvania SIDS Center, 834 Chestnut Street, Suite 200, Philadelphia, PA 19107-5127.)

Chapter 15
1. Weinstein, S.; Steinschneider, A. "The Effectiveness of Electronic Home-Monitoring Programs in Preventing SIDS." In Tildon, J. T.; Roeder, L. M.; Steinschneider, A., Eds. *Sudden Infant Death Syndrome*. Academic Press: New York, 1983; pp 719-726.
2. Spitzer, A. R.; Gibson, E. "Home Monitoring." *Clin. Perinatol.* 1991, *19*, 907-926, and personal communication.
3. Davidson Ward, S. L.; Keens, T. G.; Chan, L. S.; Chipps, B. E.; Carson, S. H.; Deming, D. D.; Krishna, V.; MacDonald, H. M.; Martin, G. I.; Meredith, K. S.; Merritt, T. A.; Nickerson, B. G.; Stoddard, R. A.; Van der Hal, A. L. "Sudden Infant Death Syndrome in Infants Evaluated by Apnea Programs in California." *Pediatrics* 1986, *77*, 451-458.
4. Kelly, D. H. "Home Monitoring for the Sudden Infant Death Syndrome: The Case For." In Schwartz, P. J.; Southall, D. J. P.; Valdes-Dapena, M., Eds. *The Sudden Infant Death Syndrome: Cardiac and Respiratory Mechanisms and Interventions*. New York Academy of Sciences: New York, 1988; pp 158-163.
5. Meny, R.; Blackmon, L.; Fleischmann, D.; Gutberlet, R.; Naumburg, E. G. "Sudden Infant Death and Home Monitors." *American Journal of Diseases of Children* 1988, *142*, 1037-1040.
6. Kandall, S. R.; Gaines, J.; Habel, L.; Davidson, G.; Jessop, D. "Relationship of Maternal Substance Abuse to Subsequent Sudden Infant Death Syndrome in Offspring." *J. Pediatr.* 1993, *123*, 120-126.

Chapter 18
1. Arnold, J. H.; Gemma, P. B. *A Child Dies: A Portrait of Family Grief*. Aspen Systems Corporation: Rockville, MD, 1983.

Suggested Reading

Arnold, J. H.; Gemma, P. B. *A Child Dies: A Portrait of Family Grief*;
Charles Press: Philadelphia, PA,1994. Explores the meaning of a child's death
to the family.

Finkbeiner, A. K. *After the Death of a Child: Living Through the Years*;
Free Press, a division of Simon & Schuster: New York, 1996. Examines the
long-term effects of losing a child. Confirms that we are tied to our children
with bonds that exist beyond death.

Fritsch, J.; Ilse, S. *Anguish of Loss: Visual Expressions of Grief and Sorrow*;
Wintergreen Press: Long Lake, MN, 1995. Expressions of emotions and
feelings about the death of a baby.

Gemmill, D. R. *Beginning Again: SIDS Families Share Their Hopes, Dreams,
Fear, and Joy*; Beachcomber Press: Escondido, CA, 1995. On starting life
again after a SIDS death, it covers and shares the thoughts of SIDS parents.

Gemmill, D. R. *Getting Through Grief: From a Parent's Point of View:
Living After Your Baby Has Died*; Beachcomber Press: Escondido, CA, 1996.
Personal story of one family's recovery from a SIDS death.

Grollman, E. A. *Talking About Death: A Dialogue Between Parent and Child*;
Beacon Press: Boston, MA, 1991. A parent's guide to explaining death to their
children. It includes a children's read-along section and a resources section.

Hacket, D.; Bevington, K. *Now Childless;* Compassionate Friends: Oak Brook,
IL, 1990. Small book on bereavement; discusses anger, how to live with new
roles, and reinvesting in life.

Ilse, S. *Single Parent Grief;* A Place to Remember: Saint Paul, MN, 1994;
612-645-7045. On facing loss as a single parent, it discusses feelings, how
others respond, relationships, special holidays, dealing with your grief, and
dating again.

Journal of Sudden Infant Death Syndrome and Infant Mortality; Roeder,
Lois, Ed.; Plenum Publishing: 233 Spring St, NY, NY 10013-1578.
Fax: 212-807-1047

Littrell, L. *A Little Friend Is Gone: A Book for Kids Dealing with SIDS*;
Colorado SIDS Program: Denver, CO, 1994; 303-320-7771.

Mehren, E. *After the Darkest Hour the Sun Will Shine Again: A Parent's
Guide to Coping with the Loss of a Child*; Fireside Book of Simon & Schuster:
New York, 1997. Poignant and refreshing true stories about surviving the
death of a child.

Morawetz, D. *Go Gently: A Parent's Grief*; Johnson, J., Ed.; Centering
Corporation: Omaha, NE, 1991. Story by a SIDS father about his personal
experience of grief.

The National Directory of Bereavement Support Groups and Services, 1996 Ed.; Wong, M. M., Ed.; ADM Publishing: Forest Hills, NY, 1996. Lists more than 1,600 community-based bereavement support groups in 11 categories and 24-hour crisis hot lines for the bereaved. Articles by bereaved individuals.

Schaefer, D.; Lyons, C. *How Do We Tell the Children? Helping Children Understand and Cope with Separation and Loss*; Centering Corporation: Omaha, NE, 1994. Discusses what children think and feel about death. Guidelines on explaining death to children. Contains age-specific information.

Schwiebert, P.; Kirk, P. *Still To Be Born: A Guide for Bereaved Parents Who Are Making Decisions About Their Future*; Perinatal Loss: Portland, OR, 1993. Discusses feelings after death, making decision about the future, medical considerations, and how to live through another pregnancy.

Sims, D. D. *Why Are the Casseroles Always Tuna? A Loving Look at the Lighter Side of Grief*; Big A and Company: Albuquerque, NM, 1992. A sensitive, humorous look at grief and advice on how to survive.

Staudacher, C. *Men and Grief*; New Harbinger: Oakland, CA, 1991. Discusses men and grief. Offers advice on how to survive. Good reference for professionals.

Temes, R. *The Empty Place: A Child's Guide Through Grief*; New Horizon Press: Far Hills, NJ, 1992. Story of a boy whose sister died. His experiences as he passes through the grieving process.

When the Bough Breaks II; Guild for Infant Survival, San Diego County: Powry, CA, 1994; 619-222-9662. Contains much information about SIDS and grief and includes poems and stories by parents and family.

Wiersbe, D. W. *Gone But Not Lost: Grieving the Death of a Child*; Centering Corporation: Omaha, NE, 1992. Good general coverage of what any parent whose child has died might want to know. Very religious, may not be for all parents.

Wolfelt, A. D. *A Child's View of Grief*; Companion Press: Fort Collins, CO, 1991. Excellent general overview of grief in children, offers helpful guidelines for the care-taking adult. Gives suggestions for involving children in the funeral. Lacks age-specific information.

This list was compiled by Elsa L. Weber, MS, CHES (with some additions by the editors of The SIDS Survival Guide*). Much of the information in this list was extracted from the California SIDS Program's Materials Resource Data Base. Telephone numbers are included for publishers that are not listed in* Books in Print 1996, *which is available in most libraries. Please see the bibliography of this book for a list of other good books and articles.*

About Joani Nelson Horchler

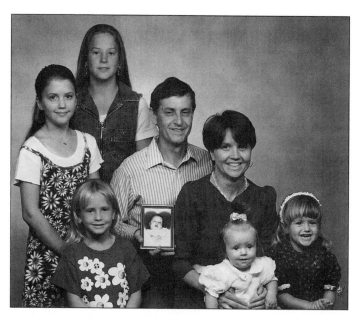

J oani Nelson Horchler has dedicated her professional career to research, writing, and public speaking. She was an associate editor and writer for *Industry Week* magazine, focusing on public policy and management issues, and has had many articles picked up by national wire services and reprinted in major newspapers such as *The Washington Post*. She has traveled internationally with the National Press Club. She was editor-in-chief of a community magazine as well as a weekly university newspaper. She has worked for United States Senator Thomas Daschle and former United States Senator James Abourezk. Joani now serves as executive director of SIDS Educational Services, a small nonprofit group dedicated to providing empathetic support to newly bereaved families. Joani and her husband, Gabe, have five daughters, Ilona, Gabrielle, Julianna, Genevieve, and Stephanie, and one son, Christian, who died of SIDS in 1991 at two months of age. (From left to right in the photo are Gabrielle, Julianna in front, Ilona, Gabe with a photo of Christian, Joani, Stephanie, and Genevieve.)

About Robin Rice Morris

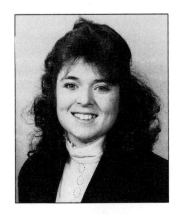

Robin Rice Morris is a writer and speaker who focuses on a variety of parenting issues, including in-home child care, the challenges and rewards of motherhood, and choosing quality children's television programming and videos. She is author of the book, *The American Nanny: A Comprehensive Guide* and the feature essayist in the book *Discovering Motherhood*. She has written the Video Reviewer's Choice column for *Sesame Street Parent's Guide Magazine* and the Perspectives column for the magazine *Welcome Home*. Robin and her husband, John, are the parents of two children, Richard and Taylor Robin.

The SIDS Survival Guide

*Information and Comfort for Grieving Family
and Friends and Professionals Who Seek To Help Them*

SECOND EDITION

Order Form

(This book may be ordered through bookstores or through this form.)

☐ Please send me_____copies at $16.95 each plus $3 book rate postage/handling for the first book and 75 cents each additional book. For special Priority Mail (usually 2-day) service, send $3.95 for the first book and $2 each additional book. Maryland residents must add 5% sales tax.

INTERNATIONAL ORDERS: $4 p/h for the first book and $1 for each additional book to be sent by surface mail to anywhere outside of the United States—Or $10 airmail p/h for the first book and $1 each additional book to be air-mailed out-side of North America, and $5.50 airmail p/h for the first book sent to Canada or Mexico and $1 each additional book. Please send international postal money orders where possible— If checks are sent, they must be in United States currency.

My check/money order for $_____ is enclosed. (Sorry, no COD or billing available.) VISA & MasterCard accepted. Call us or mail card #, signature, and expiration date.

☐ Please send me information on multiple order (5+) discounts.

Name _____

Organization _____

Address _____

City, State, ZIP _____

Phone _____

**Send check or money order to: SIDS Educational Services,
P.O. Box 2426, Hyattsville, MD 20784-0426
For more information, call 301-773-9671 or fax 301-322-2620.**

*SIDS Educational Services is a nonprofit, charitable organization
with 501(c)(3) status. Our federal employer ID # is 52-1865635.*

Honor Your Baby by Sponsoring a
SIDS SURVIVAL GUIDE
for a newly bereaved family
(or for a SIDS support group, library, hospital, emergency responder, day-care facility, etc.)

Your donation through SIDS-ES, a nonprofit charitable 501(c) (3) organization, is tax-deductible. Your purchases help this limited edition book stay in print.

Labels with your tribute will be placed on the inside cover of each book you sponsor.

If photo label is desired, include a color or b&w photo (not a negative) that is NOT your only copy. We will try to return the photo to you after we scan it onto the label. Questions? Call 301-773-9671.

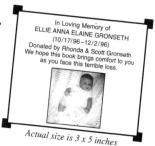

In Loving Memory of
ELLIE ANNA ELAINE GRONSETH
(10/17/96–12/2/96)
Donated by Rhonda & Scott Gronseth
We hope this book brings comfort to you
as you face this terrible loss.

Actual size is 3 x 5 inches

The SIDS Survival Guide Sponsorship Form

Your Name: _____   Organization #1: _____

Title:_____   _____

Organization:_____   Organization #2: _____

Address:_____   _____

City:_____ State:___ Zip:_____   In Memory of:_____

Phone:_____ Fax:_____   Birth date/death date: _____

Your tax-deductable sponsorship: Your relationship to baby:_____

☐ Individual Copies @ $16.95 ea: $_____

☐ Set(s) of 8 copies @ $100/set: $_____   Please write what you want your labels to say. (You may want to use the wording on the sample label above, substituting your own baby's name & dates & sponsors' names. Include separate page if necessary.)

☐ 100 Copies, a $1,000 donation: $_____

Postage/Handling $4 1st book, $2 ea. add'l $_____

(free on orders of 8 or more) **TOTAL** _____

Please indicate # of books for each:

☐ Local Library   ☐ SIDS Support Group

☐ Self (not tax-deductible) ☐ Other

Send order form with check to
SIDS-ES, P.O. Box 2426, Hyattsville, MD 20784-0426
Phone: 301-773-9671; fax: 301-322-2620; Employer ID #52-1865635
Visa and MasterCard accepted: Call or mail card #, signature, exp. date